DISEASES OF THE CANINE EYE

DISEASES
OF THE
CANINE EYE

F. G. STARTUP
Ph.D., B.Sc., M.R.C.V.S.

The Williams and Wilkins Company
BALTIMORE

First published 1969

© 1969 Baillière, Tindall & Cassell Ltd
7 & 8 Henrietta Street, London, W.C.2

7020-0242-9

Published in the United States by the Williams & Wilkins Company, Baltimore

Printed in Great Britain by
Spottiswoode Ballantyne and Co Ltd, London and Colchester

CONTENTS

COLOUR PLATES

PREFACE

During the past 20 years there has been a great increase of interest in veterinary ophthalmology, and particularly in ophthalmic surgery in the dog and cat. Some of this interest has been due no doubt to the overall increase in veterinary practice, particularly that involving the small domestic pets; other factors responsible have been the very great advances that have been made in human ophthalmology during this period, and the pioneer work in this field that has been carried out by workers in many countries.

In the past, books devoted to veterinary ophthalmology have been few in number, and it has been difficult for the practising veterinarian to obtain access to all the advances published in the world veterinary press.

The primary objective of this book is to bring together as much as possible as is known about the diseases of the canine eye in a form useful to both practitioner and student. The text provides a detailed commentary on most of the ocular conditions that are likely to be encountered in the dog, and describes almost every operation likely to be of value. The various conditions have been illustrated as far as is possible, both from my own clinical records and with the help of colleagues acknowledged elsewhere. A very full bibliography of the literature has been included so that the critical reader may find more easily references to the published work on the subject. This bibliography is no doubt far from complete, nevertheless it contains most of the published work in English and much that has been written in French, German, Italian and other languages. A few selected references from the human ophthalmological journals have been included where they are particularly relevant to the text.

As the writing of this book proceeded, it became more and more obvious that the gaps in our knowledge are considerable. Much that has been written will no doubt need considerable revision in the future, as our knowledge increases and the gaps become filled. In the meantime, I have endeavoured to present as complete a picture as possible, and have included not only work with which I am familiar myself, but also the observations of workers in many countries. It is hoped that this book will constitute a useful basis on which the reader may build his own conclusions.

F. G. STARTUP

ACKNOWLEDGEMENTS

The preparation of this book would not have been possible without the help and co-operation of many friends and colleagues; nor would it have been possible without the encouragement and tolerance of my wife. My thanks are due to my partners and professional colleagues who have provided clinical material; Mr H. G. B. Gilpin, B.Sc., who has prepared most of the black-and-white drawings; Dr W. F. Butler, Ph.D., B.Sc., M.R.C.V.S., who has both helped with the text on the vascular and nervous systems, and has prepared various illustrations (Figs. 4, 5 and 6, and Plates I and II); Dr K. C. Barnett, Ph.D., B.Sc., M.R.C.V.S., for the colour illustrations of the fundus and for the illustration of binocular indirect ophthalmoscopy; Mr D. M. Heeley, M.R.C.V.S., for the illustration of slit-lamp biomicroscopy; the late Mr A. N. Ormrod, M.R.C.V.S., for the illustration of iris cysts; Mrs B. Hood who typed and checked the manuscript and prepared the index; Miss B. Horder, B.A., A.L.A., Librarian of the Royal College of Veterinary Surgeons' Wellcome Library, and her assistants, for considerable help over many years; my senior nursing staff, for great help and encouragement over a long period, and in particular Mrs J. Dent, Miss S. Murphy, Mrs V. Norman and Miss C. Pomfret, all of whom are Registered Animal Nursing Auxiliaries; Messrs Dixey Instruments Ltd and Messrs C. Davis Keeler Ltd for illustrations of their instruments; the Editors of the *Veterinary Record*, the *Journal of Small Animal Practice* and *Aspects of Comparative Ophthalmology* for permission to reproduce extracts and illustrations from papers of mine that have appeared in their publications; W. Green & Sons Ltd, for permission to reproduce extracts from the *Encyclopedia of Veterinary Medicine*; and my publishers who have, at all times, been most patient and helpful.

PLATE I

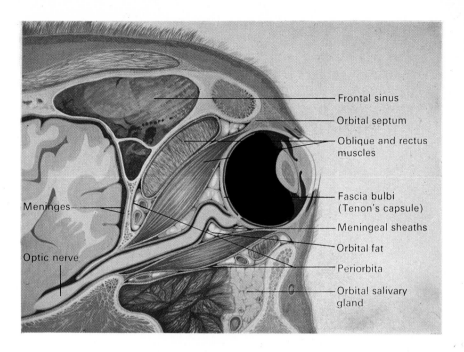

Frontal sinus

Orbital septum

Oblique and rectus
muscles

Fascia bulbi
(Tenon's capsule)

Meningeal sheaths

Orbital fat

Periorbita

Orbital salivary
gland

Meninges

Optic nerve

THE ANATOMY OF THE ORBIT

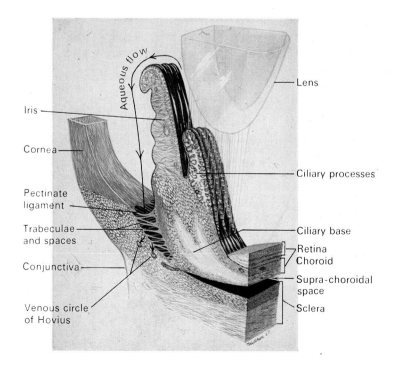

Aqueous flow

Lens

Iris

Cornea

Ciliary processes

Pectinate
ligament

Trabeculae
and spaces

Ciliary base

Retina
Choroid

Conjunctiva

Supra-choroidal
space

Venous circle
of Hovius

Sclera

THE FILTRATION ANGLE

PLATE II

THE ORBIT

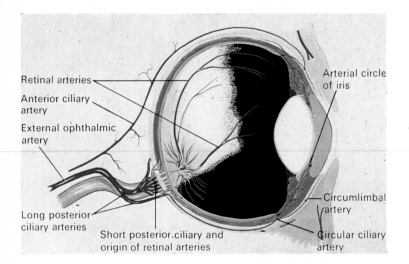

Retinal arteries

Anterior ciliary artery

External ophthalmic artery

Arterial circle of iris

THE ARTERIES

Long posterior ciliary arteries

Short posterior ciliary and origin of retinal arteries

Circumlimbal artery

Circular ciliary artery

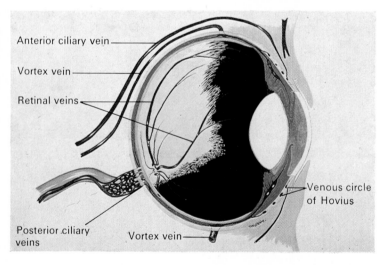

Anterior ciliary vein

Vortex vein

Retinal veins

THE VEINS

Posterior ciliary veins

Vortex vein

Venous circle of Hovius

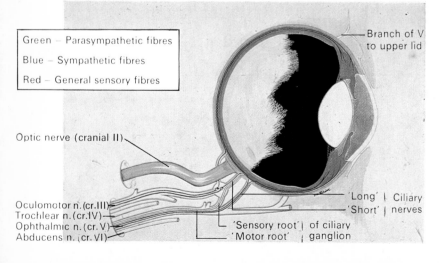

Green – Parasympathetic fibres

Blue – Sympathetic fibres

Red – General sensory fibres

Branch of V to upper lid

THE NERVES

Optic nerve (cranial II)

Oculomotor n. (cr. III)
Trochlear n. (cr. IV)
Ophthalmic n. (cr. V)
Abducens n. (cr. VI)

'Long' | Ciliary
'Short' | nerves

'Sensory root' | of ciliary
'Motor root' | ganglion

1

THE OPTICAL MECHANISM

The eye (Fig. 1) has often been compared with a camera, and this analogy is appropriate. In basic structure, both are similar. The camera possesses a lens in order to bend the rays of light entering the instrument and focus

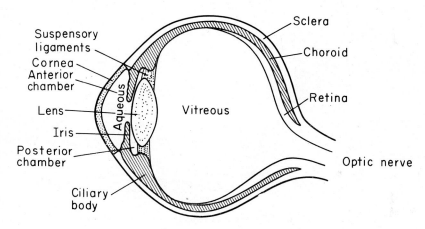

Fig. 1A. *Horizontal section of the eye.*

them upon the film; this function is performed in the eye by the refractive surfaces—the cornea and the anterior and posterior surfaces of the lens, and by the refractive media—the lens substance and aqueous and vitreous humours. Light passes through the structures of the eye to reach, and be focused upon, the retina, which corresponds to the film in the camera in that it is a light-sensitive structure. The image produced upon the retina is small and inverted. Stimulation of the retina and optic nerve produces the sensation of light. The amount of light entering the eye and reaching the retina is controlled partly by the movements of the eyelids and partly by the action of the iris.

The bending of rays of light entering the eye—*refraction*—so that these rays come to focus upon the retina, is brought about by the interruption of the rays by the refractive surfaces and media. These, in order from the outside, are as follows:

(1) The anterior surface of the cornea.
(2) The posterior surface of the cornea.
(3) The aqueous humour.
(4) The anterior surface of the lens.
(5) The lens substance.
(6) The posterior surface of the lens.
(7) The vitreous humour.
(8) The anterior surface of the retina.

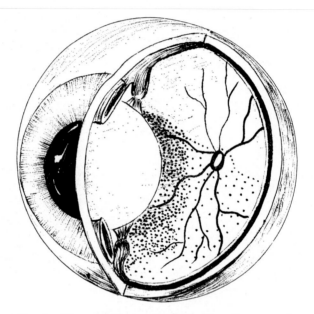

FIG. 1B. *Three-quarter view of eyeball with section removed.*

The refractive mechanism of the eye cannot be compared with a camera lens in optical perfection, but the optical aberrations that are likely to occur are compensated for by physiological factors and by the structure of the eyeball. Spherical aberration is counteracted by the curvature of the retina and the action of the pupil in conditions of good light; in such conditions the rays of light reaching the retina are confined to the more perfect axial portions of the cornea and lens. In conditions of poor light, when the pupil is dilated and the less perfect portions of the refractive system are in use, the eye is concerned in the detection of available light and movement and not with any resolution of detail.

Refraction is performed mostly by the refractive surfaces, of which the cornea is the most important; the effect of the refractive media on the rays of light is considerably less. The ability of the lens to focus rays of light upon the retina—*accommodation*—is poorly developed in the dog, partly due to the structure of the ciliary muscles and partly due to the firmness of the lens. The lack of elasticity in the canine lens and the consequent lack of accommodative power, results in the cornea being the most important

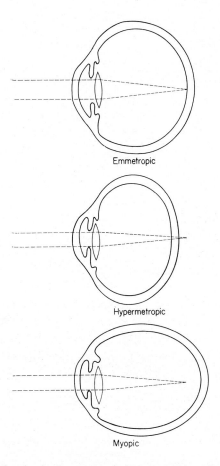

Emmetropic

Hypermetropic

Myopic

FIG. 2. *Refraction in the emmetropic, hypermetropic and myopic eye.*

refractive area. Thus the power of the cornea can be modified by the lens to only a slight extent.

The optic axis, which represents the shortest distance between cornea and retina, passes through the centre of the cornea at right angles to its surface, meeting the retina near its centre but lateral to the optic disc.

Parallel rays of light which meet the cornea perpendicularly are not refracted; those that meet the cornea at an angle are refracted and, in a normal eye, will meet at a point on the retinal surface. Such eyes are described as emmetropic, and in them the rays of light are focused on the retina and vision will be good. Eyes in which the rays of light do not meet on the retina are described as ametropic. They may be myopic (short-sighted) where the rays meet at a point in front of the retina, or hypermetropic (long-sighted) where they meet behind the retina (Fig. 2). Again, the convexity of the cornea may not be regular in all planes, resulting in images of different parts of the object being focused unevenly; such a condition is known as astigmatism.

Myopia may arise in two ways: either the length of the eyeball may be too great so that the refracted image lies at a point in front of the retina, or the refractive power of the optical parts of the eye may be too great, with the same result. Similar but opposite factors may be operative in cases of hypermetropia. Most domestic dogs are myopic and astigmatic, although those carnivorous animals that hunt by sight are usually hypermetropic. Myopia is most pronounced in the brachycephalic breeds, where variations in the curvature of the cornea and lens and variations in the antero-posterior measurements of the eyeball are most pronounced.

Histological examinations of the retina in the dog, and many other investigations, have shown that the dog is colour blind and that colours are seen as shades of grey. Vision in the dog is dominated by shape and movement and, to a less extent, brightness. Although movement is normally important, the dog is able to recognize certain objects, particularly other dogs, by shape alone. However, other factors such as the relatively large cornea and pupillary opening and the relatively wide peripheral visual field, compensate to a certain extent for the lack of colour vision and the lack of detail resolution. Under poor lighting conditions vision is further enhanced by the presence of the tapetum lucidum and the abundance of rods in the retina. Binocular and stereoscopic vision is present in the dog and, therefore, some decussation of nerve fibres in the optic nerves which allows three-dimensional objects to be observed.

Rays of light falling upon the retina stimulate a photochemical reaction, converting the light impulse into nervous impulses. These are transmitted through the retina to the optic nerve, and thence to the optic chiasma, where partial decussation of the nerve fibres take place, approximately 75% of the optic nerve fibres of each eye crossing in the chiasma. The nerve fibres continue via the optic tract to the lateral geniculate bodies in the thalamus and thence via the optic radiations to the primary visual cortex of the occipital lobe of the cerebrum, where the nerve impulses are converted into the sense of vision (Fig. 3). The eye and the optic nerve are therefore extensions of the brain, and damage to, or disease of, any part of the optic pathways may result in defective vision.

Binocular vision is, of course, important to the dog as a hunting and predatory animal. True binocular vision is present only in some of the brachycephalic breeds, but in all dogs there is some overlap of the two uniocular fields. This limits the field of vision but, on the other hand, allows the precision of vision required by a predatory creature. The two slightly dissimilar images received by the two eyes are combined into a single impression, with some degree of stereopsis, thus allowing the precise calculation of distance. The movements of the eyeball are distinctly limited, the pupil being kept horizontal whatever the position of the head. The dog,

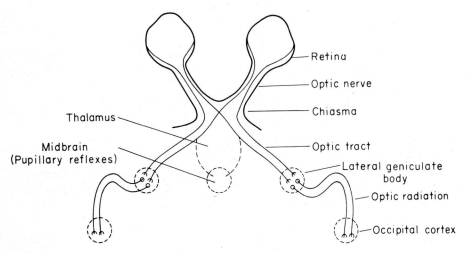

FIG. 3. *The optic pathways.*

in common with most animals, tends to follow objects by movements of the head rather than by movements of the eyeball. The compensation-fixation reflex is present, whereby a steady visual image is produced, despite movements of the body, by a linking of eye movements with posture. Ocular movement is linked with other sensations such as those of smell and gravitational change.

OCULAR ANATOMY

The detailed anatomy and physiology of each part of the eye is described in the chapter concerned with that particular part of the visual apparatus. Here we are concerned only with the general picture.

The eye is the organ of vision and, as has been seen earlier, is rather like the camera in structure and function. Each eye is roughly ball-shaped and, in the dog, is approximately 22 mm in diameter. It is contained almost wholly within a bony socket in the skull—the orbit. In the orbit it rests on a pad of fat which acts as a shock-absorber as well as protecting the optic nerve and the blood vessels of the eye, and is surrounded by muscles which hold it in place and control its movements. The exposed front part of the eye is protected by eyelids which can be closed at will.

Situated as they are, in an exposed position, it might be thought that the eyes would be subjected to repeated injuries. The eyeball, however, is able to withstand considerable violence before it becomes seriously damaged, and the movements of the head, eyelids and eyeball necessary to avoid serious damage are controlled by very well-developed instinctive reactions, both of a voluntary and an involuntary nature.

The eyeball is composed of three coats:

(1) The outer coat or sclera is the dense fibrous tissue that forms the white of the eye. It is a tough opaque membrane that protects the eye. Anteriorly there is a transparent part, the cornea, which acts as a window and allows the rays of light to enter the eye.

(2) The middle coat is the choroid which lines the whole of the sclera but not the cornea. It is a dark pigmented layer and, like the black lining of a camera, prevents the reflection of light. At the junction of cornea and sclera, inside the eyeball, it forms a muscular diaphragm, the iris, forming the coloured part of the eye. In the dog the pupil is circular.

(3) The inner coat, or retina, composed of nerve tissue. It lines the interior of the eyeball, behind the iris, and is covered with nerve endings susceptible to light. This is the receptive area of the eye and is continuous with the optic nerve.

The eyeball contains three structures: the lens, the aqueous humour and the vitreous humour. The lens is convex, like a magnifying glass, and is held in position by a ligament around its edge—the zonule or suspensory ligament—attaching it to the ciliary body. In front of the lens occupying the space between lens and cornea is the aqueous humour, a saline-like fluid that is formed constantly. The large chamber of the eye, situated between lens and retina, is filled with the vitreous humour, a jelly-like transparent substance which helps to maintain the shape of the eyeball and to keep the retina in place. The four transparent parts of the eye—cornea, aqueous humour, lens, and vitreous humour—all help to conduct rays of light from the outside to the retina.

The eyelids, which can be closed to cover the front of the eye, are lined by a transparent membrane—the conjunctiva—which is continued on the visible part of the eyeball. The third eyelid, or nictitating membrane, is well developed in the dog, and is situated at the inner angle of the eye where the upper and lower lids meet. Its purpose is both to help with the lubrication of the eye and to remove foreign matter from the cornea, and it moves across the eye when the eyeball is retracted into the orbit.

The cornea is kept moist by means of the tears which are secreted by the lacrimal gland under the upper lid. The tears flow over the eye and drain into two small openings, the lacrimal puncta, one at the edge of each lid at its inner angle, and thence into the nasal cavity.

THE VASCULAR SYSTEM

It is not possible within the scope of this book to give detailed descriptions of the vascular and nerve supply to the eye, but only to outline the principal facts. For further details, readers are referred to works listed in the bibliography.

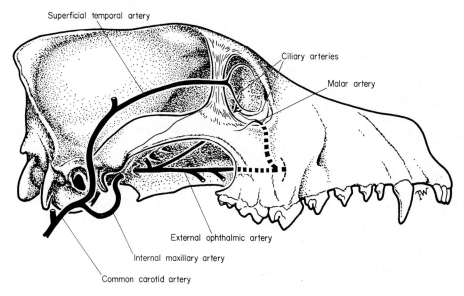

FIG. 4. *The arterial supply in the orbital region.*

Vessels of the orbit

The *external carotid artery* (Fig. 4) divides beneath the bony external auditory meatus into:

(1) The *superficial temporal artery* which courses dorsal to the zygoma to supply both eyelids.

(2) The *maxillary (internal maxillary) artery*. This gives off deep branches to the temporal region and then, after passing through the alar canal, continues along the pterygo-palatine fossa towards the maxillary foramen. In its course along the fossa it gives off:

(a) Branches to the temporal region.

(b) The *external ophthalmic artery* which gives a branch to the nasal cavity (*ethmoidal artery*) and finally divides into *ciliary arteries* near the globe of the eye. At this site, the small *internal ophthalmic artery*, which accompanies the optic nerve from the cranial cavity, anastomoses with the external ophthalmic artery.

(c) Branches to orbital structures other than the eye, and

(d) Near the maxillary foramen, a *malar artery* which supplies the region around the lower lid.

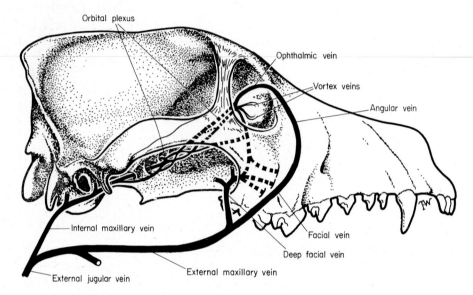

FIG. 5. *The venous drainage.*

Blood is drained from the orbital region by veins which enter the *orbital venous plexus* lying in the pterygo-palatine fossa (Fig. 5). These veins are:

(1) The *ophthalmic vein*, which enters the orbit near the medial canthus as a very large vessel, the *angular vein;* this vessel has a connection with the facial vein. The ophthalmic vein receives veins from all orbital structures.

(2) The *deep facial vein* which passes around the maxillary tubercle and is also connected with the facial vein.

(3) Vessels connected with the intracranial venous sinuses and so to the small internal jugular vein.

(4) Vessels which join the external jugular vein.

Vessels of the eye

Arteries. The *ophthalmic artery* (Fig. 4) divides to give off numerous vessels to the globe which are conveniently divided into:

(1) *Short posterior ciliary arteries*, which pierce the sclera around the optic nerve and form the capillary layer of the choroid (the *chorio-capillaris*).

(2) *Long posterior ciliary arteries*, lateral and medial, which supply the sclera, ciliary body and iris, and thus also supply the uveal tract. A vascular ring is formed within the iris (the *arterial circle of the iris*). Radial vessels supply the iris structure.

(3) *Anterior ciliary arteries*, which enter the sclera near the level of the ciliary body where they anastomose with branches of the long posterior ciliary arteries.

(4) Numerous *retinal arterioles* which arise with the short posterior ciliary arteries and penetrate the sclera around the optic nerve. Examination of the fundus reveals them as vessels which radiate from the edge of the optic disc. There are 6 to 8 major arterioles which accompany 3 to 4 major venules.

Veins. Blood is drained from the uveal tract mainly into four veins (the *vortex veins*) which leave the sclera around the equator of the globe (Fig. 5). They are assisted by *anterior* and *posterior* ciliary veins.

The *retinal venules* converge on the optic disc where they may anastomose before passing out through the sclera to join the short posterior ciliary veins, and thence the complex plexus of veins in the orbit.

NERVES OF THE EYE AND ORBIT

(1) *Somatic motor fibres.* The muscles which move the globe, except one, originate in the region of the optic foramen and orbital fissure. The three nerves supplying these muscles issue from this fissure and are called the *oculomotor nerve* (cranial nerve III), the *trochlear nerve* (cranial nerve IV), and the *abducent nerve* (cranial nerve VI).

The *trochlear nerve* innervates the superior oblique muscle whose tendon passes across a pulley-like trochlea.

The *abducent nerve* innervates the external rectus muscle, which abducts the eye, and part of the retractor bulbi muscle.

The *oculomotor nerve* innervates the remaining muscles, i.e. the superior, internal and inferior rectus muscles, the inferior oblique muscle, part of the retractor bulbi, and the levator palpebrae superioris, which inserts into the upper eyelid.

The facial musculature of the eyelids (e.g. orbicularis oculi muscle) is innervated by the *facial nerve* (cranial nerve VII).

(2) *Somatic sensory fibres* from orbital structures are found in the *trigeminal* nerve (cranial nerve V) (Fig. 6), the divisions involved being the *ophthalmic* and *maxillary nerves*.

The *ophthalmic nerve* issues from the orbital fissure and gives off the following branches:

(a) The *lacrimal nerve* to the lacrimal gland.

(b) The *supraorbital nerve* (*frontal nerve*) whose fibres innervate the tissues in the region of the upper lid.

2

(c) The *nasociliary nerve* which sends a branch to the nasal cavity (the *ethmoid nerve*) as well as a *long ciliary nerve* to the eyeball. It then continues as the *infratrochlear nerve* to innervate tissues in the region of the upper eyelid near the medial canthus.

The *maxillary nerve* passes from the round foramen along the pterygo-palatine fossa. It leaves the fossa at its rostral end and in its course gives rise to the *zygomatic nerve*. This nerve has two divisions—the *zygomatico-facial nerve* which crosses the zygoma ventral to the lateral canthus of the

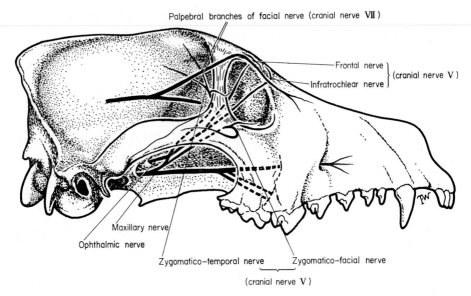

Palpebral branches of facial nerve (cranial nerve VII)

Frontal nerve ⎱
                   ⎰ (cranial nerve V)
Infratrochlear nerve ⎰

Maxillary nerve
Ophthalmic nerve
Zygomatico–temporal nerve   Zygomatico–facial nerve

(cranial nerve V)

FIG. 6. *The orbital nerves (cranial nerves II, III and IV have been omitted for clarity).*

eye where it innervates the lower lid and neighbouring tissues, and the *zygomatico-temporal nerve* which is sensory to the temporal region and the lateral canthus.

(3) *Visceral fibres.* Autonomic innervation of the orbital structures is associated with blood vessels and the cranial nerves mentioned.

(a) Parasympathetic innervation of the eyeball is mediated via the *ciliary ganglion* which is associated with the oculomotor nerve. *Short ciliary nerves* arise from the neurons contained within the ganglion and supply the iris and ciliary body. Other fibres from other sources may pass through the ganglion on their way to the eye.

(b) Sympathetic fibres arise from the *cranial cervical ganglion* and are distributed via cranial nerves and blood vessels to orbital structures.

(4) *Special sensory fibres.* The *optic nerve* (cranial nerve II) is formed from the axons of the ganglion cells of the retina. These axons converge towards the optic disc where they penetrate the sclera at the area cribrosa

and at the same time become medullated and invested with layers of connective tissue which are continuous with the meninges and which enclose an extension of the subarachnoid space. The optic nerve enters the cranial cavity via the optic foramen and forms the optic chiasma with the nerve of the other side before the axons are distributed to the lateral geniculate bodies in the brain.

2
EXAMINATION OF THE EYE

ROUTINE EXAMINATION

The routine examination of the eye should consist, as in other medical examinations, of a careful history, a physical examination, and special examinations as indicated.

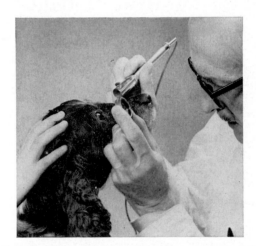

Fig. 7. *Examination of the eye with loupe and focal beam.*

Examination of the eye and its adnexa in the dog is usually possible with a minimum of restraint, but in certain cases local or even general anaesthesia may have to be employed. In some patients, manipulation of the lids and exposure of the globe may be resisted and, in addition, the powerful muscul-ature of the lids and the retraction of the eyeball into the orbit may make examination difficult. Retraction of the eyeball causes the membrana nictitans to sweep across the globe and this also hinders examination.

The eyes should first be inspected in daylight for evidence of injuries, ocular discharge or abnormal movements of the eyeball. Further examina-tion is best carried out in a darkened room, when the darkness will usually have a quietening effect on the animal and will keep the pupil dilated.

Before examination the eyes should be cleansed and any exudate removed. The animal should be placed on a table of suitable height and restrained by allowing the lower jaw to rest on the palm of the hand of an assistant, while the other hand steadies the base of the skull. This will minimize movements of the head, but in uncooperative animals, sedation or tranquillization may be required.

Certain equipment is essential for adequate examination and accurate diagnosis. Some form of electric illumination will be required, preferably in the form of a focused beam (Fig. 7); in addition the clinician will need a corneal magnifying lens or corneal loupe (Fig. 8), a condensing lens of about

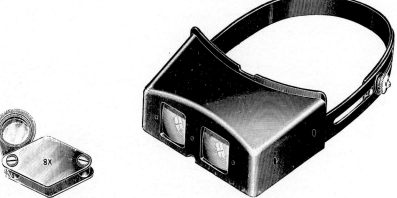

FIG. 8. *Corneal loupe.*   FIG. 9. *Binocular loupe.*

14 dioptres, and an electric ophthalmoscope. A binocular loupe may be employed (Fig. 9), thus leaving both hands free for the handling of the patient.

Drugs required during the examination will include a 2% solution of fluorescein to demonstrate corneal injuries and to test the patency of the lacrimal canals; a 2% solution of homatropine or other suitable mydriatic to dilate the pupil in certain cases; and a topical anaesthetic agent such as 4% lignocaine hydrochloride. It should be noted that cocaine is liable to injure the corneal epithelium and should be used with care.

The normal procedure is first to make a detailed examination of the adnexa and then to examine the ocular structures serially, commencing with the cornea and ending with the fundus.

Provided that the light in the examination room is sufficiently subdued and the light in the ophthalmoscope is strong, it is not usually necessary to dilate the pupil to examine the ocular media and fundus. However, in order to examine the peripheral fundus, or to study adequately incipient cataracts or retinal lesions, it is necessary to dilate the pupil to facilitate ophthalmoscopic and slit-lamp examinations.

History of the case

As in all medical examinations it is essential that an adequate history of the case is available. Special note should be made of the age of the patient as this is important as a factor in senile changes, and of the breed of the animal which is significant in many ocular conditions that have a definite breed incidence.

Clinical signs

Cases will be presented to the clinician with the owner's history of one or more of the following defects: subnormal or abnormal visual acuity; signs of pain or irritation; changes in the appearance of the lids, periorbital tissues, orbit or eye; increased lacrimal secretion, or ocular discharge, or staining of the hair around or below the eye.

Subnormal visual acuity. Points that must be ascertained include the duration of the impairment; the nature of onset; the difference, if any, in the visual acuity of the two eyes; the nature of the signs by which the owner believes the dog to have failing sight; and the presence or absence of night blindness.

Pain or irritation. The usual signs noticed are itching of the eye or eyelids with consequent rubbing at the eye by the forelimb, rubbing the eye on the ground, or scratching the eye with the hind paw. In certain cases the animal may resent being touched around the eye or may keep the eyelids tightly closed.

Changes in appearance. This may take the form of a swelling in the lids, a mass in the lids or around the eye, displacement of the eye, or discoloration. Swelling in one lid may suggest a local abscess. Swelling of both lids indicates a more generalized reaction such as blepharitis, chemosis or allergy. A mass in a lid may indicate a cyst or tumour. A mass around or behind an eye may indicate a tumour or a retrobulbar abscess.

Displacement may be associated with squint or with prolapse of the eyeball. Changes in the position of the lids may be associated with ptosis, blepharospasm, lagophthalmos, entropion, ectropion, chalazion or neoplasia.

Discoloration may be seen as a redness or congestion of the lids, orbital tissues, conjunctiva or sclera. The cornea may show colour changes associated with vascularization or opacity. Cloudiness of the anterior chamber may be noticed with intraocular infections and hypopyon. Other conditions may produce changes in the colour of the 'white' of the eye and, in jaundice, this may be yellow. Occasionally, yellowness may occur in the intraocular structures. Dark discolorations may be noted in pigmentary changes.

Discharge. Increased discharge from the eyes may be associated with epiphora or may be exudative in nature. The type and nature of the discharge must be ascertained. The duration must be noted, together with any evidence of crusting on the lid margins. Epiphora, resulting from excessive formation of tears or a blockage of the lacrimal drainage system, must be distinguished from abnormal discharges. Watery discharges not associated with redness or irritation usually indicate an epiphora, those associated with irritation usually indicate a conjunctivitis or kerato-conjunctivitis. Purulent discharges are normally associated with bacterial infections.

External examination

A general inspection is made for obvious abnormalities. The examination is greatly facilitated by the use of a well focused source of light and a magnifying loupe.

The lids are examined for evidence of injury, blepharitis, entropion, ectropion and tumours, and are then everted to allow examination of the conjunctiva and nictitating membrane. It may be necessary to examine the lymphoid tissue on the underside of the membrana, and this may be done with the aid of topical anaesthesia. Examination is made for foreign bodies and a note made of any inflammatory changes, discharges, epiphora or dryness, and changes in the clarity or colour of the cornea.

The size, shape, internal pressure and movements of the eyeballs are noted. The cornea and anterior segment of the eye are then examined under good illumination, and any changes in the cornea, anterior chamber, iris or lens noted.

Most of the common diseases of the eye may be detected by a thorough clinical examination, carried out with the minimum of equipment, under good lighting conditions.

Oblique illumination

For this procedure, a source of light is concentrated on to the anterior structures of the eye by means of a convex lens, and the illuminated spot is viewed through a magnifying lens.

The cornea should also be examined from the lateral view, or conditions such as embedded foreign bodies and anterior synechia may be missed.

Slit-lamp examination

Visualization of an optical section of the anterior segment of the eye may be obtained by use of a hand slit-lamp, either mains operated or used in conjunction with an ophthalmoscope handle (Fig. 10). The Pantoscope incorporates a device for producing a slit beam. Placed at an angle to the cornea, the beam of light from the slit-lamp, visualizing the optical section, may be viewed with the naked eye or through a loupe. Both light source and magnification are provided in the Hobbs illuminated slit-loupe (Fig. 11).

Slit-lamp examination provides a more accurate assessment of the structures of the anterior segment, and allows more accurate estimation of the depth of lesions or pathological changes.

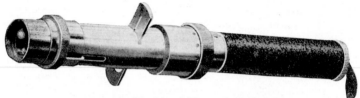

FIG. 10. *Hand inspection and slit-lamp.*

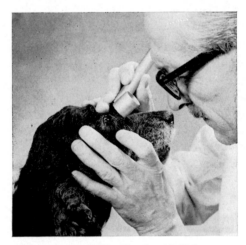

FIG. 11. *The Hobbs illuminated slit-loupe.*

Ophthalmoscopic examination

The modern ophthalmoscope is an instrument used for the examination of the posterior segment of the eye, that is the retina and vitreous body. It may also be used for the examination of the anterior structures, but the methods already described are better for this purpose.

Light can enter or leave the eye only through the pupil. The interior of the eye may be viewed by looking through the pupil along a beam of light directed through the same aperture. The ophthalmoscope reflects light from an angled mirror into the eye; as the mirror is held close to the patient's eye the rays of light from it are strongly convergent. They are bent further by the refractive media of the eye and cross the vitreous well in front of the retina, thus illuminating an area of fundus by divergent rays (Fig. 12).

The direction of rays of light in the eye is reversible. Therefore if the back of an emmetropic eye is rendered luminous, it will emit parallel rays.

If the observer, also, is emmetropic, these rays will come to focus on his retina, and he will have a clear image of the patient's fundus. If the patient is not emmetropic, it can be made so by placing a lens in front of the eye. In direct ophthalmoscopy the lens required to give a clear image of the patient's fundus has a refraction equal to the algebraical sum of the refractions of patient and observer; therefore it is possible to measure refractivity with the ohpthalmoscope. If the observer is emmetropic, the highest convex or lowest concave lens with which the patient's fundus is clearly seen is a measure of the patient's refractivity, assuming that there is no astigmatism.

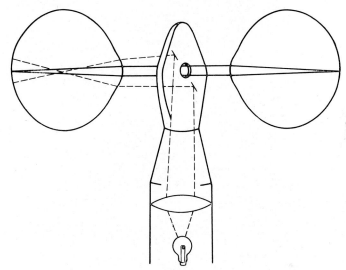

FIG. 12. *Path of rays of light in direct ophthalmoscopy.*

If the observer is not emmetropic, the necessary addition or subtraction must be made.

Direct ophthalmoscopy

This is the method that will commonly be employed in the dog, using an electric ophthalmoscope. The examination is best carried out in a darkened room and through a dilated pupil. In many cases, however, the retina may be examined satisfactorily through an undilated pupil, provided the refractive media are clear. The advantages of the direct method are that it shows greater fundus detail, there is greater magnification, the image is erect, and the equipment is easily portable. Penetration of cloudy media may be obtained by using the more powerful instruments available.

Direct ophthalmoscopy may be used to examine both posterior and anterior segments of the eye, although other methods described are to be preferred for the latter.

Many types of ophthalmoscope are available, all of which have the effect of illuminating the retina. The instrument consists of a source of light that may be derived either from a battery or from mains electricity. The light is passed through a condensing lens system, into a prism or mirror, which deflects the beam through the patient's pupil on to the retina. The observer,

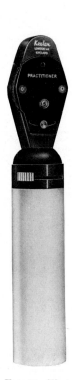

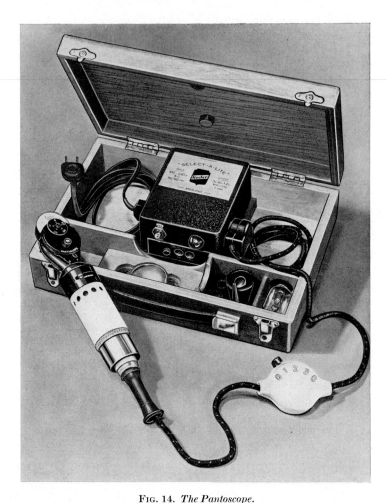

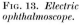

FIG. 13. *Electric ophthalmoscope.*

FIG. 14. *The Pantoscope.*

in the direct line of the reflected beam of light, observes the patient's fundus. Behind the mirror are a series of spherical lenses in a circular revolving disc, which may be selected to appear in line with the viewing aperture. The selected lens has the function of magnifying the fundus image whilst correcting the refractive errors in the patient's and in the observer's eyes. The proper lens positioned in the viewing aperture will bring into focus a clear image of the patient's fundus. The lenses differ slightly in different instruments, but usually vary from −0·5 D to −20·0 D on one side of the disc, and from +0·5 D to +20·0 D on the other (Figs. 13 & 14). The observer's vision, unless emmetropic, should be corrected by spectacles, so that the aperture marked '0' gives a clear view of the fundus provided that the patient also is emmetropic.

Some instruments incorporate other features such as filters which permit changes in the size and character of the beam produced, red-free filters, slit-apparatus and grids.

Use of the ophthalmoscope

In the dog it is sometimes difficult to maintain constant viewing of the fundus because the patient tries continuously to shift its vision. This may be

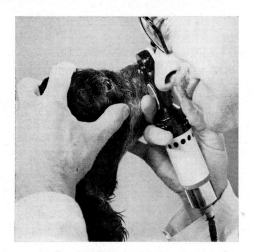

FIG. 15. *Direct ophthalmoscopy.*

largely obviated by having an assistant to hold the lids apart whilst pressing lightly with the fingers against the lateral side of the eyeball to prevent movement. The correct method, when examining the right eye, is for the observer to use his right eye and to stand on the right side of the patient. When examining the left eye, the observer stands on the left side and uses his left eye. The observer's other eye should be suppressed but not closed.

The instrument is held as close as possible to the observer's eye, in the first instance at about 25 or 30 cm from that of the patient, with the '0' or open aperture in the viewing hole. A greenish or yellowish tapetal reflex will be seen, and there will be a general view of the refractive media. It is important that the observer relaxes his own accommodation, and gazes through the eye rather than at the eye.

For a detailed examination of the fundus the instrument is brought as close as possible to the patient, thus giving the maximum magnification

(Fig. 15). As most dogs are myopic, which means that the observed image is focused on a point in front of the retina rather than directly on to it, correction must be made by altering the viewing lens. The degree of myopia is usually about 3 dioptres, and so a lens of −3 D is used to focus on the disc. The lenses are rotated until a good picture is obtained and the fundus, consisting of optic disc, tapetum lucidum, tapetum nigrum and retina, can be examined. Only a small proportion of the fundus is usually visible and it is difficult to observe the peripheral fundus by this method.

The extent of any lesion may be estimated by the ophthalmoscope. The best method is to compare the size in terms of optic disc diameters, estimating the disc as 1·5 mm width. Changes in the level of structures in the fundus, such as tumours, cupped discs or papilloedema, are measured in dioptres. An elevation of +3 D equals 1 mm, while a depression of −6 D equals 2 mm. To measure changes in elevation the instrument is focused sharply on the arterial reflex in a level part of the fundus, and the lens used is noted. It is then focused on the highest or lowest portion of the convexity or concavity and the difference in the reading is noted. Transposition of the dioptres into millimetres will give the height or depth of the lesion.

Other structures of the eye may be examined by changing the lens in the viewing aperture. By rotating the lenses through the minus range to the plus range, the structures anterior to the fundus may be examined. Vitreous opacities are seen between 0 and +8 D, the crystalline lens between +8 and +12 D, and the iris, anterior chamber and cornea between +12 and +20 D.

SPECIAL EXAMINATION

Simple indirect ophthalmoscopy

The advantages of this method are that it provides a view of a larger area of the fundus; one is able to view the peripheral fundus and, by depressing the sclera with a thimble depressor, the ora serrata and part of the ciliary body; and there is added safety to the observer. The disadvantages are the lower magnification obtained and the fact that, if the patient is restless, it is difficult to keep the beam of light centered on the eye for a sufficient length of time.

Mydriasis and semi-dark conditions will be required. A beam of light is directed into the eye, either from a mirror or by an ophthalmoscope held not less than 0·6 m (2 ft) from the patient's eye, illuminating the entire pupil. When the fundus is illuminated, a convex lens (20 D) is placed at a point about 5·0 to 7·5 cm from the animal's eye. The lens is moved back and forwards until a clear picture of the fundus is seen. The image seen is inverted, that is the upper part of the fundus appears below and the nasal part appears on the temporal side. In fact a real inverted image is produced between the observer's eye and the objective lens (Figs. 16 and 17).

As this inverted image is situated in space, it is necessary for the observer to accommodate to some extent in order to focus the image clearly. If, as with most dogs, the patient is myopic, the rays that emerge from the eye are to some extent convergent and are brought to focus nearer to the objective lens than with an emmetropic or hypermetropic patient. The degree of magnification is about 5 diameters.

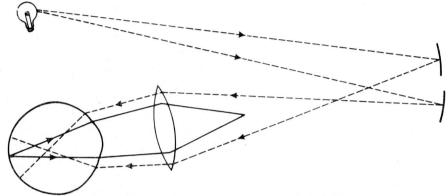

FIG. 16. *Path of rays of light in indirect ophthalmoscopy.*

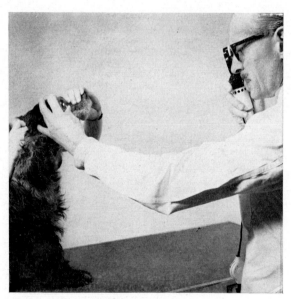

FIG. 17. *Indirect ophthalmoscopy.*

Binocular indirect ophthalmoscopy

The principles of this method are the same as those that apply to simple indirect ophthalmoscopy, in that light is reflected from a mirror through a plus lens into the patient's eye. The light rays reflect back from the fundus through the lens, forming an inverted image of the patient's fundus in space at the focal plane of the condensing lens. The observer, placing himself at a comfortable distance from the aerial image, sees this image (Fig. 18).

The source of light is carried on a headband to which is attached a pair of lenses, one for each of the observer's eyes. This aids in observing the

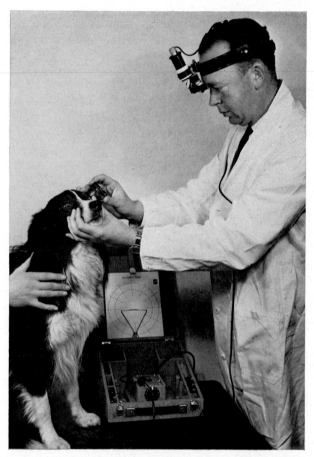

FIG. 18. *Binocular indirect ophthalmoscopy.*

image and gives a stereoscopic effect. Other advantages of this method over direct ophthalmoscopy are that the field is large, there is more illumination and better penetration of cloudy media, and the peripheral retina can more easily be examined. Both the observer's hands are free for the manipulation of the condensing lens and the control of the patient. There is an added safety factor for the observer in that he is placed further from the animal under examination. The disadvantages are that the image is inverted, magnification is not so great as with direct methods, and the equipment is somewhat cumbersome.

The location of opacities in the eye

Parallax. The position of an opacity, whether in the cornea, lens or posterior segment of the eye, may be determined by observing its apparent movement in relationship to the pupillary border when the observer's head is moved from side to side. Central opacities remain still or move only slightly in a direction opposite to that of the observer; anterior opacities move towards the pupillary border against the observer; posterior opacities move in the same direction as does the observer.

Shadow test. When the posterior part of the lens cortex is opaque but the anterior portion is transparent, oblique illumination of the eye will cause the iris shadow to fall upon the lens. In such a case a sickle-shaped shadow will appear at the opposite border if the source of illumination is transferred to the opposite side. If the whole of the lens cortex is opaque no shadow will be formed.

Biomicroscopy

Biomicroscopy, or the examination of the eye with a microscope and a special light source in the form of a slit-lamp, permits the diagnosis and evaluation of many ocular lesions that could not be determined with ordinary clinical methods. A well-illuminated and highly magnified view of the area involved is obtained.

Biomicroscopy allows the examination of an optical section of such structures as the cornea, lens or vitreous body, under a magnification of 10 to 60 diameters, using a binocular microscope (Fig. 19). The apparatus used consists of an illuminating unit and optical system, producing an intense beam of light through a slit or perforated diaphragm that can be focused on the part under observation. This unit is mounted on a stand, and may be moved to either side so that the beam may be projected into the eye from either side. A binocular microscope is mounted on another arm of the stand, and this may be focused on the illuminated area. All the components are freely movable and may be locked in any desired position, the angle between the lamp and the microscope varying from 40 to 50°. In some units both microscope and light can be focused with one control.

In a darkened room, a slit-shaped beam of light, projected at an angle upon one of the translucent structures of the eye, is visible in that structure as a brightly illuminated, sharply defined, rectangular prism. The part under examination appears as an optical section of that part and the microscope may be used to detect both normal structures and pathological changes. Optical sections of cornea, lens and vitreous body may be studied. Opaque structures such as the iris may be examined, highly magnified, under direct illumination. The retina and optic nerve may be studied by the addition to the apparatus of a prism combined with a Hruby lens (−40 D).

As the slit-lamp must be used close to the patient's eye, restraint is necessary and, in most cases, general anaesthesia will be required if a detailed examination is to be made. The dog must be positioned on its sternum, and the head must be raised and fixed at the level of the lamp. The high cost of slit-lamp microscopes, and their somewhat difficult application to the dog, makes biomicroscopy a very specialized technique rarely used under practice conditions.

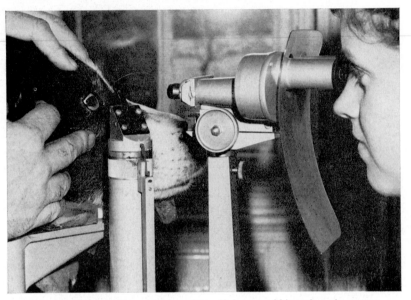

Fig. 19. *Examination of the eye with a slit-lamp and binocular microscope.*

Methods of examination in biomicroscopy

Direct illumination. This is the usual method for localizing and examining a lesion. A narrow beam of light is used, which is focused on the cornea from the temporal aspect, producing a brightly illuminated and sharp prism in the cornea (Fig. 20). The width of the slit may be altered as required and the prism is examined under the microscope. When the light is derived from the left side, the microscope is focused on the right anterior border of the prism. The anterior surface of the cornea corresponds to the point of entry of the beam into the cornea and, by adjustment of both lamp and microscope, the point where the beam emerges from the cornea, representing the posterior surface of the cornea, may also be examined. Thus both surfaces may be examined, corneal changes may be localized and studied, and the thickness of the cornea may be estimated.

Similarly both lens and vitreous body may be studied using a narrow angle of illumination for the vitreous. The iris may also be examined under direct illumination.

Diffuse illumination. This may be used for the general examination of the ocular structures.

Sclerotic scatter. By placing the light at the limbus, leaving the cornea in darkness, minute corneal lesions are illuminated by reflection.

Transmitted light. A broad beam of light focused on a reflecting surface such as iris, lens or retina, reveals small details in the transparent tissues anterior to the reflecting surface.

Specular reflection. This is the reflected light received by the observer when the angle of observation equals the angle of illumination. The reflected beam is received by one objective only and will reveal minute changes in the cornea.

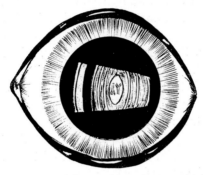

Fig. 20. *Optical section of the anterior segment seen by the slit-lamp.*

Indirect illumination. Focusing the beam on the centre of the pupil produces a dark field illumination of the iris which may reveal changes not apparent with other methods.

Biomicroscopic examination of the eye enables the early detection of many corneal changes that might not be visible by other methods. Epithelial detachment, vesicle or cavity formation, infiltrates and neovascularization may be detected, and it is possible to differentiate inflammatory changes from those due to degenerative processes. Early changes in iritis may be seen, and pigmentary deposits localized. The position and nature of lenticular opacities may be determined accurately.

Gonioscopy

Gonioscopy is the direct examination of the angle of the anterior chamber, that is the junction of the iris and cornea, an area that is concealed from view by the forward-pointing opaque edge of the scleral limbus. Examination of the angle is not possible using an ophthalmoscope unless the refractive conditions of the anterior chamber are changed by placing a contact glass over the cornea. Greater detail and magnification is obtained by using a hand binocular microscope in place of an ophthalmoscope.

Gonioscopy in the dog is carried out under general anaesthesia. The contact glass—a *goniolens*—is placed on the cornea with the membrana nictitans held outside the lens. To obtain optical continuity a suitable fluid, such as contact lens wetting solution, is placed between lens and cornea; the lens is then pushed towards the cornea to expel any bubbles of air.

The filtration angle may be examined through a circumference of 360° through the goniolens, using either a slit-lamp microscope or a hand binocular microscope and focal illuminator (a *gonioscope*). Alternatively, if other apparatus is not available, an electric ophthalmoscope may be used.

The study of the filtration angle in the dog has not, to date, been extensively reported. Gonioscopy, however, may be used in the study of filtration angles associated with the development of glaucoma, the investigation of iris tumours, and the localization of foreign bodies in the angle of the anterior chamber.

In the normal eye, the pectinate ligaments, when viewed through the goniolens, have been likened to trees in a forest, the roots having numerous branches which attach themselves to the iris border. Upwards, the trunks divide into many ramifications, ending in a darker zone of pigment, appearing like the foliage of trees (Troncoso).

In the glaucomatous eye, some or all of the pectinate ligaments may not be discernible, and adhesions may be seen of the root of the iris to the posterior surface of the cornea.

Tonometry

The determination of the intraocular pressure is termed tonometry. Intraocular pressure maintains the resistance of the eyeball to impression. Measurement of the impressibility of the tunics of the eye to deforming forces applied externally is thus a measurement of the intraocular pressure.

Two methods may be used for determining intraocular pressure—digital and instrumental tonometry.

Digital tonometry. A rough estimation of intraocular pressure may be made by placing the two index fingers on the upper eyelid over the globe to determine the tension of the eyeball, applying pressure alternately from one finger to the other (Fig. 21). A comparison should then be made with the other eye or with the eye of another animal. With experience this method can give a reasonable estimation of pressure, particularly when the intraocular tension is either quite high or quite low. It is the only method that should be employed in cases where the corneal epithelium is abnormal.

Instrumental tonometry. A far more accurate estimation of intraocular pressure may be obtained by the use of a tonometer, and this method should be used whenever possible. The tonometer (Fig. 22), which measures the corneal impressibility, records the resistance of the cornea to indentation by definite weights by the movement of a needle on a scale. A tonometer should not be used on any patient with an infected eye for fear of spreading the infection, via the instrument, to other animals. After use, the footplate should be cleansed thoroughly with a suitable antiseptic.

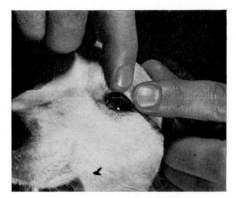

FIG. 21. *Digital tonometry.*

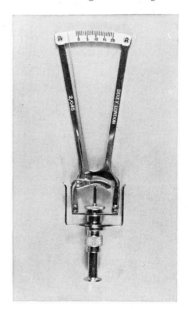

FIG. 22. *Schiøtz tonometer.*

The normal intraocular pressure reading for the dog varies from 15 to 17 mm Hg, although readings as high as 30 mm Hg may be considered to be within the normal range.

Use of the tonometer. In certain dogs it is possible to use the instrument following the instillation of a topical anaesthetic. In less cooperative patients and in those with retraction of the eyeball into the orbit or excessive rotation of the eyes, general anaesthesia will have to be employed.

The standard instrument used is the Schiøtz tonometer, the foot of which is concave to fit the normal curvature of the cornea, upon which it rests by its own weight. A metal plunger, situated in the centre of the foot, falls on to the surface of the cornea. The indentation of the cornea produced by the descent of the plunger is indicated by a lever on a scale. From the measurement on the scale, the intraocular tension (in mm Hg) may be calculated or determined by referring to a chart which converts the scale reading into mm Hg.

The dog is held so that the eye is directed upwards, the lids are separated, and the tonometer is allowed to rest by its own weight on the centre of the

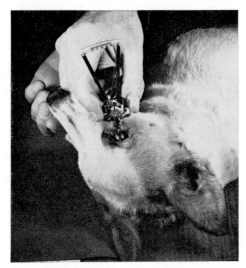

FIG. 23. *Instrumental tonometry using the Schiøtz tonometer.*

cornea (Fig. 23). It is important that no pressure is placed upon the globe by the assistant holding the head and separating the lids as any undue pressure will influence the reading. In some cases the protrusion of the nictitating membrane interferes with accurate placing of the instrument on the centre of the cornea, and readings may have to be taken with the foot-plate between the central and upper limbal area. It is not always possible, therefore, to obtain a highly accurate reading, but a good approximation of the intraocular pressure can always be made. More accurate estimation is possible if repeated readings can be made.

After use, a suitable ophthalmic antiseptic preparation should be placed in the eye to combat any infection that might have been introduced by the instrument, or any damage that might have been inflicted on the eye by the footplate.

Applanation tonometry. Applanation tonometers measure the pressure required to flatten rather than indent the cornea, the area involved being outlined by fluorescein. Such instruments are more accurate but considerably more expensive than the Schiotz tonometer and their use has not, as yet, been recorded in the dog.

Bacteriological examination

A bacteriological examination should be made in any case of internal or external ocular infection.

Direct swabs. Examination of the discharge present in the conjunctival sacs will rarely reveal the causal organism of a conjunctivitis. Direct smears from the conjunctiva are more likely to reveal micro-organisms that are normally present on the conjunctiva but which are not pathogenic. The normal bacteriology of the canine conjunctiva has yet to be established.

Scrapings. Organisms may often be identified from scrapings taken from the conjunctiva or cornea. Using a platinum spatula, scrapings may be taken from the lid margin, the conjunctiva or the cornea and a direct smear made on a glass slide. This may be stained with either Giemsa's, Gram's or Wright's stain, and examined microscopically. If necessary, cultures may be made on suitable culture material from the scraping, and the antibiotic sensitivity of the organisms established. Whereas with direct swabs it is often difficult to establish the predominant organism, scrapings will usually reveal only one or two predominant organisms and many can be promptly identified.

Alternatively a small portion of the conjunctiva may be excised under local anaesthesia, thus allowing the examination of epithelial cells for bacteria.

Anterior chamber puncture. Samples of aqueous humour for bacteriological culture may be obtained by puncture of the anterior chamber with an Amsler's needle. This needle is lancet-tipped, with a shaft stop as in a Bowman's needle and a hollow shaft. It is used attached to a tuberculin syringe.

Under topical or general anaesthesia, the eye is cleansed and antibiotic drops are instilled. A speculum is inserted and the eyeball held with fixation forceps positioned just posterior to the limbus. Using a small cataract knife, an incision about 1 mm long is made through about half the thickness of the cornea, just anterior to and concentric with the limbus in the lower temporal quadrant. The Amsler's needle is then passed through the corneal incision parallel to the anterior surface of the iris into the anterior chamber, and 0·1 to 0·3 ml of aqueous is aspirated. If the infection of the eye for which the test is being made is likely to be penicillin-sensitive, an aqueous solution of penicillin may be injected at the same time.

The aspirated aqueous may be used for Pandy's test for total protein, in which one drop of the aspirated fluid is added to 1 ml of 6% phenol solution in a watch-glass on a dark background. The amount of precipitation indicates the protein content, a faint opacity being considered normal. Similarly, a drop may be used in a Fuchs-Rosenthal counting chamber to obtain an estimation of the total cell count; or drops may be subjected to darkfield examination or hanging-drop preparations.

Corneal staining

Irregularities of the corneal surface and epithelial ulcerations are not always easily visible, even under good lighting conditions. Such erosions may be demonstrated, so that their extent and depth may be determined,

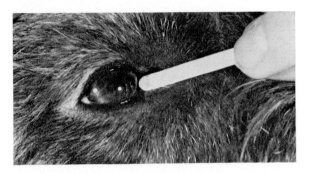

FIG. 24. *The use of fluorescein papers.*

by the installation of dyes such as fluorescein, mercurochrome or rose bengal into the conjunctival sac. Corneal staining is indicated in all cases of corneal trauma, and in other conditions when there is a possibility that the corneal epithelium is not intact.

As the corneal epithelium acts as a barrier to infection it is most important, in cases where the epithelium may be damaged, that any solution placed in the conjunctival sac is sterile. Fluorescein solutions may become contaminated, particularly with *Pseudomonas* organisms which have great affinity for, and are very destructive to, the cornea.

Technique. Fluorescein solution may be used provided that its sterility is not suspect. Solutions are best used in the form of sterile drop tubes (Guttilin, Bengue & Co) or individually packed sterile units (Minims, Smith & Nephew). One or two drops of the solution are placed in the conjunctival sac, and one or two drops of sterile water are added. A green dye solution is produced which will flow off the intact cornea but which will stain any areas over which the epithelium is missing.

Alternatively, sterile fluorescein papers may be used. A paper is wetted with sterile water or saline and this is touched on to the cornea, or the solution is allowed to drop on to the cornea (Fig. 24).

Lacrimal drainage test

Solutions placed in the conjunctival sac will normally pass into the lacrimal puncta and thence to the nasolacrimal duct and into the nose. The patency of the lacrimal system may be tested by placing a few drops of fluorescein solution in the conjunctival sac. If the dog's head is held low, the green dye will normally appear at the nostrils within 30 seconds. It must be noted, however, that in certain individuals the duct is interrupted in its length; in such cases, the dye may be transferred to the nasopharynx and may not appear at the nostrils.

X-ray examination

X-ray examination may be of value in cases of suspected orbital fractures or tumours, and may be used to locate orbital or intraocular foreign bodies. Intraocular foreign bodies may not always be visible by ophthalmoscopy, but if radiopaque, may be detected by X-ray examination. Radiopaque markers placed on the cornea may be used to help localize foreign bodies.

Functional examination

The degree of visual acuity in a dog may only be estimated. Tests for visual acuity, perimetry (the examination of the visual field), light and colour perception, and colour vision tests, are purely subjective and require the active cooperation of the patient. They are, in consequence, of no help to the animal practitioner.

The acuteness of vision may be estimated by obstacle tests, covering one eye with a bandage, or by watching the movements of the eyes in response to moving objects. Such tests are not easily applied, however, for the dog learns to adapt itself very well to failing sight and relies greatly on hearing and the sense of smell. Such vision tests should be carried out in areas as free of smells and noises as possible, using multiple obstacles.

It has been suggested, by H. B. Parry, that the degree of vision defect may be assessed as 0 to 5, representing the range from normal vision to complete blindness. The assessment may be written as 0/0 to 5/5. Such figures, however, are arbitrary and would probably be of value only to the individual practitioner who maintained records of his assessments of a wide range of cases.

Reflex activity tests

The eyes may be tested for the various reflexes associated with the cranial nerves; responses may be assessed as present or absent (0), strong (++) or weak (+), and whether or not they are bilaterally equal.

The corneal reflex (V). This determines the sensitivity of the cornea; it may be poorly developed in the brachycephalic breeds, and may be absent in cases of cerebral haemorrhage or facial paralysis. It may be tested by blowing air on to the cornea from a rubber bulb placed at the temporal aspect; or by touching the cornea gently from the side with a glass rod or brush.

The palpebral blink reflex (II). This protective blinking in response to threat may be elicited by throwing objects, such as small balls of cotton wool, towards the eye. Stimulation of the cornea and lids must be avoided, and this is best obtained by placing a sheet of clear plastic in front of the eye and throwing the balls at the plastic. Absence of the reflex may indicate either that the animal cannot see, or that the lids are paralysed (VII); the two can be distinguished by testing the corneal reflex.

The pupillary light reflex (II, III). This is determined by noting the response of the pupils to a source of light. The direct reflex may be estimated by first closing the opposite eye (to avoid a consensual reflex), and then shining a bright light into the eye to be tested; prompt pupillary constriction should take place. This reflex is initiated by the retina and travels to the oculomotor nerve via the optic nerve and the brain. The indirect or consensual reflex may be tested by observing one eye whilst the other is illuminated: both pupils should respond to light.

In cases of bilateral blindness neither direct nor consensual reflexes will be present. In unilateral blindness no direct reflex will be present in the blind eye, nor will the consensual reflex be elicited in the normal eye. However, if the oculomotor nerve in the blind eye is normal, the consensual reflex will be shown by the blind eye when the normal eye is illuminated.

The nictitating reflex (VI). This may be elicited by stimulation of the cornea, when retraction of the eye by the retractor muscle results in protrusion of the nictitating membrane.

The fixating reflex (II). This is estimated by the ability of the animal to fix the gaze on a light source, or to follow a flashing light that is moving laterally across the visual field.

Eye movements and squint are controlled by cranial nerves III, IV and VI. Nystagmus may be present in cases of cerebellar disease or lesions of the vestibular apparatus, in which case cranial nerve VIII may be involved. Ptosis may be associated with lesions of cranial nerve III, and lesions of cranial nerve II will result in changes in the fundus.

Central or peripheral lesions of the oculomotor nerve may result in *paralytic mydriasis*. In such cases, which are usually bilateral, the pupillary reflexes may be absent even though sight is present. Animals with such lesions often behave normally, except possibly in bright light, and the motor fibres of the nerve, supplying some of the extraocular muscles and the levator muscle, may remain normal.

DEVELOPMENT OF THE EYE

The development of visual acuity in the puppy is a slow, gradual process. The eyelids normally open at between the 10th and 16th days, at which time the cornea is hazy and the pupillary reflex only poorly developed, although consensual reflexes are present. The orientation of vision develops after about 25 days and the fixation and palpebral reflexes a few days later. Young puppies normally exhibit a convergent strabismus, but the resting position of the eyes becomes centralized by about the 25th day. The lens remains cloudy for the first 2 to 3 weeks.

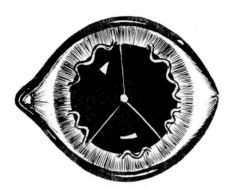

Fig. 25. *Embryonic remnants.*

Several embryonic remnants are present in the young animal, and these must not be mistaken for abnormalities (Fig. 25). The *embryonic pupillary membrane*, consisting of a fine network of filaments attached to the pupillary margin, normally disappears by the 5th week. The *embryonic hyaloid membrane*, seen as membranous adhesions near the centre of the lens, usually persists until the 4th or 6th week. The *radii lentis*, three lines on the lens in the shape of a Y, which represent the layers of cement-like substance which join the groups of lens fibres, disappear by the age of 5 weeks, but are often very obvious in later life during the development of cataract. In some breeds pigmented deposits—the *corpora nigra lentis*—are present along the radii, but normally disappear by the age of 4 weeks.

3

THE MEDICAL TREATMENT OF EYE DISEASE

The agents which have, in the past, been described and advocated for the treatment of various ocular disease conditions are many and various, and some have no place in modern ocular therapeutics. Others have been superseded by the chemotherapeutic agents, antibiotics and the corticosteroids.

EXTERNAL APPLICATIONS

Drugs may be applied to the eye in a watery vehicle, as drops (guttae) or lotions (collyria); in an oily vehicle, as oily drops, creams or ointments (oculenta); as powders; or as eye discs (lamellae).

Eye drops. Apply by raising the upper lid and allowing the drops to flow on to the eye from the 12 o'clock position, so that they spread over the cornea. If applied to the lower fornix, they quickly become mixed with tears and flow out from the eye. In any event, drugs in drop form are quickly diluted by tears and removed from the eye. This means that an effective concentration is produced for only a relatively short time and frequent repeat applications are required. Solutions, on the other hand, will have a quicker effect than ointments, and are less likely to interfere with epithelial regeneration.

To be suitable for application as drops, a drug must be soluble in a neutral solution and isotonic with tears. It must be stable in solution, non-irritant and capable of sterilization. Recently, eye drops have been made available in a solution containing a cellulosic plastic polymer (Isopto preparations, B.D.H.) which prolongs corneal contact time by coating the eye with an adherent film and by increasing the viscosity of the solution. In such a base, the drug will be held in contact with the cornea for 6 to 7 minutes as against 1 to 2 minutes with an aqueous vehicle. Such preparations have the additional advantage of being soothing and emollient on the eye.

The sterility of eye drops is essential. For this reason, use should be made of preparations in single-dose containers, or in those that deliver the drops without contaminating the remaining liquid.

Lotions. Lotions are used when it is required to irrigate the conjunctiva with a large quantity of fluid, thus allowing contact between eye and medication for several minutes. Such preparations are normally used as cleansing solutions for removing secretions from the conjunctival sacs. They are best applied, at body temperature, by an eye dropper, an undine or a rubber bulb (Fig. 26).

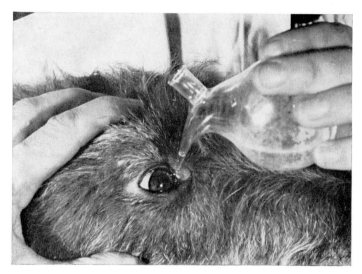

FIG. 26. *Irrigation of the eye with an undine.*

Ointments. Ointments are usually instilled into the lower fornix and spread over the cornea by gentle massage of the lids. The effect of an ointment is somewhat slower than that obtained with drops, but the prolonged contact time produces a more long-lasting effect. In certain circumstances, ointments may have some mild delaying effect on the healing process, due either to the breakdown of natural fats in the base into irritant substances, or to the clogging effect of mineral oils.

Oily solutions. These, which must be liquid at room temperature, are not commonly used because of the danger of infection.

Creams. Those containing hydrophilous fats have a soothing effect on skin, and may be employed in the treatment of periocular dermatoses.

Powders. Nowadays powders are rarely used because of their abrasive effect and there would appear to be little excuse for prescribing them for use on ocular tissues.

Electrodiaphoresis

The penetration of aqueous solutions into the conjunctiva and superficial cornea can be increased by the application of a suitable electric current. The technique, which has been described by J. F. Bone, uses a 45 volt battery, an ammeter, a potentiomenter and 2 electrodes. Using a current of 3 milli-amperes, the positive electrode is attached to the patient's body and the negative electrode, covered with gelfoam, is soaked in antibiotic solution and applied to the affected part of the eye. The electrical field produced between the negative electrode and the eye impels the antibiotic on to the ocular tissues, and results in a greater concentration of the agent in them than would have resulted from just simple diffusion. Treatment is given for 5 minutes daily. The clinical application of this method would appear to be limited, for most of the drugs that could be so used are more effectively given by subconjunctival injection.

Cleansing agents

Cleansers are used in the form of lotions, and should be employed at body temperature, using an undine. They are used to remove accumulated conjunctival discharges, thus allowing drugs subsequently introduced into the conjunctival sac to exert their maximum effect. They are also used to wash out foreign bodies from the eye.

(1) *Saline,* 0·6% is the most useful and most commonly employed agent.

(2) *Sodium bicarbonate,* 2% solution, is of value in removing grease from the conjunctival sac.

(3) *Boric acid solution* is a traditional eye cleansing agent, but its value is doubtful. It is often used, however, as a first-aid home remedy.

Lubricants

Lubricants, in the form of ointments or oily drops, are employed to relieve discomfort caused by abrasions, foreign bodies or congestion of the eye.

(1) *Liquid paraffin*—a good emollient and lubricant, but not miscible with water or water-soluble drugs.

(2) *Castor oil*—commonly used as a home remedy, but tends to decompose into irritant acids.

(3) *Cod liver oil*—a useful lubricant that has the additional value of its vitamin A content.

(4) *Methylcellulose*—probably the most useful agent of this type for it is miscible with nearly all other agents. Used as a 0·5 to 1·0% solution in normal saline.

Astringents

Astringents relieve discomfort associated with conjunctival congestion or oedema.

(1) *Zinc sulphate*—used as a 0·25% solution, often combined with boric acid. Buffered solutions (Op-Thal-Zin, B.D.H.) are less irritant to the eye and are to be preferred for the treatment of mild allergic or catarrhal conjunctival disorders. They may be combined with phenylephrine (Zincfrin, B.D.H.), and, in this form, are particularly useful in the treatment of conjunctival oedema causing blockage of the lacrimal puncta.

(2) *Silver nitrate*—used as a 1 or 2% solution, exerting an antiseptic and astringent action that results in a precipitation of protein and a desquamation of epithelium. Following its use in the conjunctival sac, its effect should be neutralized by irrigation with saline. It is of particular value in the treatment of chronic conjunctival infections.

(3) *Silver proteinate*—a useful mild astringent preparation (Argyrol, Fassett & Johnson; Argentum, The Crookes Laboratories). The use of silver preparations over many months may result in discoloration of the conjunctiva—argyrosis—which disperses only very slowly once medication ceases.

Cauterizing agents

These may be used to produce a slough of corneal epithelium or conjunctiva, and are used in the treatment of certain types of corneal ulceration, adenitis of the nictitans gland and follicular conjunctivitis. Deep penetration of the tissues is prevented by the precipitation of corneal proteins which forms a barrier to the further action of the agent.

(1) *Carbolic acid* or *phenol*—used as a pure solution.

(2) *Tincture of iodine.*

(3) *Trichloracetic acid*—used as a 25% solution, or by dipping a cotton wool applicator into crystals until the tip becomes moist.

(4) *Copper sulphate*—used as a crystal, rubbed lightly over the area (usually chronic follicular conjunctivitis) and flushed out immediately with saline.

Antiseptics

Although used formerly on many occasions, the use of antiseptic solutions has greatly decreased following the availability of chemotherapeutic and antibiotic agents.

(1) *Proflavine* 0·1% solution.

(2) *Mercuric oxide* 1% in ointment form—Golden Eye Ointment—is still commonly used as a home remedy.

(3) *Phenylmercuric dinaphthylmethane disulphonate* (Penotrane, Ward, Blenkinsop) has useful properties as a fungicide and against Gram positive and Gram negative organisms, particularly staphylococcus. It is useful in the treatment of chronic blepharitis when associated with staphylococcal infection and other pyogenic infections of the lids. It penetrates tissue well, is non-staining and bacterial resistance is not likely to develop. It may be used as a 0·033% solution (Octrane lotion) or as an ointment (Octrane gel).

Local anaesthetics

(1) *Cocaine hydrochloride*, 2 to 4%—a highly effective topical application, but largely out-of-favour because of its effect of producing corneal desiccation and slight necrosis. Slight mydriasis may follow the application of this agent.

(2) *Amethocaine*, 1%—is less effective than cocaine, but does not cause epithelial damage.

(3) *Procaine*, 2%—used for infiltration, usually combined with adrenaline to localize its effect, or with hyaluronidase when permeation is required.

(4) *Lignocaine hydrochloride* (Xylocaine, Astra-Hewlett) 4%—an effective topical application.

(5) *Proparacaine hydrochloride* (Ophthaine, Squibb) 0·5%—an extremely effective topical anaesthetic agent for ophthalmic use, producing anaesthesia within 15 seconds, persisting for 15 minutes. It does not produce local irritation nor pupillary dilatation, but open bottles must be kept refrigerated to retard discoloration.

Antihistaminics

Histamine, contained in the granular leucocytes, may be released into the tissues by trauma, by antibody-antigen reactions or by clotting. Antihistaminic agents are therefore of value in allergic ocular response and preoperatively in intraocular surgery. They may be administered orally or parenterally, in which case the depressant effect must be noted, or topically in drop form, in which case no depressant effect will be noted.

Many agents in this group are available, but mention may be made of those that are quick-acting, such as diphenhydramine (Benadryl, Parke, Davis) and mepyramine maleate (Anthisan, M. & B.), and those that are slow-acting, such as promethazine hydrochloride (Phenergan, M. & B.).

Autonomic drugs

All agents acting on the autonomic nervous system may be applied as drops or ointments, and readily pass through the corneal epithelium in effective concentrations. They may sometimes be used subconjunctivally.

(a) *Parasympathomimetic drugs.* These agents are used as miotics, and may be divided into two groups—those acting directly on the myoneural junction (pilocarpine, carbachol) and those acting as cholinesterase inhibitors (physostigmine, DFP).

(1) Pilocarpine nitrate, 1 to 2%—of limited effect in the dog, having a duration of about 6 hours.

(2) Carbachol, 0·75 to 3·00%—is poorly absorbed through the cornea, but excessive penetration, and side-effects, may occur in the presence of corneal abrasions.

(3) Physostigmine salicylate (Eserine), 0·5 to 1·0%—the most widely-used miotic, but of limited effect in the dog. It has a duration of action of around 6 hours and may cause some irritation on application. Solutions tend to turn pink due to hydrolysis and oxidation.

(4) Di-isopropyl fluorophosphonate (DFP), 0·5 to 0·10%—a powerful miotic with a prolonged action of up to 24 hours. It causes some congestion of superficial blood vessels. It must not be used in conjunction with eserine, to which it is antagonistic.

(5) Demecarium bromide (Tosmilen, Astra-Hewlett), 0·25 to 0·50%—a powerful miotic, with prolonged action.

(6) Phospholine iodide (Martindale Samoore), 0·060 to 0·125%—a powerful miotic, reaching a peak of action in 24 to 60 hours, and maintaining some activity for up to 18 days.

(b) *Parasympatholytic drugs.* These agents are used for mydriasis, and may be divided into two groups—the mydriatics (eucatropine) and the cycloplegics (atropine, homatropine, hyoscine, tropicamide)—agents which paralyse the ciliary body with resultant dilatation. Ideally, a mydriatic should dilate the pupil completely, without producing side-effects and without affecting accommodation. Rapidity of action is important and those agents with a relatively short action are normally preferable. A mydriatic should produce no irritation and no rise in intraocular pressure.

(1) *Atropine sulphate*, 0·5 to 1·0%—used as drops or ointment. The most powerful drug of this group, with a long-lasting effect, sometimes up to 96 hours, and full pupillary dilatation. Irritation may be exhibited by a small proportion of animals and, in some cases, profuse salivation will follow application to the eye—probably due to the drug travelling to the nostrils via the lacrimal duct, and then being transferred to the mouth with the tongue. Atropine is mainly used in the treatment of uveitis, corneal ulceration, deep keratitis and also postoperatively.

(2) *Homatropine hydrobromide*, 2 and 5%—produces a mydriasis of short duration, and is particularly useful for ophthalmoscopy.

(3) *Hyoscine hydrobromide*, 0·25%—a long-acting drug that may be used in cases of atropine sensitivity.

(4) *Tropicamide*, 0·5 to 1·0% (Mydriacyl, B.D.H.)—a short-acting

mydriatic and cycloplegic, with maximum effect after 20 minutes and persistence for 15 minutes.

(5) *Mydricaine No. 2* (Martindale Samoore) may be given subconjunctivally, in a dose of 0·30 ml, to prevent fibrinous clotting of aqueous in intraocular surgery, and to help in the preservation of a dilated pupil. The formula is as follows:

Procaine HCl	6 mg
Atrop. sulph.	1 mg
Adrenal. 1:1000	0·1 ml
Acid boric	5 mg
Water	to 0·25 ml

(c) *Sympathomimetic drugs.* These agents produce mydriasis but not cycloplegia. They are occasionally also used as vasoconstrictors.

(1) *Phenylephrine hydrochloride* (Lyophrin, B.D.H.)—unstable in solution, and may cause local irritation. Acts for about 3 hours.

(2) *Adrenaline hydrochloride* (Epinephrine hydrochloride)—a 1:1000 solution is occasionally used subconjunctivally to dilate the pupil. Its vasoconstrictor effect is used to decrease absorption of local anaesthetics, and to control haemorrhage from the conjunctiva. A solution of 1:10,000, introduced into the anterior chamber during intraocular surgery, may be used to help produce dilatation following extracapsular cataract extraction.

(3) *Cocaine hydrochloride.*

(d) *Acetylcholine.* May be used to produce miosis, by irrigation of the iris after delivery of the lens in intracapsular cataract surgery, thus facilitating closure of the corneal wound, and preventing vitreous presentation. It may be used in other intraocular procedures, where miosis is required, such as iridectomy. Acetylcholine is available in single-dose containers, providing a 1:100 solution in 5% mannitol (Miochol, Smith, Miller & Patch).

Vitamin preparations

(1) *Vitamin A* may be used in cases of deficiency, resulting in retinal degeneration or keratomalacia. It may be administered orally or parenterally. As an oily solution, it is of value in the treatment of corneal degenerative conditions.

(2) *Riboflavin* is of value in the treatment of corneal vascularization and ulceration, and may be given orally or by injection.

Artificial tears

A solution of methylcellulose 0·5 to 1·0% is of value in the treatment of tear deficiencies and keratitis sicca, and forms a useful base for ophthalmic solutions. Such solutions are relatively persistent in the conjunctival sac and do not interfere with epithelial regeneration. Solutions that do not interfere with the refractive index of the cornea and that provide a sterile buffered isotonic solution, are to be preferred (Isopto Plain and Isopto Alkaline, B.D.H.).

Dyes

These are used for staining and recognition of corneal abrasions and ulceration; occasionally in order to differentiate fine, white, silk sutures in the cornea and to mark the cornea for incisions.

(1) *Fluorescein*—may be used as a 2% solution, but is not compatible with any reliable antibacterial agent. Such solutions form suitable media for *Pseudomonas* organisms and care must be taken that such drops do not become contaminated. Suitable multidose containers are available (Bengue; Alcon) but contamination of the nozzle of containers must be avoided.

The risk of contaminated solutions may be avoided either by the use of sterile impregnated papers (Stercks Martin), or by the use of disposable single-dose containers (Minims, Smith & Nephew).

(2) *Mercurochrome*, 2%—provides a dye solution that is less likely to become contaminated, but which does not stain the cornea as efficiently as fluorescein.

(3) *Rose bengal*, 1%—useful for staining mucoid threads and for the visualizing of fine sutures.

ENZYME PREPARATIONS

(1) *Chymotrypsin* (Chymar, Armour)—may be used, by intramuscular injection, in the treatment of hypopyon or hyphaema.

(2) *Trypsin* (Trypvet, Evans; Tryptar, Armour)—may be used for the removal of necrotic or inspissated material from the lacrimal canals. The enzyme has a proteolytic action but does not affect living cells. The preparation is stable in powder form, and solutions will keep refrigerated for up to 3 months.

(3) *Hyaluronidase* (Rondase, Evans)—may be used to facilitate the subcutaneous infusion of drugs, or to increase the effective area of local anaesthesia. Subconjunctivally, it may be used in the treatment of hyphaema.

(4) *Urokinase* (Leo Laboratories)—activates plasminogen to form plasmin, and dissolves blood clots. May be used as an intercameral irrigation —5000 ploug units in 2 ml saline—in the treatment of hyphaema.

(5) *Alpha-chymotrypsin* (Zonulolysin, Maw; Chymar-Zon, Armour) —is used for zonulolysis in intracapsular cataract operations.

ANTICOAGULANTS

Heparin (Pularin, Evans) may be used, in a dose of 750 I.U. by intravenous injection, to prevent fibrin clotting of aqueous. It may also be used in the

4

anterior chamber, following intraocular surgery, to prevent fibrin formation, but may predispose the eye to further haemorrhage. The preoperative use of Mydricaine is to be preferred.

COAGULANTS

Systemic preparations, which decrease capillary permeability, may be used in the treatment of hyphaema, and haemorrhage occurring during intraocular surgery.

CARBONIC ANHYDRASE INHIBITORS

These are drugs which lower the intraocular pressure by inhibiting the production of aqueous.

(1) *Dichlorphenamide* (Daranide, Merck)—may be given in a dose of 25 mg every 8 hours, for a 9 to 14 kg dog.

(2) *Acetazolamide* (Diamox, Lederle)—may be given in a dose, for a 9 to 14 kg dog, of 125 mg every 8 hours for 3 doses, followed by 125 mg every 12 hours.

Other drugs that have the effect of lowering intraocular pressure include the following:

(1) *Oral glycerol*—a 50% solution in 0·9% saline and flavoured—in a dose of 1 g/kg bodyweight.

(2) *Intravenous urea* (Urovert, Baxter)—used as a 30% solution with 10% invert sugar and given in a dose of 1 g/kg bodyweight.

(3) *Mannitol*—given intravenously as a 20% solution in a dose of 2 g/kg bodyweight.

NON-SPECIFIC PROTEIN THERAPY

In the treatment of infected or indolent corneal ulceration, uveitis and purulent conjunctivitis, the use of proteins in the form of sterile milk (5 ml intramuscularly every 2 or 3 days), or typhoid-paratyphoid vaccine (15,000,000 to 60,000,000 every other day), or Omnadin (Hoechst), has been advocated to stimulate an increase in antibody content, and, therefore, an increase in natural resistance.

THE SULPHONAMIDE DRUGS

There would appear to be many sulphonamide-resistant strains of micro-organisms and they have been largely superseded by the antibiotics. They are, nevertheless, still useful in the treatment of minor eye injuries and infections. Given systemically, they penetrate the blood-aqueous barrier poorly, so that aqueous concentrations are rarely greater than 10% of the blood concentration. They have the added disadvantages that they are inhibited in the presence of pus and that most are insoluble.

(1) *Sulphacetamide* (Albucid, British Schering)—may be used as a 2·5 to 10·0% ointment or as 10 to 30% drops and penetrates the tissues reasonably well.

(2) *Sulphonamidobenzylamine propionate* (Sulfomyl, Bayer)—available as 5% drops.

ANTIFUNGAL DRUGS

The prolonged use of antibiotics facilitates fungal growth by the inhibition of the normal bacterial flora, and the use of corticosteroids enhances fungal growth by interfering with normal inflammatory reaction. Fungicides are, therefore, of increasing importance in ophthalmology, although the incidence of fungal infections of the eye is relatively low in the dog at the present time.

(1) *Penicillin*—is likely to prove effective against organisms of the *Actinomyces* group.

(2) *Amphotericin B* (Fungizone, Squibb)—is available as a 3% lotion.

(3) *Mycostatin* (Nystatin, Squibb)—is available only as a topical ointment, which may, however, be used in the eye.

(4) *Sodium propionate* (Procid, Harker Stagg)—is available as a 15% ointment or as 10% drops. It is stable, non-irritating, penetrates well into the aqueous and is also effective against a wide range of bacteria.

ANTIBIOTICS

A wide range of antibiotic drugs is available, and most of them have a place in ocular therapeutics. Resistant strains of bacteria exist to most of the available agents in this group, and the value of sensitivity tests must be emphasized.

(1) *Penicillin*—effective against Gram positive bacteria. May be given systemically by intramuscular injection, or topically in the form of drops (2500 to 10,000 units/ml) or ointment (5000 to 10,000 units/ml). Solutions tend to lose their potency when stored at room temperature, Penicillin has the advantage that it is cheap and, being relatively non-toxic, may be given in massive doses. Subconjunctivally, for anterior eye infections, it may be given in a dose of 500,000 units in 0·5 to 1·0 ml water or mixed with a 2% solution of procaine in adrenaline.

(2) *Ampicillin* (Penbritin, Beecham)—may be given orally or by injection.

(3) *Sodium cloxacillin* (Orbenin, Beecham)—may be given orally.

(4) *Phenethicillin* (Broxil, Beecham)—may be given orally.

(5) *Sodium methicillin* (Celbenin, Beecham)—may be used as 2% drops, or given by subconjunctival injection, 0·5 g in 0·5 ml saline.

(6) *Streptomycin*—effective against a wide range of organisms, including some Gram negative bacteria. Systemically, it may be given by intramuscular injection. Topically, it may be used as ointment (5000 units/g) or as drops (5000 units/ml) which lose potency at room temperature. The penetration of streptomycin into the tissues is poor, and it may be given subconjunctivally, in a dose of 0·5 g in 1 ml water.

(7) *Penicillin-streptomycin* (Crystamycin, Glaxo)—may be used as drops (1000,000 units of each/ml) or may be given by the subconjunctival route, with a single-dose vial dissolved in 1 ml water.

(8) *Chloramphenicol* (Chloromycetin, Parke, Davis)—may be given orally or by injection. This antibiotic penetrates well into the ocular tissues, and is the antibiotic of choice in the majority of conditions. It may be used as 0·5% drops or as 1·0% ointment. For subconjunctival injections, it may be used in a water soluble form (Chloromycetin succinate, Parke Davis), in a dose of 0·5 ml, of a 2·5% solution.

(9) *Neomycin* may be used topically only, because of toxic effects. Penetration into the tissues is poor, but a wide range of organisms may be affected. The drug is very soluble, and well-tolerated by local application. It may be used as 0·5% drops, as 0·5% ointment or may be given subconjunctivally in a dose of 0·5 g in 1 ml of adrenaline solution, 1:5000.

(10) *Tetracyclines* may be given orally or by intramuscular injection. These agents are not stable in solution, but are in ointment form. Penetration into ocular tissues is poor and they cannot be used subconjunctivally, for they produce irritation and local reactions. Drops are used as a 0·5% solution and ointments as 1·0%. The agents available in this group include tetracycline (Achromycin, Pfizer), chlortetracycline (Aureomycin, Lederle) and oxytetracycline (Terramycin, Pfizer).

(11) *Polymixin* is effective against many Gram negative organisms, including many strains of pseudomonas. This antibiotic is neurotoxic and should be used only for 4 to 7 days. Polymixin is often combined with bacitracin, and is available as drops, with neomycin and phenylephrine (Isopto P-N-P, B.D.H.) or with neomycin and hydrocortisone (Isopto P-H-N, B.D.H.). As an ointment, containing 10,000 units, it is usually combined with bacitracin (Polyfax, B.W.). Subconjunctivally, it may be given in a dose of 125,000 units/ml but may produce a painful reaction, unless combined with a 2% lignocaine solution.

(12) *Framycetin* (Soframycin, Roussel)—is effective against pseudomonas, has a broad spectrum, is stable in solution, but is likely to cause some inhibition of cell growth. It may be used as 1·0% drops, as 0·5% ointment or may be given by subconjunctival injection, 100 to 500 mg in 0·5 ml water.

(13) *Combined antibiotics*—a combination of antibiotics is often useful to obtain a potentiation of effect, to counteract resistant bacteria, and to combine both bactericidal and bacteriostatic forms.

ANTI-VIRAL DRUGS

Iododesoxyuridine (Dendrid, B.D.H.) is an antimetabolite that may be useful in the treatment of viral corneal ulceration. It is relatively insoluble, but may be used as 0·1% drops, applied hourly. Other agents that might prove useful in the treatment of viral conditions include systemic sulpha-dimidine or tetracycline, combined with intensive local treatment using 30% sulphacetamide solution.

CORTICOSTEROIDS

The corticosteroids decrease capillary permeability and reduce exudation, thereby reducing the effects of inflammatory reaction in the ocular tissues. In addition, they inhibit the formation of granulation tissue and inhibit the formation of new blood vessels.

The anti-inflammatory effect may be of value where the inflammation itself is self-limiting, as in allergic responses or where excessive changes in the tissues may prove harmful. These agents, however, have no anti-bacterial effect and are likely to render the tissues more susceptible to infection. Therefore, where infection is present or is likely to occur, these agents must be combined with antibiotics. They are contraindicated in cases of ulceration, and postoperatively in the immediate post-surgical period, for they will impede the healing of wounds. They have no effect on degenerative diseases, but prolonged use may result in thinning of the corneal stroma.

Corticosteroids are indicated in allergic conditions (conjunctivitis, blepharitis, keratitis); in acute uveitis due to allergy, toxins or trauma; and in diseases where it is desirable to limit exudation or tissue prolifera-tion. The corticosteroids may be given orally or systemically, or may be used topically in the form of drops or ointment at 0·25 to 1·00%. Frequent administration is necessary to obtain the desired effect. Subconjunctivally, they may be given in a dose of 5 to 10 mg in 0·25 to 0·50 ml water.

(1) *Cortisone* (Cortelan, Glaxo)—orally or by intramuscular injection.

(2) *Hydrocortisone* (Efcortelan, Glaxo)—as 2·5% ointment, 1% drops or by subconjunctival injection. (Ef-cortelan Intrathecal, Glaxo, 10 mg is a useful mode of presentation for this purpose.)

(3) *Prednisolone*—orally as tablets (Predsolan, Glaxo); as 0·5% ointment or drops (Predsol, Glaxo); combined with neomycin (Predsol-N, Glaxo) or with phenylephrine (Isopto Prednisolone, B.D.H.)

(4) *Triamcinolone*—as ointment (Adcortyl-A, Squibb) or with Graneodin (Adcortyl-A with Graneodin, Squibb). May also be given orally (Adcortyl, Squibb; Ledercort, Lederle).

(5) *Betamethasone disodium* (Betnesol, Glaxo) may be used as drops or 0·1% ointment combined if necessary with neomycin (Betnesol-N, Glaxo)·

The intra-articular form of betamethasone (Betnelan, Glaxo) is suitable for subconjunctival use, in a dose of 0·10 to 0·25 ml. Betamethasone may be given orally or by injection.

(6) *Dexamethasone* (Maxidex, B.D.H.)—available as 0·1% drops or combined with phenylephrine (Vasodex, Fassett & Johnson). Orally, it may be given in tablet form (Dexadreson, Organon; Dextelan, Glaxo).

SUBCONJUNCTIVAL INJECTIONS

In the treatment of various ocular disease conditions there are several ways in which the various chemotherapeutic agents, antibiotics, and other drugs, may be given. They may be administered orally, parenterally, or by means of local applications.

The use of the antibiotics in the treatment of eye infections is limited, firstly by the sensitivity of the causal organism and, secondly, by the toxic side-effects of some of the agents available. A third factor is the low level of ocular concentration obtained, even when blood levels are high, in the intra-ocular fluids. Fourthly, local applications are not always possible, as the agent may be relatively insoluble or locally irritating.

It will be appreciated, therefore, that the use of antibiotics or chemo-therapeutic agents is sometimes limited in the treatment of eye infections; in these circumstances, it is often important to establish the nature of the infection, so that the most effective agent may be used for treatment.

The dosages of sulphonamides and antibiotics that are required for oral or parenteral administration, in order to produce a therapeutic level at a site of infection, have been established by blood levels; such levels are adequate for any infection of the outer eye, proved or assumed to be due to any organisms sensitive to sulphonamides or to any one of the antibiotics. On the other hand, this is not so with infections of the inner eye, where it is often impossible to obtain adequate intraocular levels either by local or systemic administration.

The physiological blood-aqueous barrier prevents many substances circulating in the blood from reaching the aqueous humour; in many cases, the aqueous level is only 10% of the blood level.

Although no studies have been made in the dog, there is evidence that, of the antibiotics, chloramphenicol has the greatest penetrating power of the intact cornea, and passes readily into the intraocular fluids from the blood stream. This property would appear to be associated with the lipoid solubility and small molecular size of this particular antibiotic. As a general rule, however, the blood level of a therapeutic agent is no guide to the levels reached in any part of the eye.

The development of the subconjunctival method of administration has overcome these limitations. Intraocular levels considerably in excess of those obtained by systemic or local applications are given by this method. In this connection, it is important to remember that, using the subconjunctival method of administration, normal antibiotic sensitivity tests are not always applicable to ophthalmology. In such cases, organisms that may appear insensitive to a particular antibiotic by ordinary administration in a generalized infection may prove sensitive to subconjunctival therapy in an intraocular infection.

Certain agents, such as the sulphonamides, the tetracyclines and erythromycin are excluded because they are not readily soluble; others are likely

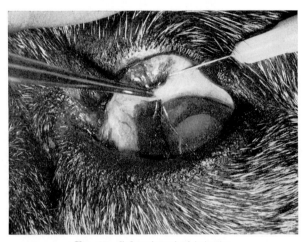

Fig. 27. *Subconjunctival injection.*

to produce severe local reaction. Agents that can be used are penicillin, streptomycin, neomycin, polymixin and chloramphenicol.

Subconjunctival injections should not exceed 1 ml in quantity and, therefore, the amount of the drug that can be given is limited by its solubility; other agents, such as neomycin, are limited by their toxicity.

Technique of injection

(1) General anaesthesia, using thiopentone sodium, or topical anaesthesia, with or without sedation, will be required.

(2) The lids are held apart with a speculum.

(3) A fold of conjunctiva is picked up with forceps, about 6 mm from the limbus.

(4) A fine needle is thrust through the conjunctiva and the injection made into the subconjunctival space. When correctly placed, the needle moves freely across the space and the injection raises a visible bleb (Fig. 27).

(5) When the injection is completed, the resultant bleb is massaged through the closed lids, so as to spread the fluid diffusely.

Subconjunctival injections are well tolerated, provided that the solution used is not too hypertonic, neither too acid or alkaline and provided that the total quantity used does not exceed 1 ml.

Penicillin

High concentrations are obtained in the aqueous, vitreous and other intraocular structures. Local reaction or pain might follow the use of highly concentrated solutions. 50,000 units will give a high but nonpersistent level; 1,000,000 units will give a very high level persisting for up to 24 hours, and this effect is increased even further if the penicillin is dissolved in 1:1000 adrenaline solution.

Streptomycin

Due to its solubility, 0·5 g is the maximum that can be given. Repeated injections may produce local reactions and may be painful. As aqueous solutions are not likely to produce a persistent level, streptomycin should be given in adrenaline solution; levels persisting for over 24 hours are then likely to be obtained.

Neomycin

Injection of 0·5 g will produce a high intraocular level for up to 48 hours, which is not prolonged by adrenaline. Due to its toxicity, repeated administration is not recommended.

Polymixin

This antibiotic is particularly useful in the treatment of *Pseudomonas* infections, in concentrations of 30,000 to 50,000 units. The addition of adrenaline makes the solution highly irritant.

Chloramphenicol

The water-soluble form may be used, as a 2·5% solution, in a dose of 0·5 ml.

The corticosteroids

The use of these agents in the treatment of certain ocular disorders, such as neovascularizations, interstitial keratitis, pannus formation and exuberant corneal granulation tissue, is well established. Certain of them may be administered by subconjunctival injection and this produces a far more pronounced effect than when given either locally or systemically. The effect is persistent for long periods.

Hydrocortisone may be given in the strength of 25 mg/ml, 0·5 to 1·0 ml being used for each injection. Prednisolone and betamethasone may also be given in this way but the quantity injected will generally be smaller.

Hyaluronidase

Hyaluronidase is sometimes employed, in the treatment of hyphaema, at a strength of 50 units/ml.

Adrenaline

A solution strength of 1:1000 may be given subconjunctivally, in a dose of 0·1 to 0·2 ml, to assist in the control of haemorrhage during the preparation of a conjunctival flap.

In all cases of subconjunctival injection, the total quantity used should not exceed 1 ml. If the maximum quantity is used, the injection should be made at several points.

PHYSICAL THERAPY

Heat. Valuable, in the form of hot compresses, as a vasodilator, it may be used to produce active hyperaemia, together with a local increase in leuco- cytes and antibodies. Although of limited value, this form of therapy may be used in any case where it is desired to promote vascularization.

Cold. In the form of cold compresses, it will act as a vasoconstrictor to reduce local oedema in cases of eyelid injury associated with swelling and pain.

Electrocautery. Of value in the treatment of trichiasis and distichiasis, and in various surgical procedures.

Beta-irradiation. The use of strontium 90 is of great value in the treatment of various superficial ocular conditions. The conjunctiva, eyelids and adjac- ent skin are more susceptible to radiation than is the cornea or iris. The crystalline lens is highly susceptible to radiation, and cataractous changes are likely to occur if this structure is irradiated. The aqueous and vitreous humours are not affected. The use of X-rays is not advocated because of the greater danger to the operator and to the patient. Beta irradiation is contra- indicated in ulcerative conditions, but disorders that are likely to respond favourably include: early pannus formation, corneal vascularization, exuberant granulation tissue and small neoplasms of the lids, conjunctiva or cornea. It is useful, also, postoperatively, in cases of corneal grafting, to prevent neovascularization.

Beta rays inhibit the proliferation of the capillary endothelium in newly- forming vessels.

It is important that the emitter used produces β-rays only, and not γ-rays. For this purpose strontium 90 with a half life of 25 years, is suitable. Half the β-rays produced will be absorbed in the first 1 mm of tissue and 97% will be absorbed in a depth of 4 mm. In the average dog, the distance between corneal surface and lens is around 4·5 mm, so the effect on the latter structure will be minimal.

Simple applicators, using strontium 90 are available, usually producing a dosage rate of 40 to 50 rep/sec (rep = roentgen-equivalent physical unit). Such emitters should be checked regularly, both for output and for safety. Small, repeated doses are likely to be more effective than single, large doses.

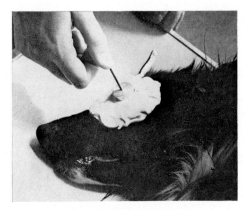

FIG. 28. *Application of beta-rays.*

Although it has been shown that the dog can tolerate 27,000 rep as a single dose over a 1 cm disc area, therapeutic doses normally given are within the range of 1000 to 10,000 rep. Applications are normally repeated at weekly intervals, for a maximum of three occasions.

For safety of both patient and operator, applications should be performed under anaesthesia. The eyelids are widely retracted. To protect the surrounding skin from radiation, a sheet of plasticine with a central hole, to expose the cornea, is passed over the eye (Fig. 28). The applicator is then held close to the eye for the required time interval. If the diameter of the applicator is small enough, it is preferable to treat only the limbal area and not the whole corneal surface.

Some tissue reaction may follow β-ray treatment initially, and the use of corticosteroid preparations for a few days after each application is recommended. Results obtained from β-ray therapy are often encouraging, particularly in those cases where the corneal vascularization is superficial or subepithelial.

Interstitial vascularization, also, often shows a satisfactory response, but, in such cases, further vascularization may follow the cessation of treatment.

4

OPHTHALMIC SURGERY

The eye presents a very specialized field of surgery. In it certain conditions, with regard to the operator, patient and the operating room, must be fulfilled if successful surgery on the eye is to be undertaken. A sound knowledge of ophthalmic anatomy and physiology is essential; also great emphasis must be placed on the all-important factors of preoperative and postoperative preparation, operating conditions, anaesthesia, drug therapy and asepsis.

Ophthalmic surgery, particularly that concerned with the intraocular structures, should not be undertaken unless the operator is keenly interested in his subject and the facilities are available. The qualities of temperament and manual dexterity that must be present in any surgeon are doubly important in the eye surgeon, whose operative field is small and where the margin between success and disaster is so little. All ophthalmic surgery must be undertaken calmly and patiently, there is no place for hasty decisions or impatience. Accurate judgement of cases where surgery is indicated and of cases where surgery is contraindicated, or where it is better to refrain from reoperating, is all-important. Preoperative planning of eye operations is essential and operative intentions must be quite clear; attention to surgical detail is also essential and any indecision or 'touching-up' is likely to end in failure. All unnecessary procedures and manipulations must be avoided.

The acquisition of skill in ophthalmic surgery and in intraocular surgery in particular, will result only from adequate practice. Refinements in skill and surgical technique will be acquired only by operating on the living eye. It is, of course, not permissible in Great Britain to obtain experience by operating on the eye of an anaesthetized experimental animal, but all techniques should be well practised on the cadaver eye. These techniques should be perfected before they are applied to clinical cases.

THE OPERATING THEATRE

In the vast majority of cases, the operating theatre that will be used for eye surgery will be used also for general surgery. Although this is often far from ideal, it can rarely be avoided. Where possible, the theatre should be located in an area where quiet can be obtained and where interruptions can be minimized. Adequate power points for ophthalmoscope, operating lights, diathermy and suction should be provided.

The operating theatre for ophthalmic surgery should be free from atmospheric particles as far as possible. This is often difficult to maintain, as the patient, the operating gowns and materials used, are all possible sources of dust, hair particles, wool and fluff. The entrance of such foreign matter into the anterior chamber at the time of operation may produce postoperative complications. For this reason, all operating gowns and drapes

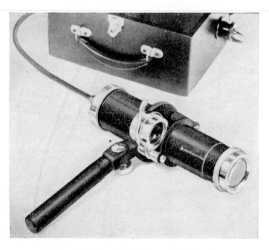

Fig. 29. *Hand-held operating lamp.*

should be of synthetic fibre rather than cotton, and polyvinyl sponges and sable brushes should be used rather than cotton wool and gauze. If operating gloves are to be worn—and most eye surgeons find that gloves do not allow the very fine sense of touch that is required—the use of talcum powder should be avoided.

Lighting

Adequate illumination is highly important. In most cases, it is best that it should be focal, with the lamp providing an area of intense illumination of about 7·5 cm diameter. Scialytic light, with an illumination of up to 1000 foot/candles is preferable, and in cases where this is not obtainable, auxiliary lights may have to be employed. Many portable, adjustable lamps are available; in certain cases, a hand-held lamp may prove beneficial (Fig. 29).

It is essential that lamps be placed so that the light does not fall directly upon the eye, but at an angle, so that the operator does not in any way obstruct the beam. Reflection from the operative field should be avoided by the use of suitable draping materials.

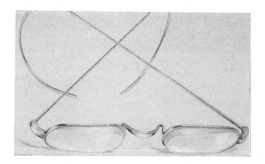

FIG. 30. *Mayou's binocular loupe.*

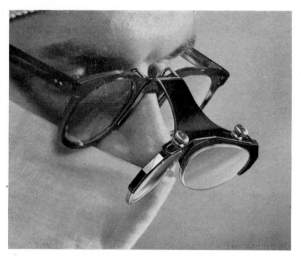

FIG. 31. *Keeler clip-on loupe.*

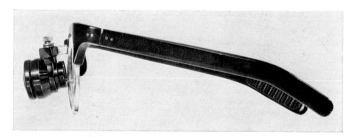

FIG. 32. *Keeler magnifying spectacles.*

In most cases, particularly when intraocular surgery is involved, it is best that the rest of the room be in total darkness. Under such conditions, where there is only a central illuminated area, additional, reduced illumination over the instrument table is required, in order to avoid unnecessary movements on the part of the operator.

Magnifying spectacles

On most occasions and particularly when intraocular surgery is to be performed, some form of magnifying spectacles will prove beneficial. Many types are available; choice will often depend on individual preferences. The most simple are the binocular loupes of Bishop Harman or Mayou (Fig. 30), which are worn at the end of the nose. Others, such as the Berger loupe, may be fitted into a headband; or in the case of the Keeler clip-on loupe (Fig. 31), they may be attached to the surgeon's own spectacles. Yet others, such as the Keeler magnifying spectacle (Fig. 32), incorporating a pair of spectacles, may include a spotlight attachment.

All spectacles must be adjusted so that they are held close to the face, and should be polished with an anti-dim compound, in order to minimize misting from the surgeon's breath.

Position of the operator

That the surgeon should be comfortable and should try not to change his position, during the operation, is an essential prerequisite of ophthalmic surgery. In most cases, it is preferable that he be seated and able to rest the forearms, particularly during the crucial stages of any intraocular operation. The eye must be just below the fingers and the table must be of the right height, so that hands and head can be held in such a position that there is adequate access to all areas and that unnecessary tiring does not take place.

Position of the patient

For most cases of intraocular surgery and many of the procedures upon the cornea, the eye is approached from above, and the surgeon is best positioned behind the patient. The dog is placed on the table; its back roughly parallel to the edge, with the upper surface of the head positioned in front of the surgeon. The anterolateral position of the orbit renders surgical manipulations difficult, and, therefore, the eye is placed on a horizontal plane by raising the nose of the dog and supporting this firmly with sandbags (Fig. 33). It is important that the supports are so arranged that they do not interfere mechanically with the movements of the surgeon's hands. Tilting of the table, as well as producing postural hypotension that is useful in many instances, renders the position of the eye rather more suitable for surgery. Adequate precautions must be taken that there is no movement of the patient due to the position of the table, and sufficient support must be provided to prevent any slip.

Instrument placement

The instruments must come easily to hand, so as to avoid unnecessary movements on the part of the surgeon that are distracting and interfere with concentration. For this purpose, a small table that can be wheeled over the operating table is the most useful. This can be covered with the same

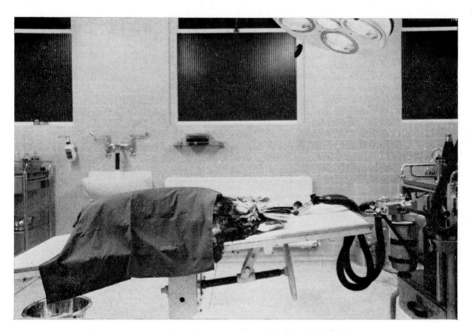

FIG. 33. *Dog positioned on operating table for ophthalmic surgery.*

drape that is covering the animal's head, thus keeping some air space beneath the drape. The animal and the instrument table should be so arranged that the minimum of movement is necessary during the course of the operation.

INSTRUMENTS

Different people must be expected to differ in their taste for certain instruments. The selection of instruments required will depend largely on personal preferences and the type of operation it is intended to perform. Normally, however, the instruments and equipment found in the average practice are neither suitable nor adequate for eye surgery; specialized equipment is required and attempts to perform the majority of eye operations without proper equipment will inevitably lead to disappointments. A multiplicity of instruments is possibly not desirable, but there is a certain minimum without which successful eye surgery cannot be performed.

Instruments must be of the best quality—a perfect edge is of the utmost importance on all cutting instruments and suturing needles. Upon the condition and perfection of the sharp instruments might depend the whole success of the operation, for very rarely is there a chance to make a second incision.

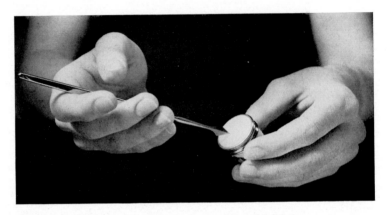

FIG. 34. *Testing a knife on a kid-covered drum.*

Ophthalmic surgery instruments must be carefully maintained and well looked after. Points and edges must be perfect, and all delicate instruments should be kept in a rack; the point of a cataract knife may be ruined if it comes in contact with another instrument or with a tray or dish. Rust and corrosion will ruin cutting edges. Since most operating areas tend to be damp from steam, great care must be taken to see that all instruments are thoroughly dried after use, possibly by the use of a hot-air oven and that they are adequately oiled before storage.

The selection of sharp instruments

All points and edges should be examined before each operation to ensure that they are perfect. The conventional method used is the kid-covered drum, where the point of a knife should perforate the drum easily by its own weight or with the slightest movement. The edge should cut the kid easily (Fig. 34). No ophthalmic instrument, except those used for splitting, such as Tooke's knife and Desmarre's scarifier, can be too sharp.

Alternatively, the edge and point of an instrument may be checked under a microscope, using oblique illumination and a magnification of about

× 90. Any instrument that shows evidence of distortion, or bluntness, or rust should be rejected.

The sterilization of sharp instruments

The sterilization of instruments with perfect cutting edges, without in any way affecting the edges, presents some difficulties. Three methods are available, and these are listed in order of preference.

(a) *Dry heat.* Electric ovens are available and the recommended sterilization time is 1 hour at 160 °C (320 °F). A further period of a half hour is required for the instruments to be raised to the required temperature, then a further

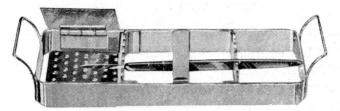

FIG. 35. *Sterilizing rack.*

half hour for cooling to take place before the instruments can be handled. To avoid damage to points, cutting instruments are best arranged in special racks (Fig. 35) or in individual tubes. The dry heat method causes very little damage to cutting edges but is time-consuming and, if any amount of eye surgery is planned, requires a large stock of instruments.

(b) *Boiling in AC.10.* In this method, a film of oil is placed on the metal surfaces which does not impede sterilization. Blades are dipped in AC.10 for 15 seconds, and then placed in an ordinary sterilizer containing 2% w/v of AC.10 in 2% sodium carbonate solution. Five minutes is required for sterilization, thus instruments can be quickly prepared between operations. Although the method has the advantage of speed, allowing a smaller stock of instruments to be maintained, it has two disadvantages. First, instruments are greasy and will require wiping with sterile gauze before use; secondly, corrosion will occur after repeated sterilization.

(c) *Chemical sterilization.* Various proprietary preparations are available for the cold sterilization of instruments. The method is, however, the slowest and probably the least effective of all. Long periods are normally required for effective sterilization, but sharp instruments may be left permanently in certain solutions if desired. Careful cleaning is essential before the instruments are placed in the solution and they should be rinsed in sterile water and dried with sterile gauze before use.

The sterilization of blunt instruments

Blunt instruments may be sterilized in a hot-air oven, an autoclave or by boiling. Boiling in distilled water requires a period of 2 hours to produce sterility; boiling in 2% sodium carbonate solution reduces the effective time to 5 minutes.

It is far easier to handle small and delicate instruments if they are dry, particularly if rubber gloves are worn. For this reason, facilities for drying instruments that have been boiled or placed in chemical solutions should be available, using sterile materials. Provision should also be made for the surgeon to dry his hands on a sterile towel after scrubbing-up.

DRESSINGS AND SWABS

Ordinary surgical gauze and cotton wool swabs are suitable for operations on the external structures, but their use in operations involving the interior of the eye is best avoided. Polyvinyl sponge, obtainable in strips, is more suitable as a swabbing medium. This may be cut into a variety of shapes, producing swabs of various sizes suitable for all procedures. The use of sable brushes, which are obtainable in a sterilizable form, is also to be advocated as a means of both cleaning the operative area and keeping the cornea moist. Irrigation of the site with saline from a syringe or undine also helps to keep the area clean and free from foreign material.

In the absence of infection, the less the eye is dressed after operation the better. The use of complicated dressings and shields is normally not possible on the dog and bandaging is often difficult. Sometimes it is possible to adequately cover the eye with a bandage after surgery. This is best accomplished using a gauze pad held in place with a continuous strip of elastic adhesive bandage (Elastoplast 1 or 2 in. bandage).

Protection from light after surgery allows the eye to be in a state of rest; therefore, provided that the eye can be bandaged without causing interference by the patient and provided that there is no pressure exerted on the globe by the dressing, there is some advantage in affording protection in this way. The method described by A. N. Ormrod is to be preferred, in that pressure on the globe is avoided. In this, a strip of adhesive elastic bandage, 3 in. wide, is laid adhesive side downwards on a smooth surface and a roll of gauze of $\frac{3}{4}$ in. diameter applied to the non-adhesive side of the bandage, parallel and close to the long edge. By rolling the edge a padded tube, with the adhesive side outwards, is produced. This is formed into a circle and the ring applied to encircle the eye. A piece of thin card is placed over the ring and the whole is firmly attached to the head by bandages, the adhesive nature of the ring helping to prevent movement of the ring and bandage-slip. An alternative is to use thick chiropodist's felt, cut to form a ring of suitable size to encircle the eye. This is applied to the head with the adhesive side on the skin, and held in place with bandages. Again, in this method, undue pressure upon the eye is avoided.

DROPS AND LOTIONS

The sterility of drops and lotions used during eye surgery, particularly when intraocular procedures are involved, must be maintained. Individual bottles, with pipettes, are acceptable provided that they are sterilized on each occasion. Alternatively, sterile droppers delivering one drop at a time, such as Bengue's Guttilin, may be used, but in this case, it is difficult to ensure the sterility of the outside of the container and the nozzle.

Aqueous drops of various eye preparations may be prepared, and placed in Ballantyne's tubular bottles, normally within a cruet-like container of six, and the whole may be sterilized. In Ballantyne's container, each bottle is coloured differently, so that different solutions may be easily distinguished.

Most ophthalmic solutions can be sterilized by boiling, but adrenaline solution should be sterilized by autoclaving. Eserine can only be sterilized by bacterial filtering. In addition, suitable chemical preservatives and bactericides should be added.

It will be seen, therefore, that it is easier and preferable to use ready-prepared sterile solutions, particularly during intraocular surgery. Single-dose units, with sterile contents and sterile containers (Steri-Units, B.D.H.) are available and recommended for this purpose.

The only lotion likely to be required is sterile normal saline or balanced salt solution. This may either be sterilized by autoclaving or purchased in a sterile pack.

THE SELECTION OF INSTRUMENTS

Speculum. The conventional type of speculum is satisfactory for some operations in the dog, particularly those involving the cornea and superficial structures; but, in cases involving intraocular surgery, a speculum, however constructed, obstructs the operation field and renders many of the manoeuvres difficult to perform. In addition, most types of speculum tend to move easily away from the lids or slip in position.

Many types of speculum are available and of these, patterns such as Clark's (Fig. 36), with light arms are to be preferred to those with solid blades. The small wire adjustable speculum, for example the D.P. (Fig. 37), is of value, particularly as the thin arms cause little obstruction to the operation site. All specula, however, tend to cause pressure against the globe, which in many cases is contraindicated.

Lid retractors. Retractors for manipulation of the lids and palpebral opening have the advantage that they are easily adjustable and tend to cause less obstruction to the field. Castroviejo's lid clamps (Fig. 38) are useful, but tend to slip easily from the lids unless carefully adjusted.

Hand-held lid retractors are often helpful, and the small pattern of Desmarre (Fig. 39) is the most useful. Vierheller's spring retractor (Fig. 40), attached to lid sutures, is generally the best method of lid retraction in the

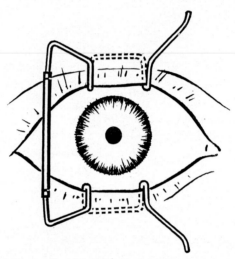

FIG. 37. *D.P. wire speculum.*

dog. This retractor, consisting of a coiled hub of spring wire, with two arms, is very satisfactory. Each arm, about 4 in. long, has a looped end to which lid sutures may be tied. Using this appliance, the degree of tension exerted on the lids is easily adjustable, there is no mechanical interference to the operation field, no pressure is created upon the globe and the retraction may be quickly released by cutting the suture of either lid.

Forceps. Fine fixation forceps (Fig. 41) with 1/2 or 2/3 teeth are useful for the manipulation of the lids, nictitating membrane and so on, but bruising and tearing of the conjunctiva and skin must be avoided. Similar forceps with a locking device (Fig. 42) are extremely valuable for manipulation of the eyeball and nictitating membrane, allowing structures to be easily held away from the operational site.

Fine plane forceps (Fig. 43), without teeth, are used for holding tissues lightly and these inflict little damage on the conjunctiva when used to manipulate it for suturing.

Forceps that can fix a structure and at the same time be used for holding a needle for suturing will be required. A suitable type is Jayle's forceps (Fig. 44) which is straight, has 1 and 2 oblique teeth and a block behind the teeth designed to hold even fine suture material or fine needles. Using this

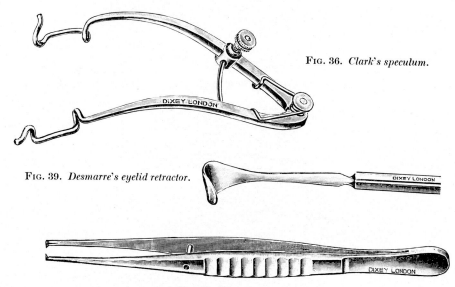

Fig. 36. *Clark's speculum.*

Fig. 39. *Desmarre's eyelid retractor.*

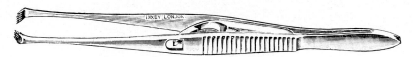

Fig. 41. *Fine fixation forceps.*

Fig. 42. *Fixation forceps with locking device.*

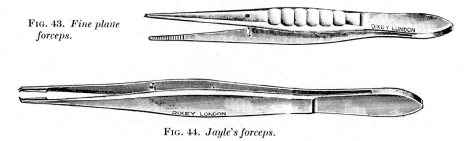

Fig. 43. *Fine plate forceps.*

Fig. 44. *Jayle's forceps.*

Fig. 45. *St. Martin's forceps.*

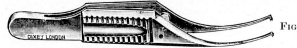

Fig. 46. *Barraquer's corneal forceps.*

type of forceps with a suitable needle-holder, sutures may be tied without being touched manually.

For corneal surgery, the size of the forceps used will depend largely on the size of needles and suture material. Of the various patterns available, St. Martin's (Fig. 45) are useful of the larger type, and Barraquer's (Fig. 48)

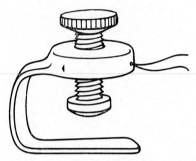

FIG. 38. *Castroviejo's eyelid clamps.*

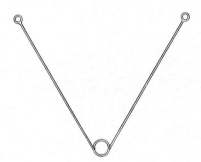

FIG. 40. *Vierheller's eyelid retractor.*

for very fine work. Rycroft's suture forceps (Fig. 47) are helpful in manipulating fine threads and for tying knots. These have no teeth, and no hatching on the face of the blocks through which fine sutures could slip.

Fixation of the globe to prevent rotation during cutting procedures is often difficult, particularly in the dog, where the loose conjunctiva often interferes with adequate immobilization of the globe. Forceps with a wide base with spaced settings of sharp teeth, such as the Barraquer-Llovera forceps (Fig. 48), are useful in this connection. Alternatively, the von Mandach forceps (Fig. 49) have non-tooth jaws which accurately interlock to grasp a wide fold of conjunctiva and subconjunctival tissue, and these have no tendency to puncture or tear the conjunctiva.

Cross-action forceps, of the 'Bulldog' pattern, will be found useful for the manipulation of fine threads and to secure sutures so that they do not become muddled. Whitfield's cilia forceps (Fig. 50) are used for the removal of unwanted hairs from the palpebral edge.

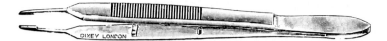

FIG. 47. *Rycroft's suture forceps.*

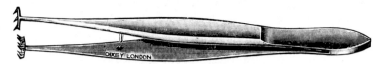

FIG. 48. *Barraquer-Llovera fixation forceps.*

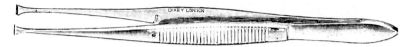

FIG. 49. *von Mandach forceps.*

FIG. 50. *Whitfield's cilia forceps.*

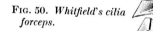

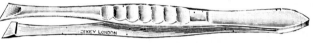

FIG. 51. *Arruga's needle-holder.*

FIG. 52. *Castroviejo's needle-holder.*

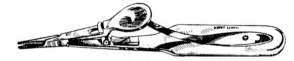

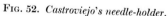

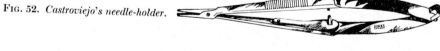

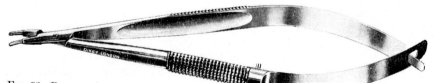

FIG. 53. *Barraquer's needle-holder.*

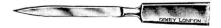

FIG. 54. *von Graefe's cataract knife.*

Special types of forceps will be required for operations upon the iris and lens, and for corneal graft work, and these will be described later.

Needle-holders. These instruments, for eye surgery, must be capable of firmly retaining fine needles, must be comfortable, light and well-balanced, and must have an efficient and reliable locking mechanism. Of the various types available, those of Arruga (Fig. 51) and Castroviejo (Fig. 52) will be found suitable, both having ingenious and efficient release mechanisms. For very fine work, the needle-holder of Barraquer (Fig. 53), without a locking device, is sometimes to be preferred.

Knives. For 'coarse' surgical work on the lids, the Bard-Parker knife, with either a no. 15 or a no. 11 blade, has many uses. Cataract knives are of many patterns; the knife of von Graefe (Fig. 54) has the point in the midline of the blade, whereas that of Smith (Fig. 55) has the point in line with the back edge of the blade. Allowance, in the former, must be made when making the counter-puncture in a cataract incision. All cataract knives must be long enough to transfix the cornea easily, and a long thin blade is preferable to a short broad blade.

To secure a perfect edge on every occasion, for general eye surgery, the fragment holder of Barraquer (Fig. 56), which firmly grips small pieces of razor blade, broken to the desired shape and size, may be used. Alternatively, disposable blades are available ('Beaver' blades); the range includes three miniaturized handles of different shape, cataract blades, keratome blades and other blades designed specifically for ocular surgery.

Hooks. Sharp hooks, such as Stallard's scleral hook (Fig. 57) or Gillie's hook, are of value for manipulation and retraction. Tyrell's blunt iris hook (Fig. 58) may be used for retraction of the iris at the pupillary margin, or wherever it is desired to retract without damage to the tissues concerned. A strabismus hook (Fig. 59) is useful to obtain artificial proptosis.

Scissors. Fine scissors, straight and curved, both with sharp points and with blunt points, will be required for various procedures. For fine man-oeuvres and delicate work, spring scissors (Fig. 60) are to be preferred for their ease of use and because they can be used easily by either hand and at any angle. Special scissors are required for corneal sectioning, and miniature scissors for the removal of sutures are essential for very fine work.

Electrocautery. An electrocautery unit is essential for many procedures, and any apparatus that is flexible, and allows the use of fine electrodes, will prove suitable. For fine work, the small, battery-operated models have much to commend them (Fig. 61).

A diathermy apparatus is also extremely useful on many occasions, and of these, the Manchester ophthalmic diatherm (Fig. 62), specially designed for eye work, and having a maximum coagulating current of 150 mA, is possibly the most useful.

Needles and suture materials. For general work around the eye and eyelids,

FIG. 55. *Smith's cataract knife.*

FIG. 56. *Barraquer's fragment holder.*

Razor *blade fragment.*

FIG. 57. *Stallard's scleral hook.*

FIG. 58. *Tyrell's iris hook.*

FIG. 59. *Strabismus hook.*

FIG. 60. *Spring action scissors.*

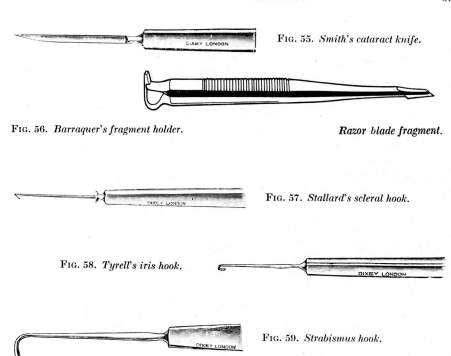

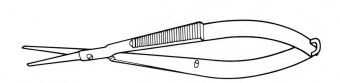

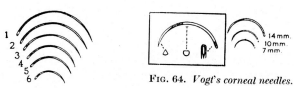

1
2
3
4
5
6

FIG. 63. *Curved eye needles.*

14 mm.
10 mm.
7 mm.

FIG. 64. *Vogt's corneal needles.*

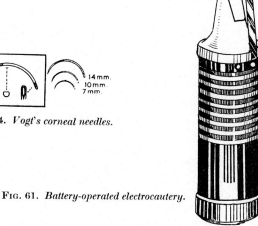

FIG. 61. *Battery-operated electrocautery.*

eye needles, straight, half-curved or curved. Nos. 1 to 6, are the most useful (Fig. 63).

For corneal suturing, many patterns are available, and choice will largely depend on individual preferences. Corneal needles are normally curved, having a triangular anterior portion with lateral cutting edges, and the spine on the convexity of the needle—such as the Vogt needle (sizes 7, 10 or 14 mm) (Fig. 64) and the Vogt-Barraquer needle (sizes 5, 7 or 10 mm). Needles which have the spine on the concavity of the curve are likely to cut out when passing through corneal tissue. Other needles, such as the Jameson

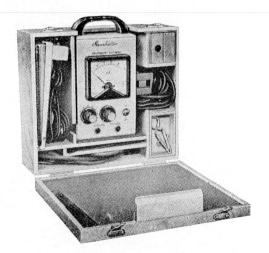

FIG. 62. 'Manchester' ophthalmic diatherm.

Evans' (Fig. 65), are flatter in vertical section, with sharp side edges, allowing the needle to split the corneal lamellae easily; rotation of such a needle, however, allows it to cut out.

Most corneal needles have eyes, but eyeless atraumatic needles with a fixed thread are obtainable—for example, Stallard's eyeless corneal needle. The larger the radius of curvature, the greater will be the amount of corneal tissue taken in by the needle.

For general work around the eye and eyelids, black braided silk is most suitable, and this can be obtained in sizes ranging from English gauge 3/0 to 2 (U.S.P. equivalent 6/0 to 2/0). Ophthalmic sutures, with eyeless needle attached, can be supplied in catgut or black or white silk, single or double needles, in any size required.

For corneal suturing, Kalt's silk is normally employed, having a size equivalent to 0·09 to 0·10 mm. For very fine work, particularly with corneal grafts, Barraquer's 5-strand virgin silk, 0·04 mm thick, may be used, and this may be obtained either in the pure state, or dyed blue for ease of handling.

Miscellaneous. Artery forceps will be required, and either mosquito forceps of $4\frac{3}{4}$ in or Spencer-Wells forceps of $3\frac{1}{2}$ in will prove suitable.

A measuring device is of value on many occasions, and Castroviejo's calipers (Fig. 66) are probably the most useful.

For irrigation of the anterior chamber, or for general flushing procedures, an anterior chamber irrigator (Fig. 67) will be required. Alternatively, single-dose units (Steri-Units, B.D.H.) containing balanced salt solution may be used.

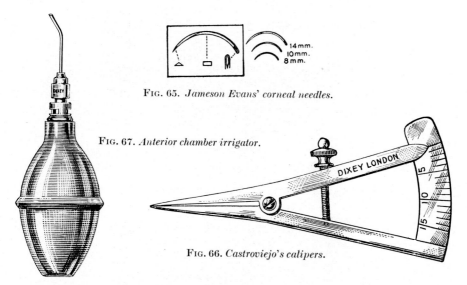

FIG. 65. *Jameson Evans' corneal needles.*

FIG. 67. *Anterior chamber irrigator.*

FIG. 66. *Castroviejo's calipers.*

PREOPERATIVE PREPARATION

The head of the patient must be adequately supported, particularly if the table is tilted to provide postural hypotension. For this purpose, sandbags are normally employed, and should be completely covered with plastic material, to provide ease of cleansing and to ensure that the contents of the bags cannot leak on to the operation site.

The operational site must be rendered as aseptic as possible, and the area around the eye, approximately 5 cm in width, is clipped as close as possible, and the eyelashes removed (Fig. 68). When intraocular surgery is to be performed, this clipping is carried out on the day before the operation, to avoid the accumulation of hair and debris in the conjunctival sac just prior to surgery. In those cases in which prior clipping is not possible, contamination of the conjunctival sac may be avoided by filling the palpebral fissure, and covering the eye, with a thin strip of polyvinyl sponge that has been soaked in normal saline solution. The conjunctival sac is subsequently irrigated with saline to remove any particles that may have penetrated the protection.

After clipping, the lids and surrounding skin are well cleansed, using soap and water, care being taken that soap does not enter the conjunctival sac. The skin is then dried and sterilized by the application of an antiseptic and antimycotic solution, such as 4% mercurochrome. Alternatively, particularly when it is desired not to stain the skin around the eyes, a

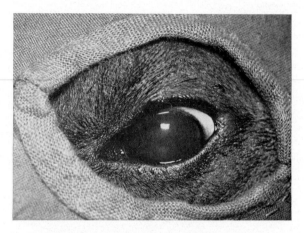

Fig. 68. *Preparation of the operation site.*

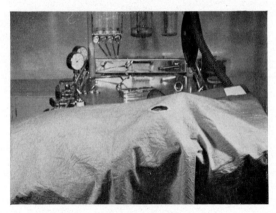

Fig. 69. *Draping the operation site.*

1:2000 solution of Hibitane in 70% alcohol may be employed. In all cases, the entry of such antiseptic solutions into the conjunctival sac must be avoided.

Preoperative flushing of the conjunctival sac may be required to remove any hair particles, and a few drops of chloramphenicol solution should then be instilled.

The operational site should be surrounded with sterile drapes, leaving only the minimal area exposed, but bearing in mind that a temporal cantho-tomy will be required in some cases. The use of specially prepared drapes, with a central oval opening corresponding to the size of the operation site, is to be recommended (Fig. 69). Drapes should be dyed dark green, to avoid dazzle from reflected light.

To minimize the area of lid and surrounding skin exposed during the operation, W. G. Magrane suggests the use of rubber dental dam. A strip of this dam is sterilized in the usual way. A small slit is cut in the centre of it sufficiently large to allow the insertion of a speculum and to expose the eye itself, whilst the remainder of the rubber sheet covers the eyelids (Fig. 70).

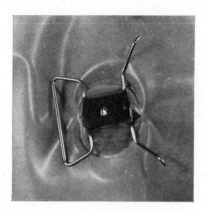

FIG. 70. *The use of rubber dental dam for draping.*

5

ANAESTHESIA FOR OPHTHALMIC SURGERY

Most ophthalmic operations in the dog are carried out under general anaesthesia. In certain circumstances, however, topical applications to the cornea may be used or local infiltrations employed. Retrobulbar and auriculopalpebral blocks are of some use on special occasions.

TOPICAL APPLICATIONS

In an eye free from congestion, the installation of 2 to 4% cocaine hydrochloride solution on four occasions at intervals of about 3 minutes, will produce complete anaesthesia of the cornea and conjunctiva. In congested eyes, the addition of a few drops of 1:1000 adrenaline solution will enhance the effect. Under cocaine, however, the corneal epithelium is likely to become dry, cloudy and easily injured and, for this reason, cocaine, although highly effective, is less commonly used at the present time.

Proparacaine hydrochloride (Ophthaine, Squibb) is a highly effective topical application for surface anaesthesia and is to be preferred. A 4% solution of lignocaine hydrochloride is also effective.

This form of anaesthesia affects only the superficial structures of the eye not the deeper parts. Its use is therefore confined to minor operations upon the conjunctiva or cornea, such as the removal of foreign bodies or the eversion of the nictitating membrane in order to examine the nictitans gland.

LOCAL INFILTRATION

Local infiltration, using 2% procaine, usually with the addition of adrenaline to localize the effect, is sometimes employed in lid surgery. In such cases, restraint may be assisted by the use of suitable tranquillizers or sedatives. Slight head movements during the course of the operation and the distortion of the tissues produced by the infiltration, are contraindications to this method and usually general anaesthesia will be found preferable.

Paralysis of the orbicularis muscle may be obtained by local infiltration with procaine or lignocaine, and this may be used, in conjunction with general anaesthesia, where it is desired to keep the plane of anaesthesia at a light level, yet have adequate relaxation of the periorbital muscles. For this purpose, a $1\frac{1}{2}$ in no. 26 S.W.G. needle and a dental syringe is employed, and the technique is as follows. The needle is inserted about 1 cm posterior to the lateral canthus and is passed downwards and backwards towards the zygomatic arch. A few drops of anaesthetic solution are injected. The needle is then directed to pass deeply through the upper lid, about 6 mm from the

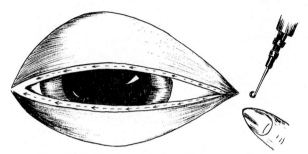

Fig. 71. *Infiltration of the lid with local anaesthetic.*

tarsal edge, anaesthetic solution being injected as it is inserted. Without withdrawing the needle completely, it is similarly redirected to anaesthetize the lower lid (Fig. 71).

RETROBULBAR BLOCK

It is unlikely that this form of anaesthesia will be employed in the dog, except as an aid to relaxation in light-plane general anaesthesia. In elderly patients, however, where a deep level of general anaesthesia may be considered dangerous, it will allow adequate relaxation of the ocular muscles.

A $1\frac{1}{2}$ in no. 26 S.W.G. needle is used and the amount of anaesthetic injected is normally 1·0 to 1·5 ml. A 2% solution of lignocaine is usually employed, and the addition of 6 to 10 units of hyaluronidase per ml ensures better anaesthesia. Longer needles may produce damage to the orbital structures, and shorter ones are unlikely to reach the structures to be anaesthetized. The needle is inserted through the conjunctiva at the outer third of the lower eyelid and into the gap between eye and orbital margin, the injection being made as the needle advances at a tangent to the globe. The needle is directed so that it eventually lies behind the globe, aimed at the apex, within the conical space formed by the recti muscles (Fig. 72). The main part of the injection is then completed. Anaesthesia takes about 10 minutes to become complete, by which time the extraocular muscles are paralysed and relaxation complete.

As Tenon's capsule is penetrated by the needle, the eye will be deflected towards the needle, causing a slight depression of the globe. This movement of the globe is to be expected. On occasion, an orbital vein may be damaged by the needle, producing a retrobulbar haemorrhage. This will produce

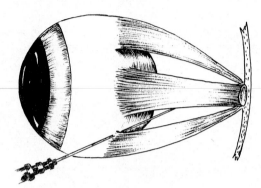

FIG. 72. *Retrobulbar block.*

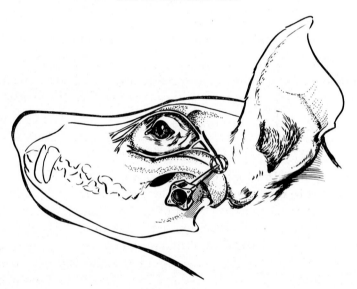

FIG. 73. *Auriculopalpebral block.*

proptosis and subconjunctival swelling and haematoma, and may be avoided by continuous injection as the needle advances, so that vessels are pushed out of the way by the stream of solution. A severe retrobulbar haemorrhage may mean the postponement of the operation, or the injection of 50 units of hyaluronidase into the orbit may reduce the swelling effectively.

Following retrobulbar block, the eye remains fixed and central in position, rotation and retraction being avoided. The technique may be usefully employed, therefore, for retinal photography and some operations on the lower segment of the cornea. Intraocular pressure decreases following the use of this block, producing a somewhat softer eye, a factor which may be of advantage in the surgery of hypertensive eyes.

AURICULOPALPEBRAL BLOCK

The technique of blocking the auriculopalpebral branch of the facial nerve does not produce analgesia of the eye or of the lids. It does, however, prevent closure of the eyelids and this may prove useful during and after intraocular operations and to prevent blepharospasm.

Either procaine hydrochloride or lignocaine hydrochloride may be used, and 1 ml of the solution is injected under the subcutaneous fascia in the region of the nerve. The point of insertion of the needle is found where the zygomatic arch dips sharply inwards (Fig. 73).

The dose employed of all local analgesic drugs must be carefully controlled to avoid toxic reaction, and care must be taken that accidental intravenous injection is avoided.

GENERAL ANAESTHESIA

Intravenous thiopentone is suitable for both short and minor operations. Although intravenous barbiturate anaesthesia provides an excellent depth of anaesthesia and good relaxation, it has proved unsuitable for intraocular techniques. Even with adequate premedication and postoperative sedation, the recovery period often proves turbulent. Postoperative excitement, which at times can be violent, may jeopardize the success of the operation or may result in failure.

The difficulties of conducting, say, cataract surgery, under local anaesthesia, even with adequate sedation, are great. Morphine is likely to produce postoperative restlessness and vomiting. These factors and the impossibility of providing suitable restraint, that will neither interfere with the operator nor with certainty prevent any sudden movement on the part of the animal, contraindicate the use of local anaesthesia for intraocular surgery in the dog.

The objections which, in the past, have been held against inhalation anaesthesia in ocular surgery, have now been largely eliminated. The increased haemorrhage that could be expected from an anaesthetic-induced congestion, and the septic and mechanical embarrassment of a face-mask, are factors which have been eliminated by the introduction of endotracheal administration. Postoperative nausea, vomiting and excitability have been eliminated, party by the introduction of new anaesthetic agents and partly by the use of new drugs for premedication. The development of 'balanced anaesthesia' in the dog has removed many of the hazards; nevertheless,

6

cases will be met showing occasional head movements, straining or sudden vomiting. Such complications may cause serious damage, open the operative wound or cause prolapse of the intraocular structures. The aim, therefore, must be a quiet and smooth induction, adequate anaesthesia of a depth that is suitable during the whole of the operating period, and a smooth recovery, unassociated with either vomiting or excitement.

A mask constitutes a great mechanical interference to manipulation and instrumentation, particularly as the position of the operation field in ocular surgery, in relationship to the mask, makes the task of the anaesthetist difficult. The use of endotracheal intubation, following induction with thiopentone, eliminates these difficulties.

Ether provides an adequate depth of anaesthesia but has certain disadvantages. Excessive mucous secretions can be controlled, in part at least, by giving atropine preoperatively. The vascular congestion produced by ether may cause embarrassment, or may result in excessive haemorrhage during the operation. The vasodilatation of scleral vessels can be controlled, to a certain extent, by the use of adrenaline drops.

Halothane has proved to be a useful agent for anaesthesia in ophthalmic surgery. The depth of anaesthesia is readily adjustable, with a wide margin of safety, even in the poor-risk patient. The postoperative period is normally quiet, with no postoperative excitement, nausea or vomiting. In cases where no premedication is employed, recovery from anaesthesia is rapid; in those cases in which premedication is used, a more prolonged recovery period is experienced, but this is normally quiet and free from postanaesthetic narcotic excitement. Muscular relaxation is adequate, and there is suppression of salivary secretions. Halothane has a hypotensive effect, particularly when the drug is administered in high concentration, venous dilatation is marked, but capillary seeping is reduced. Although such hypotension may increase the risks of severe haemorrhage during general surgery, where some degree of haemorrhage is, in any case, to be expected, it is of great value in intraocular surgery, where a bloodless field is so often required and is, in fact, an essential factor for successful surgery.

Halothane has proved to be an excellent anaesthetic agent for use in ocular surgery, allowing the three main requirements to be attained—a quiet induction, adequate maintenance and a smooth postanaesthetic period. It has the additional advantage that, being non-inflammable and non-explosive, it may be safely used when electrocautery or diathermy are required.

ANCILLARY PROCEDURES

Premedication

Adequate, and suitable, premedication will be required for all the more lengthy procedures, in order to assist with smooth induction, adequate relaxation without too great a depth of anaesthesia and freedom from post-operative excitement. Many suitable agents are available, but, of these, chlorpromazine or acetylpromazine are probably the most useful in obtaining consistent results. These should be given about one hour prior to operation, and atropine should be given simultaneously. The combination of promethazine and chlorpromazine, for premedication, may be used to give the greatest tranquillizing effect combined with a marked antihistaminic effect. This may be of particular value in preventing miosis following corneal section, due to the release of histamine-like substances from the severed tissues.

Anaesthesia may be reinforced by the use of pethidine intravenously immediately following intubation. The use of this drug, in a form combined with levallorphan tartrate (Pethilorfan, Roche Products) to counteract the respiratory-depressant effect of the pethidine, will further reduce the amount of volatile anaesthetic agent required for maintenance.

The method of general anaesthesia of choice for ophthalmic surgery may be summarized, therefore, as follows—premedication with chlorpromazine or acetylpromazine, with or without the addition of promethazine and atropine, one hour prior to operation; induction with thiopentone sodium; intubation, possibly followed by intravenous pethidine; and maintenance with oxygen, nitrous oxide and halothane. In order to maintain the general anaesthesia on a light plane, surface anaesthesia, infiltration of the orbicularis and retrobulbar block may be employed. The value of the relaxant drugs should also be borne in mind. Following the administration of one of these drugs, the voluntary muscles become progressively paralysed, starting with the extraocular muslces and the orbicularis, thence to the muscles of the head, neck, trunk and limbs, and finally to the muscles of respiration. This sequence, and the fact that the minimal doses affect the muscles of the eyeball and lids, is of particular advantage in eye surgery. It must be stressed, however, that relaxants should never be given to the conscious patient and must only be administered after general anaesthesia is complete. Intubation and the facilities for controlled respiration are essential These methods should only be used in the presence of a qualified anaesthetist.

It is essential that the postoperative course should be as smooth as possible and it is here that the tranquillizers and pethidine play an important part.

The reduction of haemorrhage

In all surgical operations on or around the eye, and particularly in intra-ocular procedures, the avoidance of unnecessary haemorrhage is important, and, in some cases, essential.

In plastic surgical procedures, such as entropion operations, adrenaline may be infiltrated into the operation site. Care must be taken, however, that cardiac arrhythmia is not produced by using the technique in combination with certain anaesthetic agents that sensitize the myocardium to the action of adrenaline.

Haemorrhage during anaesthesia may be minimized by the use of postural hypotension. This may be accomplished by tilting the operating table so that the head is higher than the general level of the body, thus promoting free venous drainage from the area. In all cases it is important to avoid airway obstruction, producing a rise in venous pressure, and endotracheal intubation is essential. A rise in venous pressure may also be produced by straining, coughing, vomiting and respiratory depression. Coughing may be avoided by the use of local analgesic sprays before intubation and the use of analgesic lubricants for tubes. Cyclopropane should be avoided because of its tendency to produce postoperative vomiting.

Controlled hypotension

The deliberate lowering of arterial blood pressure, combined with postural hypotension, produces ischaemia at the operation site. Ischaemia of the eye, however, results also in ischaemia of the brain, and care must be taken not to elevate the head to a point where the cerebral blood supply is impaired to a dangerous level. Controlled hypotension also results in marked lowering of the intraocular pressure, producing a soft eye. The production of controlled hypotension is not without danger, and should not be used except by an anaesthetist experienced in the technique, who has the necessary facilities available.

Hypotensive techniques should not be employed in hypertensive dogs, such as Greyhounds, or heart failure may result, neither should they be used in cases of hepatic or renal disease.

For details of these techniques, the reader is referred to various publications on anaesthesia. Briefly, however, the technique mostly in use depends on adequate premedication, using tranquillizers and atropine, anaesthesia induction with thiopentone sodium followed by intubation and maintenance with nitrous oxide—oxygen—halothane in a semi-closed circuit. Intraarterial blood pressure is monitored from the femoral artery, the pressure being displayed on an oscilloscope or recorder, and hexamethonium bromide is given intravenously. Postural hypotension is employed, and the level of blood pressure is controlled by altering the concentration of halothane. The aim is to reduce the systolic blood pressure to 70 to 80 mm Hg, but not to levels below this.

6

THE EYELIDS

ANATOMY AND PHYSIOLOGY

The eyelids are two movable folds of skin, upper and lower, which are able to close and cover the eye. In the dog, most of the movement takes place in the upper lid, the lower lid being relatively poorly developed. The functions of the lids are—to protect the eye both from injury and from excessive light, to help in the removal of foreign matter from the cornea, to spread the lacrimal fluid over the cornea and to move the lacrimal secretions towards the lacrimal drainage channels.

The lid is covered, on its outer surface, by skin, which shows a stratified squamous epithelium and numerous small hair follicles. The hairs on the two lids point in opposite directions, away from the palpebral orifice. On its inner surface, the lid is lined by the palpebral conjunctiva. Skin and conjunctiva meet at the lid margin. At the free margin of the lid are the eyelashes and certain small glands.

The skin of the lids is relatively thin, and contains small sebaceous glands, small sweat glands and pigment cells. Beneath the skin is a subcutaneous layer of loose connective tissue, containing many elastic fibres, which is loosely adherent to the underlying muscle.

The shape of the lid is maintained by a curved plate of dense white fibrous connective tissue, the tarsal plate, situated between the muscles and the conjunctiva. The tarsal plate, which is not well-developed in the dog, extends to the lid margin and, embedded within it are a number of alveolar glands—the Meibomian glands (Fig. 74).

Each Meibomian gland has a straight central duct, which opens on to the inner lid margin. Numerous small orifices are present, arranged in a single row along the margin. The secretion of the Meibomian glands, which is viscous in nature, lubricates the lid edges and helps to prevent the overflow of the lacrimal secretions.

Located around the palpebral orifice, situated in the subcutaneous connective tissue, and extending almost to the edge of the lid, is the orbicularis oculi muscle, which, acting like a sphincter, draws the eyelids

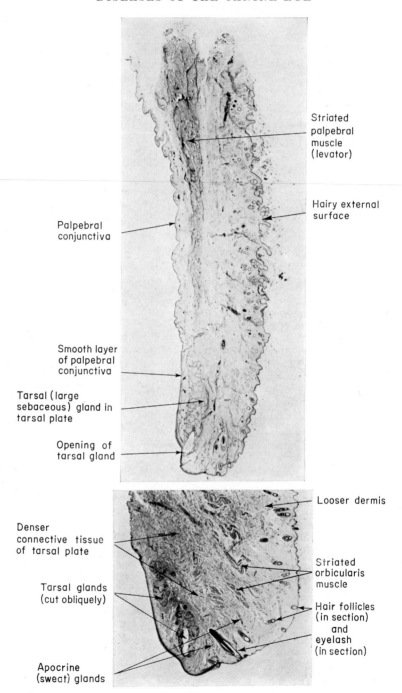

Striated
palpebral
muscle
(levator)

Hairy external
surface

Palpebral
conjunctiva

Smooth layer
of palpebral
conjunctiva

Tarsal (large
sebaceous) gland in
tarsal plate

Opening of
tarsal gland

Looser dermis

Denser
connective tissue
of tarsal plate

Striated
orbicularis
muscle

Tarsal glands
(cut obliquely)

Hair follicles
(in section)
and
eyelash
(in section)

Apocrine
(sweat) glands

FIG. 74. *Vertical section through the upper eyelid.*

together. This muscle is well-developed in the dog. The shape of the palpebral orifice, when closed, is maintained by two palpebral ligaments, nasal and temporal, which prevent the aperture from assuming a circular shape. The orbicularis oculi is innervated by the seventh cranial nerve.

The upper lid may be raised by fibres of the levator palpebrae muscle, innervated by the third cranial nerve, which pass through the connective tissue to be inserted on to the anterior surface of the tarsal plate.

Also well-developed in some dogs is the corrugator supercilii muscle, which, with the orbicularis oculi, acts in pulling the eyebrows inwards and downwards. It is divided into two parts, medial and lateral, of which the former is the larger, and inserts in to the upper medial lid margin. It is innervated by the seventh cranial nerve.

Situated in the lid margin of the upper lid, but almost absent in the lower lid, are the eyelashes or cilia. These are heavy, curved hairs with no erectile muscles, arranged in two or three irregular rows.

Associated with the eyelashes are large sebaceous glands, the glands of Zeis, and, between the hair follicles, large sweat glands, the glands of Moll, which open near the cilia, anteriorly to the ducts of the Meibomian glands.

The sensory supply of the upper lid is by the ophthalmic branch of the fifth cranial nerve, and that of the lower lid by the maxillary branch.

CONGENITAL ABNORMALITIES

Ablepharon, or absence of the lid, is rare, and, when it occurs, is usually associated with an under-developed eye.

Ankyloblepharon. This condition, in which the eyelids are fused together, is, of course, normal for the first 10 to 15 days of a pup's life. Occasionally, cases are seen in which the eyelids fail to open, and in some

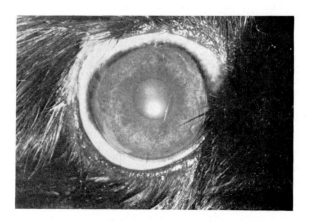

FIG. 75. *Coloboma of the eyelid.*

cases surgical intervention may become necessary. Cases also occur in which infection develops within the closed or partly-closed eyelids.

Symblepharon. Adhesion of the lid, in part or in toto, to the eyeball is known as symblepharon.

Coloboma. A notch in the margin of an eyelid or coloboma (Fig. 75), is uncommon but may be complicated by epiphora and will require plastic surgery.

Blepharophimosis. Narrowing of the palpebral opening or blepharophimosis (Fig. 76), may be seen occasionally, especially in the Chow, Collie and Shetland Sheepdog.

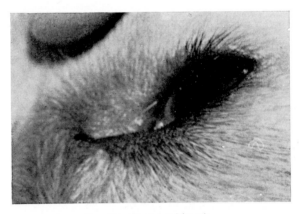

Fig. 76. *Blepharophimosis.*

In the Bull Terrier, blepharophimosis may occur as a congenital defect, and, in some cases, may be associated with other ocular changes, such as heterochromia, or with deafness.

Epicanthus. A fold of skin connecting the upper and lower lids, covering the nasal canthus (epicanthus), may be treated by simple excision or multiple ligation.

Ptosis, trichiasis, distichiasis, entropion, ectropion and *atresia of the lacrimal puncta* may also be congenital.

INJURIES TO THE EYELIDS

Abrasions of the eyelids are common in the dog as a result of accidents and fights, and even trivial injuries may produce severe oedema or ecchymosis. More severe contusions may lead to greater leakage of blood into the subcutaneous tissues, and may be associated with subconjunctival haemorrhage. Sometimes the underlying bone may be fractured and this may be associated with subdermal emphysema.

Minor abrasions and contusions require little treatment other than simple wound dressing, but in every case, careful examination should be made of the remainder of the eye to exclude any corneal injury. In the presence of marked chemosis, general anaesthesia may be required if a worthwhile examination is to be made.

Wounds of the eyelids resulting from fights and accidents, are also common in the dog and may be accompanied by excessive lacrimation and, sometimes, epiphora. Wounds may be at right angles or longitudinal to the lid margin and are often complicated by loss of part of the lid. Wounds at the nasal canthus may cause damage to the lacrimal puncta or canal, and the subsequent healing may result in occlusion or malpositioning of the puncta. Other wounds, on healing, may result in either entropion or ectropion.

Treatment will, of course, vary with the position and nature of the damage, but simple wounds, parallel to the lid edge, may be sutured with fine nylon. Suturing should be carried out at the earliest opportunity, and it is important that these sutures pass only through the skin edge, and that penetration of the tarsal plate and puckering of the wound be avoided.

Wounds involving loss of lid substance are best sutured without trying to replace the missing tissue, except in those cases that are very full in the lid. At a later date irregularities can be remedied by plastic surgery. Subsequent wound infection should be treated by antibiotic therapy and the use of topical anaesthetic ointments to prevent interference by the patient.

The commonest sequel to wounds of the eyelids is a V-shaped notch through which tears will overflow. In some cases, there is sufficient lid to spare to allow suturing after preparing fresh edges. In other cases, the wound may be sutured by relieving tension, either by means of a counter-incision at the side of the V, allowed to heal as an open wound, or by performing a canthotomy.

Burns and scalds involving the lids are not common in the dog, but occasionally lime or disinfectant are the cause of considerable damage or sloughing. Treatment of burns is normally by saline irrigations and local antibiotics, but routine plastic operations may be required at a later date. If the cornea is exposed, an immediate tarsorrhaphy should be performed or the cornea should be covered with a conjunctival flap.

DISTORTIONS OF THE LID MARGINS

The lid margins may be distorted by being inverted (entropion) or everted (ectropion). Either of these conditions may be congenital in origin, and there is evidence that they are hereditary in certain breeds. In acquired cases, the distortion may be produced mechanically through scar tissue, or functionally through spasm or weakness of the muscles controlling the lid. Where there is mechanical distortion, the lid will turn inwards if the conjunctival surface is affected and outwards if the skin is scarred. Of the functional types, spastic distortions are generally associated with acute inflammatory lesions, whereas atonic distortions, usually affecting the less rigid lower lid, are more often an accompaniment of senility, with slackness of the tone of the skin and musculature and thickening of the conjunctiva from chronic infection.

ENTROPION

The inversion or rolling inwards of the lid margin, and the irritation produced either by the edge of the lid, the hair of the lid, or the eyelashes, will lead to some degree of conjunctivokeratitis, which, in some cases, may be severe.

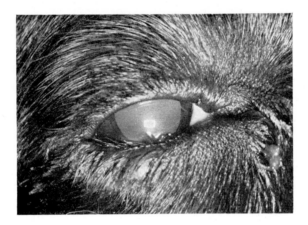

FIG. 77. *Congenital entropion.*

(1) *Congenital entropion* is seen most commonly in the Chow, Bloodhound, Labrador Retriever, Bullmastiff, Springer Spaniel, Papillon and Pomeranian. It is also seen frequently in the Cocker Spaniel, often in association with an ectropion in another part of the same lid. In the Chow, it is usually associated with a small palpebral opening and a shortened lid. In the Bullmastiff and Bloodhound, it may be associated with excessive folds of loose skin over the head. It is usually bilateral, may affect both upper and lower lids, and will often affect the various lids to differing degrees (Fig. 77). The lower lids are more commonly affected than the upper, and the lateral margins more commonly than the nasal border.

(2) *Acquired entropion* may be associated with the cicatricial contraction of wounds of the eyelid, or with cicatricial contraction of the palpebral conjunctiva or subconjunctival tissues in cases of severe or chronic conjunctival infection. The upper lid is more commonly affected in this type of inversion.

Spastic entropion is seen in cases of persistent blepharospasm, usually resulting from foreign bodies in the conjunctival sac, or with chronic conjunctivitis or keratitis (Fig. 78). The irritation from the inturned lid edge and eyelashes tends to aggravate the inflammatory process and this, in turn, accentuates the degree of entropion. The lower lid is more commonly affected. Other cases will occur where there is atrophy of the eyeball, or whenever there is marked sinking of the eyeball due to absorption of the retrobulbar fat.

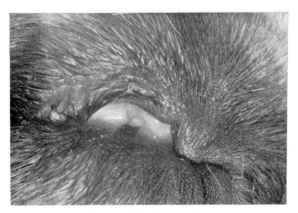

FIG. 78. *Spastic entropion.*

Atonic entropion, produced by lack of tone in the tarso-orbital fascia, is seen occasionally in old dogs, particularly in the Cocker Spaniel.

Clinical signs

The signs exhibited will vary according to the degree of the entropion, but will be accompanied by lacrimation and possibly irritation. Severe cases will cause blepharospasm which, in turn, will produce entropion of a greater degree, and may lead to conjunctivitis, keratitis and corneal ulceration. The position of the lacrimal puncta may be upset, leading to marked epiphora.

Treatment

This is based on the surgical eversion of the lid. Many operations have been devised for the correction of this condition, and each will have its value in specific cases. Successful results in all cases of entropion depend on the selection of the most suitable type of operation, and its accurate application; such selection can be based only on clinical experience.

Skin-and-muscle operation. This is the orthodox operation, adopted in most cases of congenital entropion, and in many cases of acquired spastic or atonic inversion (Fig. 79).

The operation consists of the removal of an elliptical portion of skin and orbicularis muscle, parallel to the lid, and of such a size as to correct the deformity when the wound is sutured and the lid thus drawn outwards to its normal position. The subsequent healing of the wound and cicatricial contraction will then keep the lid in its normal position. Critical judgement of the site and area to be removed is most important for good results, so that there is no tendency to produce an ectropion, while the condition is being satisfactorily corrected, and to minimize the degree of the visible scar.

The operation is best performed under general anaesthesia. Some surgeons prefer the use of local anaesthetic infiltration, maintaining that it is difficult

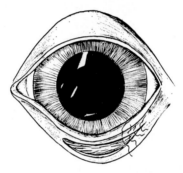

FIG. 79. *Skin-and-muscle operation for entropion.*

to assess the incision accurately when the animal is anaesthetized and the eyeball has rotated. However, the infiltration of an anaesthetic solution along the proposed line of incision also produces some distortion of the tissues, affecting the degree of inturning shown; in addition, the restraint necessary in many animals makes the application of an accurate incision and adequate suturing difficult. It is usually preferable to assess the line of the incisions before anaesthesia is induced, and then perform the operation on the unconscious animal.

The elliptical portion of skin is best removed by first outlining the site with a scalpel incision, and then removing with curved scissors and forceps. One incision is made about 4 mm from the tarsal edge, and parallel to it; the other curved incision is made at a point estimated to remove sufficient skin to correct the deformity when sutured. The orbicularis muscle is then picked up, and, generally, the full length is removed to correspond with the skin wound; other surgeons prefer to take multiple snips from the body of the muscle. Haemorrhage is usually profuse, and may be controlled with pressure swabs or the application of adrenaline solution; larger vessels may need to be clamped or, on occasion, ligated.

The wound should be sutured with very fine nylon sutures, drawn only sufficiently tightly to approximate the wound edges. Some postoperative swelling is usual around the operation site, and sutures tied too tightly will tend to cut-out. Multiple sutures should be used, firstly as a safeguard against self-inflicted damage, and secondly to minimize the subsequent visible scar.

Where considerable blepharospasm is present, producing a spastic state, it is advisable to use a topical anaesthetic preparation for several days before the operation, in order to eliminate the effect of the blepharospasm, and thus enable a finer judgement to be made of the extent of the incision necessary.

Canthoplasty operation. In those breeds, such as the Chow, which normally

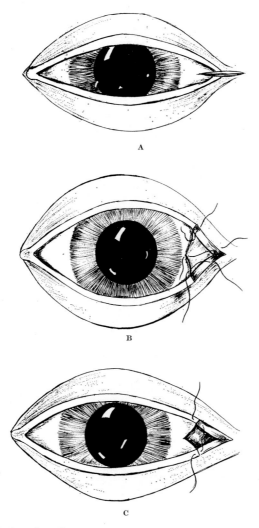

FIG. 80. *Canthoplasty and canthotomy.* A, *the line of incision;* B, *suturing for canthoplasty;* C, *suturing for canthotomy.*

have a small siit eye, the orthodox operation may result in a round palpebral orifice. In such cases, it is preferable to carry out a moderate skin incision, and, at the same time, to lengthen the orifice by incision at the temporal canthus (Fig. 80).

The skin at the temporal canthus may be incised in an outward direction with pointed scissors, tensing the skin before the incision is made. The incision is made in the horizontal plane, for approximately 2 to 3 cm. Tension is applied to the skin at the lateral canthus by the surgeon's forefinger and one blade of the scissors is passed into the conjunctival sac. Haemorrhage is often profuse and must be controlled before the operation is continued. Digital pressure over gauze is sometimes sufficient, but because of the difficulty that is sometimes experienced in obtaining good healing of a canthotomy incision, the use of haemostatic pressure along the line of the incision, before this is carried out, is not recommended. Infiltration of the line of incision with adrenaline may be employed, or the haemorrhage may be controlled simply and speedily by the use of coagulation diathermy.

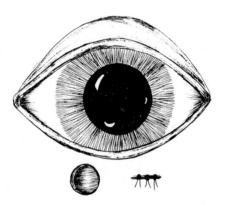

FIG. 81. *Trephine operation for entropion.*

After incising the skin, the underlying conjunctiva is picked up and severed in a similar way. One suture of fine nylon or cotton thread is inserted into the angle so formed, uniting skin and conjunctiva, and two sutures are placed through skin and conjunctiva on either side of the incision.

Trephine operation. Small corrections to lid edge deformities may be made by using trephine incisions at the points where correction is required. Trephines of 3 to 12 mm diameter may be used and circular areas of skin are removed, together with a small portion of orbicularis muscle. This method is applicable only to the lower lid, and the edge of the trephine incision is kept close to the lid margin. Correction is obtained by suturing the trephine incisions horizontally (Fig. 81).

Advancement flaps. Dixon's operation, using advancement flaps, in which the skin is split, allows the skin to be moved at will to any new position that the case may require.

An incision is made in the eyelid farther away from the margin than in the classical operation, and a narrow strip of skin is removed. The skin between the wound and the margin of the lid is then undermined, leaving a narrow strip on the margin of the lid intact to ensure the blood supply, and leaving the fat attached to the skin and raised with the flap. The skin of the lid now slides over the underlying structures to its new position, the extreme edge of the lid rolling outwards. This method gives more accurate correction and avoids stretching and puckering.

Using this technique, it is possible to make a single incision, undermining the wound, and drawing the skin away until the lid is in the correct position. The excess skin is then trimmed away and the flap fitted accurately into its new site. Any tension resulting at the outer canthus can be relieved by making a V incision, with the point away from the eye, undermining and suturing the wound as a Y.

In cases where there is an entropion at the inner canthus, and ectropion in the centre of the lid, a rotation flap is used. In this case, a curved incision is made, as a sharp curve below the entropion and straight below the ectropion. The skin is undermined and a small triangular piece of skin is removed at either end of the wound. Suturing is started at the inner canthus, where the apex of the triangle is drawn down to the long outer curve. The flap is then rotated outwards until the remaining side of the triangle can be fixed to the outer curve. The edge of the flap is now stretched to the outer curve, so that the fitting of a wide flap into a narrow opening will correct the entropion and the ectropion at the same time.

Operations for cicatricial entropion. If there are only a few inturned lashes, epilation may prove adequate.

Where contraction of the conjunctiva alone is responsible for causing the lashes to impinge on the cornea, correction may be obtained by the use of a buccal mucous membrane graft, inserted behind the line of the lashes.

Operations for atonic entropion. Entropion associated solely with abundant loose skin may be corrected by excision of the redundant skin or, in the case of the lower lid, a Y–V operation may prove effective.

Those cases associated with excessive loose folds of skin on the head may require the excision of some of the loose skin before the entropion can be satisfactorily corrected; or may benefit from a sling operation, in which a bridge of skin is transposed from the upper lid to the lower lid.

ECTROPION

Ectropion is the reverse of entropion, being the eversion of the lid with exposure of the conjunctival surface. It will, of course, affect the lower lid only. This eversion leads to stagnation of tears in the lower fornix and, in many cases, eversion of the lacrimal punctum so that lacrimal drainage is affected. Infection of the conjunctiva is likely to occur, and the subsequent congestion may aggravate the malpositioning of the lid margin. Overflow of tears is likely, with the production of excoriation of the skin of the lower lid. If uncorrected, chronic inflammatory changes in the conjunctiva are likely, with the formation of granulations (Fig. 82).

This condition may be congenital in the case of such breeds as the Spaniels, Hounds and Mastiffs, where it is associated with excess skin of the lids and excessive length of the palpebral fissure. Acquired cases may be cicatricial, spastic or atonic in origin. Cicatricial ectropion may result from scarring of

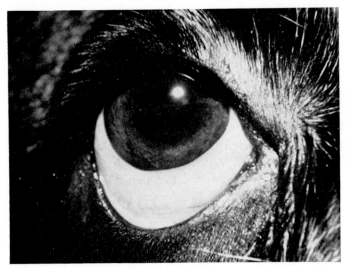

Fig. 82. *Ectropion.*

the skin of the eyelid from burns, trauma or inflammation. Spastic ectropion may result from spasm of the orbicularis in those cases in which the overlying skin is tight or where some degree of proptosis, thrusting the lid margins forward, is already present. Atonic ectropion may occur in old animals, due to loss of tone in the skin and musculature or in cases of lagophthalmos due to paralysis of the orbicularis muscle.

Treatment

Various operations have been devised for the correction of ectropion, mostly designed to shorten the offending lid and so correct the eversion.

Cicatricial ectropion. Acquired ectropion, resulting from cicatricial contraction, will usually require the application of skin grafts for its correction. In the dog, local flaps are to be preferred, which may be of the sliding, rotation or transposition variety.

Atonic ectropion. In mild cases, correction may often be obtained by removing a portion of the conjunctiva lining the eyelid at the site of the ectropion, and allowing the subsequent cicatricial contraction to pull in the lid. In other cases, the conjunctiva may be shrunk by the application of a 2% solution of silver nitrate, or by the use of a cautery, burning a series of small holes parallel to and about 4 mm from the lid margin. More severe cases will require one of the operations described below.

Lateral tarsorrhaphy. A tarsorrhaphy (suturing together of the lids) will normally be permanent when used to correct an ectropion, and will be applied at the outer canthus. Simple removal of the epithelium of the lids, opposing the raw surfaces and suturing together, will invariably be followed

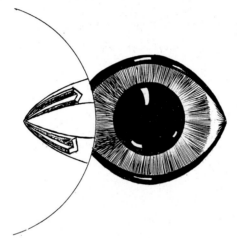

Fig. 83. *Lateral tarsorrhaphy.*

by a breakdown of the wound from interference by the patient. In the dog, a better technique is to cut a step from each lid margin, so that the two portions overlap and may be sutured antero-posteriorly. The lid is first split over the required area, then the posterior part is removed from the upper lid and the anterior part from the lower lid (Fig. 83).

Wedge resection. A part of the entire thickness of the lid may be removed and the wound subsequently sutured, or a length of the rim of the lid at the temporal canthus may be removed, the remainder being sutured to the palpebral angle. Less distortion will occur if the lid is split along the affected area, and a wedge of tarsus and conjunctiva removed; a similar wedge-shape area of skin is removed at the outer canthus, the skin is undermined and, after trimming, is sutured into the wedge-shaped area, thus reducing the length of the lower lid.

Trephine operation. Similar trephine incisions may be made below the centre of the eyelid, as described for the correction of entropion, but, in

7

this case, should be sutured perpendicularly instead of horizontally (Fig. 84A).

V-Y *operation.* An alternative method is to make a V incision in the lower lid, with the point downwards, and to suture this wound as a Y, combining this technique, if necessary, with a canthotomy (Fig. 84B, C).

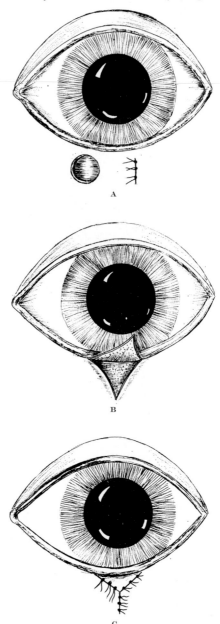

FIG. 84. A *Trephine operation for ectropion,* B V-Y *operation for ectropion—the incision,* C *suturing.*

Sling operation. In those dogs with excessive folds on the head, associated with an entropion of the upper lid and an ectropion of the lower lid, a sling support may be used, transposing a bridge of skin from the upper to the lower lid (Fig. 85).

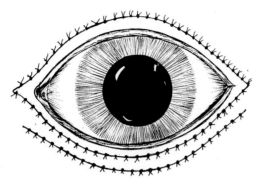

FIG. 85. *Sling operation for ectropion.*

OTHER ABNORMALITIES

Symblepharon

The adhesion of the lid to eyeball, due to loss of opposing conjunctival surfaces, may be congenital or may result from caustic burns. Treatment is usually disappointing, for the removal of the scarred conjunctival tissue is invariably followed by further adhesions.

Ankyloblepharon

Adhesions between the lid margins may be congenital or may result from adherent lesions of both lid edges. Division of the adhesion is usually simple.

Trichiasis

In the condition of trichiasis, the eyelashes arise from their normal position at the edge of the lid, but are wrongly angulated or misdirected so that they impinge on either the conjunctiva or on the cornea. The palpebral fissure and the Meibomian glands are normal (Fig. 86).

Trichiasis, which is most commonly seen in the Pekingese, may be congenital in origin; in other cases, the misdirection of the eyelashes may be acquired from blepharospasm or mild entropion.

The abrasion of the cornea by the eyelashes produces excess lacrimation and irritation. This may lead in time to either a conjunctivitis or a keratitis and eventually to superficial corneal vascularization or ulceration.

Treatment can be in the form of epilation, carried out with cilia forceps, but this can only afford temporary relief and will require repetition every few weeks or months. Recurrences can sometimes be avoided by the use of electrolysis—inserting a cathode needle at a current of 2 mA for a few seconds into each hair follicle—thus destroying the hair root. A very fine epilation needle is required, together with good magnification. The cornea may be protected from accidental damage during the operation by inserting a padded tongue depressor under the treated lid. In most cases, the procedure will need to be repeated several times before all lashes are removed.

Orthodox entropion operations may be employed, removing a strip of skin and orbicularis muscle just sufficient to result in redirection of the

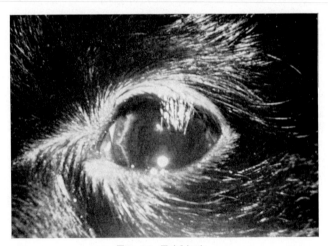

FIG. 86. *Trichiasis.*

lashes. In the absence of any entropion, however, such an operation produces a mild ectropion, resulting in some disfigurement.

Alternatively, and preferably, a radical operation can be performed by incising along the edge of the lid on either side of the row of offending lashes, directing the angle of the incisions so that a V-shaped piece of tissue, containing the lashes and their roots, is removed. Provided that the two parallel incisions are kept as close together as possible, no suturing is required, and the result is normally excellent. In some cases, one or two sutures of very fine silk may be required to appose the edges of the wound.

Distichiasis

Distichiasis signifies a double row of eyelashes along the margin of the lid. One row is situated in the normal position, the other—which may be partial or complete—arises from the Meibomian gland openings on the posterior eyelid border. The lashes from this inner row curve inward and impinge on the cornea. Either or both lids may be affected and the abnormal lashes are usually small and non-pigmented. The upper lid is more commonly involved and the number of abnormal lashes may vary from one to twenty or so (Figs. 87, 88).

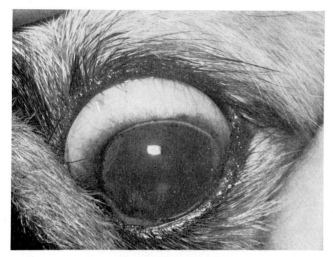

FIG. 87. *Distichiasis.*

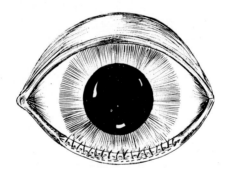

FIG. 88. *Operation for distichiasis.*

Distichiasis is, in most cases, a congenital abnormality, the breeds most commonly affected being the Pekingese and Poodle, although cases have been reported in the Bedlington Terrier, Boxer and Alsatian. Inherited factors are probably involved. Other cases may be acquired, some observers reporting that the spontaneous eruption of cilia in this position is possible, at any age, in response to continued irritation.

As in trichiasis, stimulation of the eyeball by the abnormal lashes may result in lacrimation, irritation, photophobia and mild conjunctivitis. In cases where the cilia are strong, or the irritation prolonged, keratitis may result which, in advanced cases, may terminate in corneal ulceration.

The diagnosis of distichiasis is sometimes difficult unless conditions of adequate illumination and magnification are employed; in many cases, the abnormal lashes are very fine and unpigmented and difficult to see. A few cases may be associated with other congenital malformations such as entropion, blepharophimosis, microphthalmos or atresia of the lacrimal puncta.

In cases where only a very few abnormal lashes occur, treatment may be by repeated epilation, although the very fine nature of the cilia in some cases makes the procedure difficult. The procedure will need to be repeated at regular intervals, although, in a very few instances, the abnormal cilia fail to regrow after several repeated removals. Electrolysis may be employed in some cases, although recurrence is common unless a very careful technique is employed. In many cases, the lashes involved are of such a fine nature as to make the application of the epilation needle impossible. In other cases, excessive scarring from repeated electrolysis may result in distortion of the lid margin.

The most satisfactory results will be obtained by the surgical removal of the offending lashes. As in the case of trichiasis, two parallel incisions are made into the lid margin, one on each side of the Meibomian gland orifices, and a V-shaped portion of the lid margin, containing the Meibomian glands and their lashes are removed. Care must be taken not to interfere with the lacrimal puncta; only the minimum amount of tissue necessary should be removed. Healing is normally rapid and uneventful, and providing that the incisions are not carried too deeply, scarring and contraction is minimal.

DERANGED MOVEMENTS OF THE EYELIDS

Blepharospasm

This is a tight closure of the eyelids, due to involuntary spasm of the orbicularis muscle, sometimes affecting the associated facial muscles. It is usually produced as a reflex response to trigemial irritation, and may result from foreign bodies, entropion, corneal abrasions, keratitis or acute conjunctivitis. The condition itself may produce a keratitis, sometimes ulcerative, due to the mechanical rubbing of the edge of the lid against the cornea.

Treatment will consist of the removal of the cause and the relief of spasm by the use of anaesthetic preparations. The spasm may be arrested by the injection of procaine into the facial nerve, and all cases should be treated urgently to avoid corneal damage. Those cases that cannot be corrected by simple means may be relieved by the injection of warm sterile liquid paraffin under the skin of the eyelid, to evert it; or by the insertion of sutures, without the removal of any skin, to hold the lid in its normal position. In a few cases a canthotomy may be necessary or this may need to be made permanent as a canthoplasty.

Blepharoptosis or Ptosis

The drooping of the upper lid, may be congenital in origin; or associated with neoplasia of the lid; or with cerebral tumours; or may be traumatic in origin, due to paralysis of the levator muscle resulting from damage to the third cranial nerve.

Congenital ptosis. A congenital drooping of the upper lid is uncommon in the dog, but occasional cases may be met. The degree of ptosis varies from complete closure of the lid, usually unilateral, to a slight asymmetrical appearance of the two lids. Some cases may be associated with blepharophimosis.

Acquired ptosis. A weakness of the levator muscle may be exhibited in the following circumstances.

(1) *Myasthenia gravis*, a disease associated with progressive muscle fatigue, usually commencing in the levator palpebrae and extraocular muscles, has been reported in the dog; this, when it occurs, will exhibit ptosis. The muscular weakness is presumed to be due to a curare-like block at the myoneural junction; this diagnosis may be confirmed by testing the reaction of neostigmine, which abolishes the block. Treatment also employs this drug, given orally, together with atropine to reduce any possible side-effects.

(2) *Muscular dystrophy*, in the form of myotonia atrophica, is occasionally encountered in the dog, particularly the Alsatian breed, associated with progressive atrophy of the temporal and masseter muscles. In such cases, ptosis may be found. No treatment is available.

(3) *Horner's syndrome*—the Claude Bernard-Horner syndrome (p. 131)—is associated with a low-grade ptosis.

(4) *Neurogenic lesions*, affecting the motor paths to the levator muscle, will result in ptosis. Unilateral ptosis, associated with a dilated pupil, may result from some cerebral lesion. Bilateral ptosis, associated with a constricted pupil, may result from mid-brain lesions. Lesions of the peripheral nerves may be associated with local orbital disease.

(5) *Mechanical lesions* of the lids, such as oedema, neoplasia or haematoma, may result in ptosis.

Lagophthalmos

Lagophthalmos or inability to close the eyelids, will result in excessive drying of the cornea, leading to keratitis sicca and corneal ulceration. This condition may be due to injury to the seventh cranial nerve and subsequent paralysis of the orbicularis muscle. Other causes may be prolapse of the nictitans gland, tumours of the lids or of the orbit, exophthalmos, corneal injuries or lacrimal gland infections.

Treatment must be aimed at the removal of the cause when possible and, in cases where the remedy cannot be applied immediately, the cornea must be kept moist by constant bathing and the application of either liquid paraffin or artificial tears. In some cases, it will be found beneficial to suture the lids together and, when this is done, it is best to apply the sutures over a gauze pad.

Closure of the palpebral fissure

This may take the form of a congenital blepharophimosis, or the closure may be traumatic in origin resulting from cicatricial contraction of an eyelid wound. In those cases in which the eyeball is normal underneath, canthoplasty may be performed, thus enlarging the palpebral opening.

INFLAMMATION OF THE EYELIDS

Periorbital dermatitis

Dermatitis of the lids and skin around the eyes is common in the dog and may occur as an extension of specific skin disease affecting the face. Alternatively it may be secondary to a conjunctivitis or other eye disease, or may be largely self-inflicted.

Many lesions affecting the lids are aggravated by rubbing on the ground or with the forelegs. Such irritation is likely to increase tear production, so that the skin easily becomes excoriated and a simple irritation may result in a marked reaction. In addition, the rubbing may produce oedema of the eyelids, or chemosis, and so worsen the condition.

Irritant dermatitis may result from allergy to various plants or, on odd occasions, from certain drugs such as penicillin and atropine, applied to the eye; from chemicals accidently splashed on to the eyelids; or from various soaps and shampoos used in bathing. Mild cases may produce a slight oedematous reaction in the lids only, whilst more severe cases will show all the signs of an erythema or eczema, and, if infected, will become pustular.

Treatment will depend on the removal of the cause, where known, cleansing of the skin with saline and the application of simple dressings, such as zinc oxide ointment, or calamine in either lotion or cream form. Severe cases may require the use of antihistamine or corticosteroid preparations.

Infective dermatitis may result from primary or secondary lesions and may be a manifestation of a systemic condition, or may be purely local in origin. Secondary dermatitis may follow epiphora associated with dacry-ocystitis, conjunctivitis, infection of the nictitans gland, trichiasis or distichiasis, lacrimal duct occlusion, entropion, ectropion, deformities of the eyelids or corneal dermoids. Systemic cases may be associated with either the distemper complex or virus hepatitis (Fig. 89).

Bilateral periorbital ulceration, associated with either a staphylococcal or a streptococcal infection, may be seen in dogs of any breed (Plate III, Fig. 1, facing p. 104). The initial lesions are usually at the mucocutaneous margin of each inner canthus, and the lesions may progress to surround the eye.

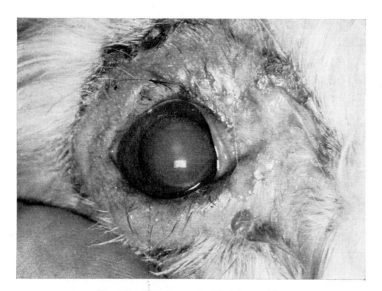

FIG. 89. *Infective periorbital dermatitis.*

On occasion, the palpebral margins and lash follicles may be destroyed, and the labial folds and nasal mucocutaneous margins may also show ulceration. In some cases, the margins of the prepuce or vulva may also be affected.

Treatment will depend on the removal of the cause in those cases that are secondary in origin, and the treatment of any specific systemic disease. Local treatment will consist of cleansing with saline and the application of suitable chemotherapeutic or antibiotic preparations. In some cases, the use of these drugs systemically will be required. Steps must be taken with the use of suitable sedatives to prevent further self-inflicted damage. Some protection may be obtained by bandaging the feet, and in particular the dewclaws. Results in the treatment of periorbital ulceration are often disappointing, but combined antibiotic-corticosteroid-enzyme therapy is often of value.

Parasitic dermatitis of the eyelids may occur as an extension of such disease from the surrounding skin. In the dog, this may take the form of demodectic or sarcoptic mange, or of dermatomycosis, the fungi involved being either trichophyton or microsporum. On rare occasions, either pediculosis or myiasis may effect the eyelids.

The treatment of parasitic affections of the lids will follow the general lines adopted for these diseases. Particular care must be taken, however, that dressings used either do not come in contact with the eyes or, if they do, that they are such that they will not cause harm to the ocular structures. When applying dressings, the eye may be protected with ointment and low-melting point petroleum jelly is particularly useful for this purpose.

Blepharitis

Inflammation of the margins of the eyelids may be associated with specific diseases, dietary deficiencies or local infections. Two types may be recognized, a non-ulcerative or squamous form and an ulcerative form.

Squamous blepharitis exhibits a hyperaemia of the lid margin together with scales that collect around the lashes; there may be some oedema of the margin (Plate III, Fig. 2, facing p. 104). Irritation is usually mild, but self-inflicted trauma may result in thickening of lid margin—tylosis—or dermatitis of the surrounding skin.

Ulcerative blepharitis results in suppuration around the lashes, the discharge forming crusts which tend to cause the eyelids to adhere together (Plate III, Fig. 3, facing p. 104). Irritation is usually marked and photophobia may be present.

Blepharitis may be caused by seborrhoea of the lid margin; by staphylococcal infection, particularly in the ulcerative form, often associated with some debilitating disease; irritation from chemicals or dressings; or may be self-inflicted in the presence of some other irritative eye disease.

Treatment will consist of the cleansing of the lid margins, using saline or olive oil, followed by the application of antibiotic preparations. Antibiotic sensitivity tests may be performed to isolate the causal organism. As the staphylococcus is usually involved, response will normally be obtained from the use of penicillin initially followed by one of the other drugs of this type, such as chloramphenicol or neomycin. Prolonged courses are usually required before a satisfactory response is obtained, and applications must be made frequently so that the contact of the antibiotic is maintained. Corticosteroids may be used to control congestion and irritation, but must be combined with some antibacterial agent. At the same time, attention must be given to any associated conjunctivitis, dermatitis or lacrimal occlusion.

Oedema of the eyelids

Oedematous conditions of the eyelids may be caused by trauma, conjunctivitis, infection or allergy—particularly to pollen, stinging insects and toads.

Treatment will depend on the removal of the cause, and the use of antibiotic and antihistaminic preparations.

Hordeolum

A hordeolum or external stye is an abscess which starts in the sebaceous gland of a lash follicle (Fig. 90). The infective organism usually involved is the staphylococcus. The style is painful and appears as a localized, reddened swelling at the lid margin, in the line of the lashes. A yellow spot appears in a day or two, in the centre of the swelling, and from this a lash is usually seen to project. Oedema of the lid is sometimes present, there is usually lacrimation and sometimes blepharospasm.

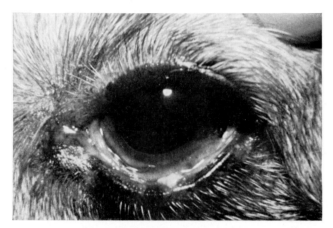

FIG. 90. *Hordeolum (external stye).*

Treatment consists of hot compresses, incision of the abcess when pus presents, and antibiotic ointments. In cases of repeated recurrence, the use of a staphylococcus toxoid or an autogenous vaccine may be considered.

Chalazion

The terms chalazion, internal stye, meibomian cyst and tarsal cyst are usually used synonymously, to signify cystic swellings occurring anywhere in the tarsal plates. More correctly, a meibomian cyst signifies a quiet cystic swelling; an internal stye signifies an inflammatory cystic swelling; and chalazion signifies a hard fibrous swelling (Fig. 91).

A chalazion may be found in either lid, usually the upper, and appears as a small, globular, hard swelling beneath the skin of the lid. It will usually be situated about 3 mm from the lid margin, well separated from the line of the lashes. On eversion of the eyelid, a red discoloration, sometimes with a yellow centre, is seen on the surface of the conjunctiva.

The swelling is due to an accumulation of lymphoid tissue within one of the Meibomian glands, as a result of chronic inflammation following obstruction of the duct of the gland.

Treatment is surgical and consists of making a vertical incision over the centre of the conjunctival aspect of the swelling. The affected part of the lid may be compressed with a meibomian clamp, which both holds the lid everted and, by means of its inner blade, surrounding the cyst, controls the haemorrhage. Following incision, the contents of the cyst are removed with a curette.

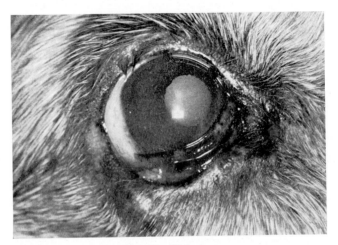

FIG. 91. *Chalazion.*

Cysts of the eyelids

Retention cysts may form in the glands of Moll, and will show as small vesicles on the lid margins. They will usually cause no irritative signs but, if necessary, may be removed by excision of the top of the vesicle.

Sebaceous cysts may occasionally be seen in the skin of the eyelids and may be excised if troublesome. Similarly, cysts may be found forming in the glands of Zeis and these, also, may be excised if necessary.

NEOPLASIA OF THE EYELIDS

Papillomata are common, and may occur as strawberry-like growths on the lid margin, or as the senile type of wart, either on the lid margin or on the skin of the lids (Fig. 92). Melanosis is frequently seen and irritation to the cornea may occur where there is contact between the tumour and the eye. Treatment is by simple excision or cautery.

Melanomata are uncommon and usually benign. Malignant melanoma has been reported. Such tumours are likely to ulcerate and may later affect the orbital tissues, or even the frontal bone.

Carcinomata are not common but may be seen in older animals, and may involve the membrana nictitans. Squamous-celled, basal-celled and adeno-carcinomata have been recorded. Excision is possible in some cases, but

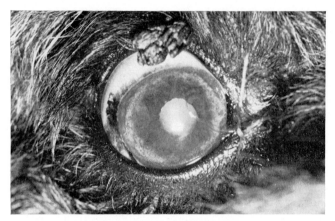

FIG. 92. *Papilloma of the eyelid.*

enucleation of the eye may be necessary. Some value may be attached to the use of β-ray therapy in these cases.

Basal-cell carcinomata are found more commonly than squamous-cell types. Sebaceous adnexal carcinomata of meibomian origin tend to remain localized; other adnexal carcinomata tend to be slowly progressive and invasive, and may result in extensive damage (Fig. 93).

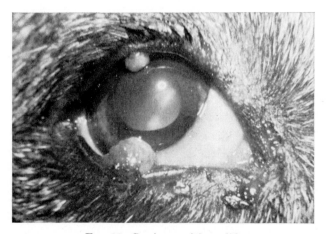

FIG. 93. *Carcinoma of the eyelid.*

THE NICTITATING MEMBRANE

ANATOMY AND PHYSIOLOGY

The nictitating membrane, membrana nictitans, or third eyelid, is situated at the nasal canthus, in the angle of the palpebral fissure, behind the external eyelids. At rest, only the free edge is visible, but it is able to move laterally and diagonally across the eye, to cover most of the surface of the cornea. Movements of the nictitating membrane across the eye are controlled not by muscular activity but by action of the retractor bulbi. Retraction of the eyeball into the orbit causes the membrane to move into a higher position. Similarly, external pressure exerted upon the eyeball, causing the post-orbital pad of fat to be compressed, will result in the membrane sweeping across the eye.

The purpose of the membrane is twofold—to exclude and remove dust and foreign bodies from the cornea, and to assist in the retention of moisture and lubrication.

The nictitating membrane is composed of a T-shaped plate of hyaline cartilage, covered on both surfaces with epithelium. The horizontal member of the plate is parallel with the edge of the membrane, and the plate is slightly concave in order to match the shape of the cornea. The epithelium is continuous with the bulbar conjunctiva on one side, and with the palpebral conjunctiva on the other. Elastic tissue is plentiful within the structure; the free edge often shows complete or partial pigmentation. Many lymphatic nodules are contained within the membrane, and diffuse lymphatic tissue occurs beneath the epithelium.

Surrounding the posterior end of the nictitating membrane, and completely concealed by that structure, is the nictitans gland or Harderian gland. In the dog, this gland, which is pinkish in colour, is small but thick. It is surrounded by fat and attached by connective tissue to the surrounding structures. The Harderian gland is a compound alveolar gland, acting as an accessory to the lacrimal gland. The secretion passes to the conjunctiva through many minute ducts.

Some confusion exists over the terminology used for the glands of the nictitating membrane. In some species, the gland is double, the two parts being connected by an isthmus. The deeper part, which does not exist in the dog, is properly called Harder's gland, or the Harderian gland. It is suggested that the superficial part should be termed the nictitans gland.

DISEASES OF THE NICTITATING MEMBRANE

Injuries. The third eyelid is frequently torn or lacerated in accidents and fights. On occasions, haemorrhage may be profuse and local applications of adrenaline solution may be used to control bleeding. Simple wounds may

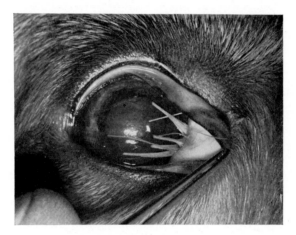

Fig. 94. *Foreign body (grass seed) beneath the nictitating membrane.*

be sutured, using fine, interrupted sutures of silk. At other times, where the laceration is extensive, amputation of the injured areas may be required. Whenever possible, it is advisable to preserve as much as possible of the membrane and the nictitans gland.

Foreign bodies. Foreign material will travel between the membrane and the cornea, resulting in inflammatory changes in the conjunctiva, often with excessive conjunctival oedema, lacrimation and blepharospasm. The most common foreign body encountered in this area is the grass seed (Fig. 94). Examination and detection is sometimes difficult, owing to spasm of the orbicularis muscle, and local anaesthetic applications will probably be required both for examination, and for the removal of the foreign body. Pointed grass seeds will often become embedded in the thickness of the membrane and their removal can, on occasions, prove difficult.

Displacements of the nictitating membrane. Whilst, normally, only the free edge of the membrane is visible, the membrane can become excessively prominent under certain conditions. Similarly, hypertrophy of the membrane may be exhibited. The membrane may be involved and thickened, in consequence, in conjunctival inflammatory reactions or where the nictitans gland is infected. Tumours involving the membrane may cause displacement and, in certain breeds, prolapse of the nictitans gland is not uncommon.

Excessive prominence of the third eyelids will be seen in debilitating disease, due to absorption of the retrobulbar fat and subsequent sinking of the eyeball (Fig. 95). The condition is invariably bilateral and half of each

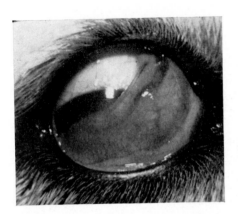

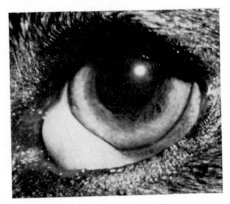

Fig. 95. *Excessive prominence of the nictitating membrane.*

Fig. 96. *Congenital prominence of the nictitating membrane.*

eyeball may be covered by the membrane. Any condition producing generalized emaciation will result in prominence of the membrane. This may be particularly noted in association with virus diseases and with cestode infestations. Similarly, the membrane may become more prominent in any inflammatory condition affecting the conjunctiva or cornea.

Congenital prominence is seen in such breeds as the Boston Terrier and Boxer (Fig. 96), often associated with exophthalmos, and the membrane may be trimmed to improve appearance. Total removal may lead to chronic conjunctivitis, due to destruction of conjunctiva and the formation of a sac. Again, a condition is encountered from time to time where the free edge of the membrane is folded over upon itself, producing a thickened edge that may cause considerable irritation (Fig. 97). In such cases, trimming of the folded edge is indicated.

Hypertrophy of the membrane may follow conjunctivitis, and may affect one or both eyes. Such a condition is seen particularly in the Labrador

PLATE III

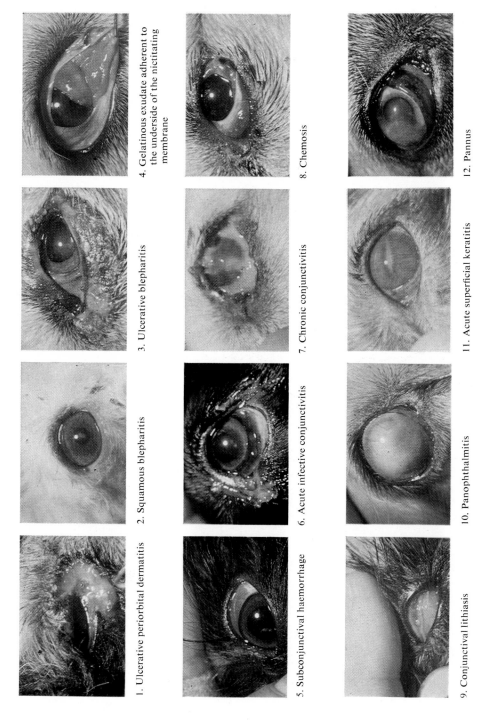

1. Ulcerative periorbital dermatitis

2. Squamous blepharitis

3. Ulcerative blepharitis

4. Gelatinous exudate adherent to the underside of the nictitating membrane

5. Subconjunctival haemorrhage

6. Acute infective conjunctivitis

7. Chronic conjunctivitis

8. Chemosis

9. Conjunctival lithiasis

10. Panophthalmitis

11. Acute superficial keratitis

12. Pannus

Retriever and the Great Dane, and may cause considerable discomfort and necessitate the removal of part or all of the membrana.

Tumours of the third eyelid, such as epitheliomata, endotheliomata, carcinomata and sarcomata have been recorded (Fig. 98). In such cases, particularly where malignancy is suspected or proven, total removal of the third eyelid at the earliest opportunity is indicated.

Prolapse of the nictitans gland occurs particularly in the Bulldog, Bull Terrier and Boston Terrier, but may be observed in any breed (Fig. 99). The

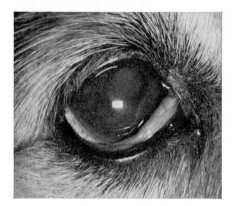

FIG. 97. *Folding of the edge of the nictitating membrane.*

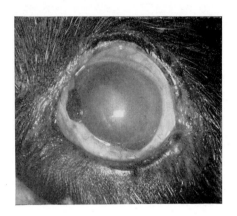

FIG. 98. *Epithelioma of the nictitating membrane.*

prolapse is caused by swelling and hypertrophy of the gland, or adenitis, the gland becoming oedematous and projecting beyond the edge of the third eyelid as a round, red mass. Treatment is by excision of the gland.

Inflammatory conditions. The conjunctiva covering the third eyelid will, of course, be involved in any conjunctival inflammatory state, and will be treated along with the generalized conjunctivitis. The diffuse lymphatic tissue occurring beneath the epithelium of the membrane, on the underside of this structure, is frequently involved in inflammatory changes, particularly of the follicular type. These changes may be mild, often associated with excessive lacrimation, but little other visible sign (Fig. 100); in other cases, acute inflammatory reactions, sometimes associated with a dense, gelatinous exudation adherent to the underside of the membrana, may be exhibited (Plate III, Fig. 4, facing p. 104).

Adenitis of the nictitans gland is often associated with excessive tear production. In such cases, the gland may be enlarged and erythematous, with a follicular conjunctivitis in the overlying conjunctiva. Histologically, such glands may show hypertrophy and hyperplasia of the secretory tissues, cyst formation and interstitial oedema. Overflow of tears results from increased tear production and obstruction to the puncta by the swollen

8

gland pushing the membrana forward. Some cases show a reddish-brown discoloration on the face, forming a tear streak, where pigment in the tears has become discoloured on exposure to light (Fig. 101). Such a condition may be treated by cauterization or surgical excision of the nictitans gland.

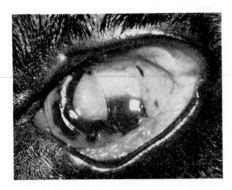

Fig. 99. *Prolapse of the nictitans gland.*

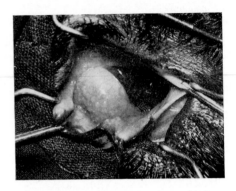

Fig. 100. *Adenitis of the nictitans gland.*

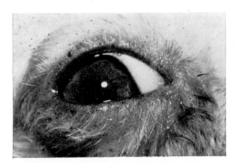

Fig. 101. *Tear streak resulting from adenitis of the nictitans gland.*

Cauterization of the membrana

Inflammatory changes involving the lymphatic tissue may be treated by phenol cauterization. Under anaesthesia, the membrana is withdrawn and the underside exposed. The cornea is best protected during cauterization by the liberal application of low-melting point petroleum jelly. The under surface of the membrana is dried with swabs of cotton wool. A small piece of cotton wool is then wound on to a carrier or probe, tightened, and dipped into a solution of pure carbolic acid (phenol B.P.) Excess solution is removed by gently squeezing the swab in gauze, then the surface of the membrana is rubbed all over with the phenol. The area of application must be carefully controlled and evidence of adequate application is afforded by the white appearance of the treated tissue. The area is then once again dried with cotton wool swabs, covered with petroleum jelly and allowed to return to its normal position. No after-treatment is required, but the process may need to be repeated in 7 to 14 days.

Plasma cell infiltration of the membrana

Plasma cell infiltration of the nictitating membrane, of unknown aetiology, has been reported from Germany in the Alsatian and Dobermann. Changes take place in the edge of the membrane, consisting of raised rolls of tissue, grey-red to grey-blue in colour, 3 to 4 mm thick. No acute inflammatory reaction is exhibited and the cornea is not affected. Histological examination reveals large numbers of plasma cells and a picture similar to that of conjunctival plasmoma in man. In many cases, rapid improvement follows topical or subconjunctival corticosteroid therapy; in advanced cases, some trimming of the membrana may be required. There is some tendency to relapse after a considerable period.

Removal of the nictitans gland

Whenever possible, it is advisable to remove as little as possible of the membrana. Total removal leads to the formation of a sac in the conjunctiva at the medial canthus, and this, in turn, may result in interference with the

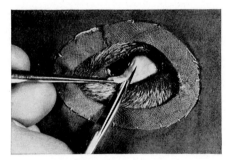

FIG. 102. *Trimming of the edge of the nictitating membrane.*

lacrimal drainage system, and a chronic conjunctivitis. In cases where only the free edge of the membrana is involved in some abnormal condition, it is advisable to remove only this portion, and to leave the bulk of the membrana intact. Similarly, the nictitans gland may be removed without destroying the overlying membrane.

Any surgical interference with the nictitating membrane is usually accompanied by considerable haemorrhage and this may, to a certain extent, be controlled by injection of adrenaline solution into the surrounding conjunctiva preoperatively. The blood supply to both the membrana and the nictitans gland is quite extensive, and some difficulty may be experienced in controlling the resultant haemorrhage.

Removal of the nictitans gland is accomplished by first everting the membrana, and maintaining this position by the application of rat-tooth clip forceps. An incision is made over the gland, through the conjunctiva, and the gland may be dissected away with scissors. Haemorrhage may be controlled by the use of adrenaline drops or by packing the area with thin strips of gauze soaked in adrenaline solution. Such an application for a few minutes is normally satisfactory, but on some occasions, it may be necessary to apply electrocautery to the bleeding points. In many cases, it is possible to clamp the vessels of the nictitans gland with haemostats, before they are incised. In all cases, it is important to control haemorrhage before the retraction of the remaining tissue into the fornix makes control sometimes extremely difficult.

Areas of thickened or prominent edge of the membrana may be trimmed by grasping with toothed forceps and removing the unwanted tissue with fine, curved scissors. Only as much as is necessary should be removed, and haemorrhage may be controlled in the suggested manner (Fig. 102).

8
THE ORBIT

ANATOMY

The orbit is the cavity within the skull which encloses the eyeball, together with the muscles, vessels and nerves associated with the eye. It is continuous with the temporal fossa behind. This bony cavity separates the eyeball from the cranial cavity, and serves to protect the eye, whilst suspending it by muscles and membranes. The muscles, in addition, provide the eye with movement, whereas the membranes as well as offering additional protection to the eye, restrict its movements. The various blood vessels and nerves associated with the eye gain entrance to the orbit by means of various foramina.

In the dog, five of the facial and cranial bones—the frontal, lacrimal, sphenoid, palatine and zygomatic—help to form the outline of the orbit; a sixth bone, the maxillary, is also concerned, external to the periorbita and the true orbit (Fig. 103).

In order to permit a wide gape for the seizing of prey, and to permit the jaw to close firmly, the orbit is not closed by a complete bony ring in the carnivorous animals. The bony ring ends, on one side, at the zygomatic process of the frontal bone, and on the other side, at the frontal process of the zygomatic bone. The gap is bridged by a strong fibrous ligament—the orbital ligament—which allows complete closure of the orbit without undue rigidity.

The shape of the orbit, in the dog, is to some extent influenced by the type of head present in the breed concerned—dolichocephalic or long-headed, mesaticephalic or medium-headed, or brachycephalic, or short-headed.

Orbital foramina

Orbital fissure—entrance for the third, fourth and sixth nerves, the ophthalmic division of the fifth, and the orbital vein.

Optic foramen—entrance for the second (optic) nerve and the internal ophthalmic artery.

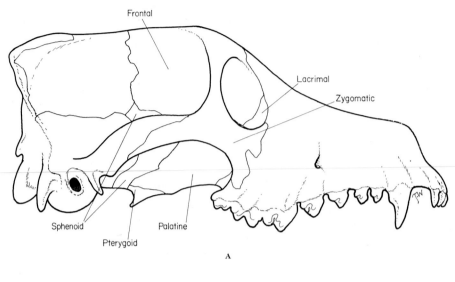

Frontal

Lacrimal

Zygomatic

Sphenoid   Palatine

Pterygoid

A

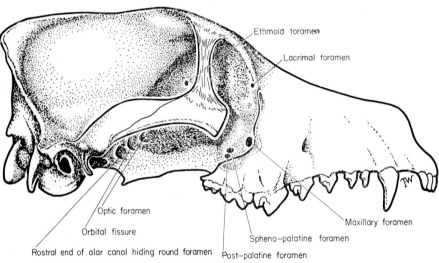

Ethmoid foramen

Lacrimal foramen

Optic foramen

Orbital fissure

Maxillary foramen

Spheno-palatine foramen

Rostral end of alar canal hiding round foramen   Post-palatine foramen

B

FIG. 103. *The orbital region.* A *the bones,* B *the foramina (note that part of the zygomatic bone has been removed for clarity).*

Round foramen—entrance for the internal maxillary artery and the maxillary nerve.

Ovale foramen—entrance for the mandibular division of the fifth nerve and the middle meningeal artery.

Ethmoid foramen—entrance for the ethmoidal artery and vein.

Maxillary foramen—entrance to the infraorbital canal, giving passage to the intraorbital nerve, artery and vein. At the anterior end of the canal is the infraorbital foramen.

Sphenopalatine foramen—passage for the sphenopalatine vessels and nerve.

Postpalatine foramen—passage for the palatine artery and vein.

Alar foramen—the posterior entrance to the alar canal, which forms, with the canal for the maxillary nerve from the cranium, the round foramen. The alar canal carries the internal maxillary artery.

Lacrimal fossa—a shallow fossa in the lacrimal bone which holds the lacrimal sac. From this passes the nasolacrimal canal into the ventral nasal meatus.

Periorbital tissues

The majority of the eyeball and its attached muscles is surrounded by a dense connective tissue membrane, Tenon's capsule. Some blood vessels are present in this membrane. Superior to this, continuous with the periosteum of the facial bones at the orbital rim, and with the dura of the optic nerve at the optic foramen, is a membrane composed of loose collagenous bundles, connective tissue cells and elastic fibres, the periorbita. The periorbita lines the bony wall of the orbit and completely surrounds the orbital contents. It is loosely attached to the bones wherever the surface is smooth, but is firmly attached at the suture lines, the foramina, the lacrimal fossa and the entrance to the optic nerve.

The periorbita thus separates the orbital contents from the bony wall of the orbit and from the infraorbital and temporal areas. At those places where the various vessels and nerves supplying the ocular tissues penetrate the periorbita, this membrane forms a sheath around them. At the anterior aspects, it is firmly attached to the orbital margin and merges with the eyelids. Deposits of fat occur around the periorbita where it is not firmly connected to bone. All the posterior tissues of the eye are included within the cone formed by the periorbita, but the lacrimal gland lies outside this cone.

The extraocular muscles

The eye is suspended within the orbit by the conjunctiva, the palpebral ligaments and the extraocular muscles.

The muscles of the eyeball are seven in number—the four recti, or straight muscles, the two oblique muscles, and the retractor (Fig. 104).

The four recti muscles, which are flat, and, in the average dog, of approximately 9 mm width, are designated according to their position—lateral, medial, superior and inferior. They have their origin from around the orbital apex at the optic foramen and diverge as they pass forward to the eyeball, to be inserted in the sclera, with thin flat tendons, in front of the equator. The superior and inferior recti muscles rotate the eyeball about a transverse axis, moving the cornea upwards and downwards. The medial and lateral recti rotate the eyeball about a vertical axis, turning the cornea inwards and outwards. The superior, inferior and medial recti are innervated by the third cranial nerve; the lateral by the sixth nerve.

The superior oblique muscle arises at the orbital apex, from between the superior and medial recti, passes obliquely across, and is inserted between

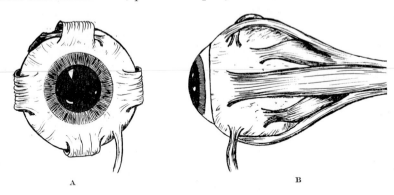

A   B

FIG. 104. *The extraocular muscles.*

the tendons of the lateral and superior recti. It is innervated by the fourth cranial nerve. The inferior oblique muscle has its origin near the lacrimal fossa, curves around, and is inserted into the sclera near the insertion of the lateral rectus muscle. It is innervated by the third cranial nerve. The oblique muscles rotate the eyeball about a longitudinal axis.

The retractor bulbi muscle, which withdraws the eyeball into the orbit, originates at the rear orbital wall and is usually divided into four parts; of these, two insert on either side of the superior rectus, and two on either side of the inferior rectus, into the posterior half of the globe. Innervation is by the sixth cranial nerve.

The levator palpebrae muscle, the action of which is to raise the upper eyelid, is a long, thin band, lying above the superior rectus, which originates between the superior rectus and the superior oblique and is inserted, by an expanded tendon, between the fibres of the orbicularis oculi.

Associated structures

As the orbital floor is not completely bony, several vessels and nerves, not serving the orbital structures, are separated from the orbital contents only by the periorbita. These include the sphenopalatine nerve, ganglion and artery, the infraorbital nerve and artery, the deep facial vein, and the zygomatic gland.

The zygomatic or dorsal buccal, salivary gland, lies against the internal surface of the anterior part of the zygomatic arch, and is in contact with the periorbita on its superior aspect. The deep facial vein lies between the gland and the periorbita, and below the gland is separated from the maxillary nerve and artery by fat.

Also situated in the orbital region are the lacrimal and orbital or nictitans glands.

CONGENITAL DEFORMITIES

Congenital deformities of the skull are uncommon in the dog, but are occasionally encountered, especially in the Pekingese. In such cases, the orbit may be involved, resulting in an under-development and consequent protrusion of the eye or squint. Some cases of under-development of the orbit may be associated with congenital hydrocephalus, where the orbit is shallow, or with microphthalmos. In cases where the foramina are constricted, retinal atrophy may be present. Enlargement of the orbit may be associated with buphthalmos.

INJURIES TO THE ORBIT

The orbit may be involved in injuries received from street accidents, kicks, blows, dog fights and gunshot wounds. The degree of injury will range from simple contusion or abrasion of the skin in the orbital region to fractures of the orbital ring.

Fractures of the orbital ring, which may be associated with fractures of other bones of the skull, may be simple or compound. Depressed fractures may cause an exophthalmos and fractures involving the floor of the orbit may result in optic atrophy, due to injury to or pressure on the optic nerve.

Treatment of simple wounds is straightforward and should follow the pattern of careful toilet, debridement and dry dressings. Chemosis and conjunctivitis may follow, and a careful search must be made for damage to other ocular structures. Subcutaneous emphysema is a common complication and any infection should be treated with antibiotics.

Simple fractures are best left alone, but any depression should be corrected if possible by elevation. In compound fractures, loose fragments of bone should be removed and steps taken to prevent infection.

Intraorbital haemorrhage rarely occurs in the dog as a spontaneous complication of some haemorrhagic disease, but may be seen following trauma, usually associated with fracture of the orbital walls. Cases may also occur following retrobulbar injections or with strangulation. Haemorrhage of any degree will produce a proptosis, the degree varying with the severity of the haemorrhage. If the haemorrhage occurs within the muscle cone, the eye will be forced forwards. If the haemorrhage occurs outside the muscle cone, the eye will be deviated to the side opposite to that of the haemorrhage. In severe cases, there may be evidence of pain or loss of vision due to pressure on the optic nerve. In most cases, the haematoma will be cleared spontaneously within a few weeks.

ORBITAL FOREIGN BODIES

Wild barley awns are a cause of abscess formation in the postorbital fat, and will enter this area either through the pharynx or, more commonly, from beneath the nictitating membrane. The abscess will burst either through the supraorbital fossa, or through the conjunctiva or externally through the eyelid. Irreparable damage may be caused to the eyeball or the optic nerve, and treatment must depend on antibiotic therapy and drainage of the abscess at the earliest possible moment.

Other orbital foreign bodies are rare, but, on occasion, needles may pass through the hard palate or through the pharynx and may lodge in the supraorbital fossa. Shot and airgun pellets are sometimes found in the orbit. Although located by radiography, such foreign bodies may prove difficult or impossible to remove.

DISEASES OF THE ORBIT

Diseases of the orbital structures, other than the eyeball itself, are not common in the dog. Those that do occur are associated with the structures around the orbit or with disease of bone and soft tissues. Any swelling that may develop in the surrounding soft tissues is likely to push the eyeball forwards, causing an exophthalmos, where the eyeball alone protrudes in a forward direction, or a proptosis, where the eyelids and orbital contents are also involved.

Orbital neoplasia

Many types of tumours have been recorded involving the orbit and eyeball, but they are comparatively uncommon. Those most commonly seen would appear to be melanotic sarcomata, originating in the uveal tract, and epitheliomata, originating in the conjunctiva. Metastasis appears to be rapid in both these types. Fibromata, papillomata, sarcomata, osteosarcomata and carcinomata have also been recorded. Lipomata occasionally occur between the extrinsic muscles.

Clinical signs are likely to be proptosis or exophthalmos, with displacement away from the tumour site, squint, venous congestion of the lids, conjunctiva and retina, pain, prominence of the nictitating membrane, exposure keratitis, dilatation or eccentricity of the pupil, and loss of vision due to pressure on the optic nerve. Diagnosis is often difficult until the case is advanced. In those cases where there is no evidence of involvement of the orbital bones, or of metastasis, exenteration of the orbit offers the only hope of preserving life.

Orbital cellulitis

Acute inflammation of the orbital tissues, not uncommon in the dog, must always be regarded as serious. Vision may be damaged by pressure on the optic nerve or through exposure keratitis, septic absorption will always take place because of the rigid orbital wall, and the risk of the spread of infection either to the ocular contents or to the meninges is always present. Most cases arise either from postorbital foreign bodies, or from septic foci in teeth or accessory nasal sinuses.

The signs exhibited are invariably acute, and include oedema of the eyelids, chemosis, proptosis, fever and immobility of the eyeball. Oedema of the surrounding tissues is usually present, together with marked pain, particularly noticeable on jaw opening. Fluctuation may be noticed above the upper lid. Corneal ulceration may result from exposure.

The treatment consists of full doses of systemic antibiotics, combined with local heat treatment by hot bathings. Any fluctuating swelling should be incised and drainage may sometimes be secured by extraction of the last upper molar tooth.

Eosinophilic myositis

Eosinophilic myositis presents signs that are, in many ways, similar to those exhibited in cases of orbital cellulitis. This disease, of unknown aetiology, is characterized by an increase in the eosinophil count, and by symmetrical swelling of the masseter, temporal and pterygoid muscles. There is usually some degree of exophthalmos, due to pressure from the enlarged muscles on the retrobulbar tissues, chemosis, and hypertrophy of the nictitating membrane. The jaw may normally be opened to its full extent, but this procedure usually proves painful. In some cases, however, the jaw cannot be opened to its fullest extent, even under general anaesthesia.

The acute phase of the disease, which may involve one or both eyes, normally lasts for 10 to 21 days. Repetitive attacks are likely to occur, some cases may recover spontaneously, and others may prove fatal.

Eosinophilic myositis would appear to be confined to the Alsatian and Weimaraner. Little is known regarding the treatment of this condition, but the corticosteroids and ACTH appear to be of value. Recovered cases are likely to exhibit atrophy of the affected muscles, and atrophy of the peri-orbital tissues may result in enophthalmos.

9

THE CONJUNCTIVA

ANATOMY AND PHYSIOLOGY

The anterior surface of the eyeball, as far as the limbus, and the inner surface of the eyelids, are lined with a thin, transparent mucous membrane, the conjunctiva. This membrane folds upon itself to line the two structures, forming a fornix. At the lid margin, the conjunctiva is continuous with the skin of the eyelid, and, at the limbus, it is continuous with the corneal epithelium. The conjunctiva aids the suspension of the eye within the orbit and acts as a barrier to foreign bodies.

The conjunctiva is divisible into two parts, the bulbar conjunctiva which covers the eyeball and the palpebral conjunctiva which lines the eyelids. The ducts from the lacrimal and auxiliary glands enter at the fornix, where the two parts fold over against one another, and pour their secretions into the palpebral area.

Except for the area immediately posterior to the limbus, the bulbar conjunctiva is loosely attached, whereas the palpebral portion is firmly anchored to the tarsal plates of the eyelids. Behind the limbal attachment of the conjunctiva is the attachment of Tenon's capsule to the globe.

The conjunctiva consists of an epithelium and a connective tissue substantia propria. The epithelium has a stratified squamous character at the lid margin, and is thin over the tarsal plates. The epithelium of the bulbar conjunctiva is somewhat thicker, again becoming of a stratified squamous nature at the limbus. Some goblet cells are present in the palpebral conjunctiva, but the bulbar portion is much less glandular.

The substantia is composed of a thin layer of fine connective tissue fibres, firmly united with the epithelium in the tarsal area, whereas it is of a more elastic nature in the bulbar portion.

Deep and superficial blood vessels—derived from the anterior ciliary vessels—occur in the conjunctiva, more being present in the palpebral area than in the bulbar area, and in greater profusion at the fornix than at the limbus. Numerous lymphatics also occur, and the membrane is innervated by branches from the ciliary nerves.

The conjunctiva passes over the nictitating membrane, covers the caruncle and passes into the lacrimal canals. In the area of the caruncle and nictitating membrane, it possesses numerous small accessory lacrimal glands, and the deeper layers contain pigment cells.

CONJUNCTIVAL INJURIES

Lacerations of the conjunctiva usually heal rapidly. If extensive, they may be sutured by direct sutures of thin silk.

Chemical burns are uncommon in the dog, but occasional cases of lime burning will be met, usually associated with coexistent injury to the cornea. Acid burns tend not to penetrate the conjunctiva, because of the precipitation of the epithelial proteins, whereas alkalis penetrate more deeply and produce greater fibrosis by virtue of their dissolving action on proteins.

Treatment of chemical burns should consist of immediate and very thorough irrigation with water or saline, and the neutralization of any embedded lime particles with 5% ammonium tartrate solution. Antibiotic applications should be used to control secondary infection, and cortisone to reduce the inflammatory exudate and limit the fibrosis. Atropine and anaesthetic preparations may be used to control pain and irritation.

Extensive burns affecting the conjunctiva may result in a symblepharon, the adhesion of the eyelid to the eyeball. Such injuries are thus best treated by the use of an amniotic membrane graft, placed over the injured area and sutured to the adjacent cornea. Division of the adhesions associated with a symblepharon is often followed by fresh adhesions, and in an attempt to prevent this, the raw surfaces may be covered, as far as is possible, with conjunctival flaps or with grafts taken from buccal mucous membrane.

DISTURBANCES OF THE CONJUNCTIVAL CIRCULATION

Hyperaemia of the conjunctival vessels may result from local irritation, such as foreign bodies, or may be associated with rubbing of the eye on the ground or with the paw, or with the early stages of systemic virus infection. A passive hyperaemia may be caused by an obstruction to venous outflow. When associated with a discharge, a conjunctivitis will be present.

Conjunctival hyperaemia must be distinguished from ciliary or circumcorneal hyperaemia. Ciliary hyperaemia will be apparent only near the limbus, and, as the vessels are deeper, they will be less readily distinguished, and may appear only as red flush. Conjunctival hyperaemia will be apparent over the whole of the bulbar and palpebral conjunctiva and the vessels will be more easily apparent.

In conjunctival hyperaemia, the vessels are engorged, especially in the palpebral area. In the bulbar area, the vessels are markedly noticeable against the white sclera. Treatment consists of removing the cause of the irritation.

Subconjunctival haemorrhage is uncommon in the dog, but, when it does occur, is invariably associated with trauma. No irritative signs are shown, but the haemorrhage is apparent as a red patch against the white sclera (Plate III, Fig. 5, facing p. 104). Absorption takes place in the course of a week or so, and no local treatment is necessary. Some cases may be associated with cranial fracture.

Conjunctival oedema or chemosis, although common in the cat, is seen less often in the dog. It occurs particularly when a conjunctival foreign body, such as a grass seed, is present, and may also be apparent after other irritations or allergy. On occasion, it may be so marked that the cornea is completely concealed beneath oedematous folds of conjunctiva, which may protrude between the lids (Plate III, Fig. 8, facing p. 104). Chemosis is likely to be marked in any case where there is orbital obstruction to venous drainage.

CONJUNCTIVITIS

Inflammatory changes within the conjunctiva are, without doubt, the commonest affliction of the eye in the dog. Several types have been recognized in the past, and these have been classified according to the gross signs present. Thus, acute and chronic, catarrhal and purulent types, and combinations of these, have been described. Today, a more logical classification, based on aetiology, is more commonly used.

Acute infective conjunctivitis

Most organisms responsible for conjunctivitis produce, in the initial stages, a simple catarrhal form, but depending on the severity of the infection, an acute infective conjunctivitis may be catarrhal, mucopurulent, or purulent (Plate III, Fig. 6, facing p. 104). Such a bacterial conjunctivitis may be caused by a wide variety of organisms, and although the normal and abnormal flora of the conjunctival sacs in the dog has been little studied, several bacteria, at least, are known to be responsible.

Those organisms that have been isolated as responsible for conjunctival inflammation include coagulase-positive staphylococci, haemolytic streptococci, *Pseudomonas pyocyanea*, *E. coli*, *Moraxella lacunatus* and *Neisseria flava* II. Cultures from the normal conjunctiva will prove sterile in a large proportion of cases, whereas nonpathogenic staphylococci, streptococci and diphtheroids will be found in other instances. Many cases of clinical acute conjunctivitis will also yield sterile cultures. In some instances, fungal infections may be involved and cultures on special media may be required.

Acute infective conjunctivitis may arise as a primary infection, or may be secondary to some generalized bacterial or virus infection. Infection may enter the conjunctiva from direct trauma; or from injury caused by such conditions as entropion, ectropion or trichiasis; or from foreign bodies.

Clinical signs. Acute conjunctivitis is characterized, initially, by increased lacrimation, the tears at first being clear and watery, and later mucoid or mucopurulent in nature. The conjunctiva is congested, appearing pinkish or red, sometimes swollen and sometimes oedematous. Chemosis may be present in very acute cases. Some photophobia may be present, but irritation, except in the presence of a foreign body, is not particularly marked. Marked photophobia or blepharospasm may indicate the onset of a keratitis. If the discharge becomes purulent, there is a tendency for this to exude from the eye and mat the lashes, causing the eyelids to adhere together.

The blood vessels that are engorged in conjunctivitis are the surface vessels derived from the palpebral branches of the ophthalmic artery. These vessels, which are arranged in spirals and folds, must be distinguished from the anterior ciliary vessels, which run in parallel straight lines. The latter vessels, which are visible when engorged, forming a circumcorneal ring, are rarely involved in conjunctivitis, but will become conspicuous in ciliary infections, interstitial keratitis and glaucoma.

Diagnosis. Swabs may be taken from the conjunctival sac to determine the causal organisms, making a smear of the exudate. By this method, many types of bacteria may be demonstrated, and it is sometimes impossible to determine the predominant organism. More accurate information may be gathered by the use of conjunctival scrapings, using a small platinum spatula, and performing what is virtually a limited biopsy of the conjunctival cells. By this method, only one or two organisms may be found to predominate. The results of treatment may also be evaluated to a certain extent by scrapings, particularly in low-grade infections, in which the presence of bacteria and leucocytes may indicate the desirability of a change of therapy.

On some occasions, swabs taken from apparent cases of infective conjunctivitis prove sterile. In such cases, this may be due to the selection of unsuitable media, and the possibility of fungal infections should be considered. In all cases where conjunctival swabs are employed, plating on media should be carried out before the lysozyme in the conjunctival secretions may have effect on any bacteria that may be present.

Treatment. The treatment of acute conjunctivitis is aimed at clearing the condition quickly, in order to prevent the spread of the infection to other structures of the eye. Young animals, particularly, should be examined carefully for the presence of virus infection.

Whenever possible, any exciting cause should be removed, followed by flushing of the conjunctival sac with saline. Friction from gauze or cotton wool should be avoided as far as possible, as well as the spread of any infection from one eye to the other if the condition is unilateral. Foreign bodies, which are often lodged under the nictitating membrane, can be removed under local or general anaesthesia.

In simple cases, the application of a soothing ophthalmic ointment will be sufficient; in other cases, antibiotics, in ointment or drop form, will prove necessary. Under ideal conditions, the appropriate antibiotic or sulphonamide is selected after culture and sensitivity tests, but in most cases, an agent such as chloramphenicol or neomycin, will be given empirically.

In cases where there is marked irritation, topical anaesthetic preparations may be used, particularly where blepharospasm is present. It must be remembered that cocaine may have a damaging effect on the superficial epithelium of the cornea and on the substantia propria, and lignocaine hydrochloride is probably the agent of choice. Corticosteroids, preferably prednisolone or betamethasone, used as ointment or drops, may be of value in suppressing the exudate phase of the inflammation. The effect is suppressive, not curative, and other therapeutic agents must be used simultaneously. In no instance should corticosteroids be used in acute bacterial infections unless chemotherapeutic drugs are included.

Chronic conjunctivitis

Chronic forms of conjunctivitis may occur from infection with resistant organisms, or more often from constant reinfection from infected foci in the surrounding skin, the Meibomian glands or the lacrimal ducts. Other cases may be associated with interstitial keratitis or keratitis sicca, and, in most cases, there is occlusion of the lacrimal drainage, causing stagnation of infected material in the lower fornix.

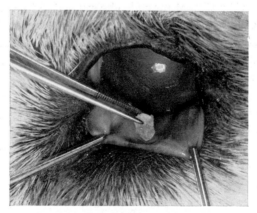

FIG. 105. *Copper sulphate cauterization.*

A viscid and tenacious discharge is usually present, together with some hyperaemia and, in many cases, periorbital dermatitis due to the overflow of secretions (Plate III, Fig. 7, facing p. 104).

Chronic conjunctival infections are often resistant to treatment and may, due to the tissue changes that have taken place, prove very difficult to manage. The essential first step is to exclude any underlying cause, such as entropion, ectropion, or lacrimal obstruction, and any possible foci of reinfection. Antibiotics should be given to control any infection and, thereafter, astringents such as zinc sulphate or silver proteinate may be employed. Copper sulphate crystal cautery (Fig. 105), on both the palpebral and bulbar conjunctiva, followed by irrigation, has been recommended; or irrigation with 1 to 2% silver nitrate solution, followed by saline neutralization, may be helpful.

Follicular conjunctivitis

Follicular conjunctivitis is characterized by enlargement of the follicles on the inner surface of the membrana nictitans, and, occasionally, on the palpebral and bulbar conjunctiva (Fig. 106). This may lead to a hypertrophic inflammation of the conjunctiva, in which subconjunctival lymphatic proliferation is associated with the formation of lymphatic follicles and vascular papillae. This, in turn, may result ultimately in pannus and eventually lead to corneal ulceration.

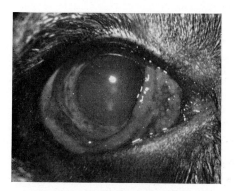
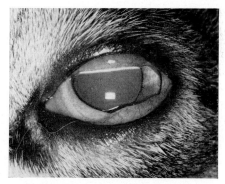

Fig. 106. *Follicular conjunctivitis.*   Fig. 107. *Allergic conjunctivitis.*

The medical treatment of follicular conjunctivitis consists of the use of zinc sulphate or a light copper sulphate cautery, followed by corticosteroids. Beta-ray therapy has also been used with success. For treatment of the condition affecting the membrana nictitans, cauterizing the inner surface of the membrane with copper sulphate, followed by irrigations and the application of copper sulphate ointment subsequently, has been suggested. On other occasions, the follicles may be wiped off vigorously with gauze,

9

again followed by copper sulphate ointment; or phenol cautery may be used; or, the follicles may be dissected away with fine scissors. In refractory cases, the membrana may be removed.

Allergic conjunctivitis

Non-specific allergies of the conjunctiva are common in spring and summer months, usually associated with allergy to pollens or grasses. Occasional cases of allergy are met due to sensitivity to various drugs that have been instilled into the eyes.

The irritative signs are usually acute, with engorgement and oedema, profuse lacrimation and intense irritation (Fig. 107). If the epiphora is marked, the skin of the lower lid may become eczematous.

Although the responsible allergens can rarely be determined, rapid response usually follows the application of antihistaminic preparations. The corticosteroids may also be of value.

Parasitic conjunctivitis

The parasite, *Thelazia californiensis*, has been reported as occurring in the dog in the State of California, Oregon, Arizona and Nevada in the U.S.A. The life cycle is not known.

Worms of this species, white in colour, may occur in the conjunctival sacs, lacrimal ducts, under the nictitating membrane, or on the cornea. Signs of ocular irritation—lacrimation, conjunctivitis, photophobia and eyelid oedema—may occur. The worms may be seen as they move across the cornea and may be removed with forceps, under topical anaesthesia, or inactivated with 1% silver nitrate solution and flushed from the conjunctiva with saline.

Thelazia callipaeda has been reported in the dog from India and China.

PTERYGIUM

A pterygium is a degenerative condition of the conjunctiva, rare in the dog, probably arising from a peripheral degeneration of the cornea with fragmentation of Bowman's membrane and the underlying corneal stroma. The stroma of the affected part then becomes replaced by vascular connective tissue from the limbus, and over this, conjunctival epithelium replaces the corneal epithelium.

The pterygium appears as a flattened triangular-shaped prominence of thickened conjunctiva, sometimes white in colour and sometimes vascular. It lies parallel to the palpebral fissure, with its base situated in conjunctival tissue and its rounded apical head growing towards the corneal centre. Pterygia are more commonly seen on the nasal side, and their bases may extend as far as the inner canthus (Fig. 108).

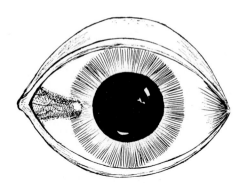

FIG. 108. *Pterygium.*

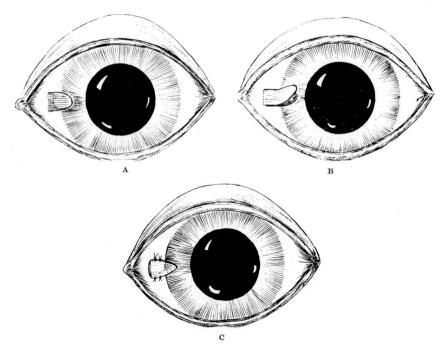

FIG. 109. *D'Ombrain's operation (stages A, B, and C).*

Pterygia normally produce no irritation unless particularly large, and only if they encroach on the pupillary region will sight be affected. If the inward growth of a pterygium does impair vision, attempts at removal may be made, but recurrence after simple excision is usual. For this reason D'Ombrain's operation (Fig. 109) is normally practised in human surgery.

This involves incision of all the diseased tissue beneath the conjunctival epithelium, posteriorly from the apex, leaving a perilimbal strip of sclera 4 mm wide, denuded of epithelial covering. This method allows the corneal epithelium to completely cover the denuded area of the cornea before the growth of conjunctival epithelium is able to reach the limbus.

D'OMBRAIN'S OPERATION

By holding the pterygium at the limbus with a hook, and the adjacent conjunctiva with forceps, a horizontal incision is made with scissors in the conjunctiva on either side of the pterygium. The incision is carried down as far as the sclera, and is continued from the limbus towards the canthus. This area is then undermined with scissors as far as the surface of the sclera.

After shaving the apex of the pterygium from the cornea, using a Tookes' corneal dissector, together with a thin layer of corneal tissue, the apex of the pterygium is held taut vertically and the diseased subepithelial tissue is dissected away with scissors from under the conjunctival epithelium. Lastly the epithelium, from over the head, neck and part of the body of the pterygium, is excised so as to leave an area of sclera, approximately 4 mm wide, exposed. The remaining edges of the conjunctival incisions are sutured with silk sutures.

DERMOID

A dermoid is an embryological defect, consisting of some of the structures of normal skin. It is composed of fibrous tissue, hair follicles, sebaceous glands, sweat glands and fat, and usually has hairs projecting from its surface. Usually oval in shape and with a convex surface, it is embedded in the conjunctiva, usually at the corneal margin, sometimes extending well on to the surface of the cornea (Fig. 110). Other cases may be purely conjunctival in location. Although a somewhat uncommon defect, seen in many different breeds of dog, it is perhaps most commonly encountered in the Alsatian. A dermoid will usually cause considerable irritation, with a resulting conjunctivitis and pannus formation, and occasionally interstitial keratitis.

Treatment consists of dissecting the dermoid away from the conjunctiva (Fig. 111). Great care is necessary when removing that part embedded in

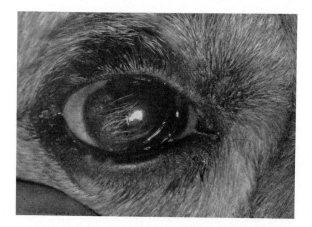

FIG. 110. *Dermoid.*

the cornea, as penetration of the cornea must be avoided. On the other hand, the dissection must be carried deeply enough to remove all hair follicles. The wound may be repaired by undermining the adjacent conjunctiva and fashioning a conjunctival flap to cover the defect. This is sutured in position with fine silk sutures, and if continued on the corneal surface, will remain adhered to the cornea when the sutures are removed. Such a small adherent flap will cause no trouble, and with the removal of the dermoid and the irritating hair growth, the signs of discomfort will abate.

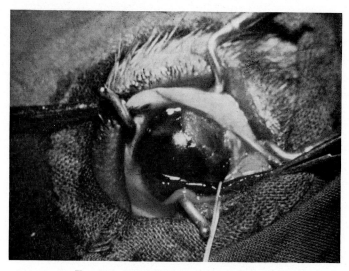

FIG. 111. *Operation for removal of dermoid.*

CONJUNCTIVAL CYSTS AND TUMOURS

Concretions (or lithiasis) occasionally occur in the palpebral conjunctiva. They usually appear in the upper lid, in older animals, and show as small

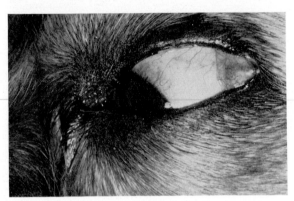

FIG. 112. *Conjunctival cyst.*

white or yellowish spots when the lid is everted (Plate III, Fig. 9, facing p. 104). Occasionally they become calcareous and, if they project beyond the epithelial surface, may lead to irritative signs. Treatment consists of the incision of the epithelium over the concretion and the evacuation of the contents.

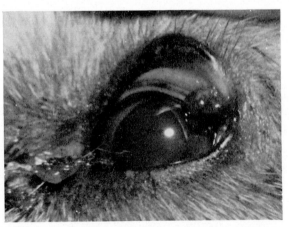

FIG. 113. *Conjunctival adenoma.*

Conjunctival cysts are uncommon, but occasionally appear as typical cystic swellings on the bulbar conjunctiva (Fig. 112). Treatment consists of the removal of the overlying cyst wall.

Conjunctival tumours are rare. Those most commonly encountered include lipomata, adenomata (Fig. 113), papillomata, fibromata and lymphomata. If desired, they may be excised, although the underlying cornea, if this is involved, will remain opaque. They are usually found in the limbal area.

Malignant tumours, in the form of melanomata or epitheliomata, although very uncommon, may occasionally be seen in the limbal area, and are likely to spread to the intraocular structures. Removal is rarely possible, and the desirability of enucleation of the eye before the onset of metastasis must be considered.

OPHTHALMIA NEONATORUM

Occasionally, new-born puppies are seen with a purulent condition of one or both eyes. This infection sometimes causes the eyes to become open at an earlier age than is usual and at other times the opening is delayed. In such cases, the lids appear markedly swollen, and a purulent exudate may escape from a small separation in the closed lids. Left untreated, most cases will result in corneal involvement, with resultant scar formation, or panophthalmitis and phthisis bulbi.

Treatment consists of forcible lid separation at the earliest opportunity, using blunt-pointed scissors, cleansing and release of the exudate behind the lids, and topical antibiotic treatment.

10

THE EYEBALL

DESCRIPTION

The eyeball, situated in the orbit, is essentially spherical, and lies suspended by means of the extraocular muscles, and periorbital membranes, in fat that largely fills the orbital cavity. It is light-proof, except for the anterior transparent surface, and all of it, except this part, is separated by only a few millimetres from the orbital walls.

The angle at which the two eyes are set in the orbits varies considerably with different breeds, and the angle between the visual axes varies from 20 to 50°. The shape of the palpebral orifice, also, shows considerable variation in various breeds, and may be round, elliptical or oblique. Again, the size of the eyeball shows great variation. The cornea is slightly more curved than the rest of the globe, so that the antero-posterior length is normally slightly greater than the other measurements. The average antero-posterior measurement is approximately 24 mm, whilst the vertical and horizontal diameters are approximately 22 mm although there is a wide range on either side of these figures. The average weight of the eyeball is 4 to 8 g.

The eyeball consists, in the main, of three separate concentric layers, containing a transparent jelly, the vitreous body. The outermost layer, the sclera, is wholly protective in nature, whilst the innermost layer, the retina, is the light-sensitive membrane. Between these two is the nutrient layer, consisting of the choroid, and the intraocular muscles, ciliary body and iris, that control the movements of the pupil and accommodation.

CONGENITAL ABNORMALITIES

Anophthalmos, or complete absence of the eyes, is rare. Some parts of the eyes are usually present, or the orbit may contain fibro-fatty tissue (Fig. 114).

Cryptophthalmos, a condition in which the chiasma, corpora quadrigemina and optic nerve are normal, but in which the eyeball is either absent or seen as a small, pigmented cyst, may be either unilateral or bilateral. It has been recorded in the Old English Sheepdog and the Fox Terrier.

Microphthalmos (Fig. 115), a congenital condition in which the optic cleft fails to fuse, so that the eye remains small and may be cystic. It may be

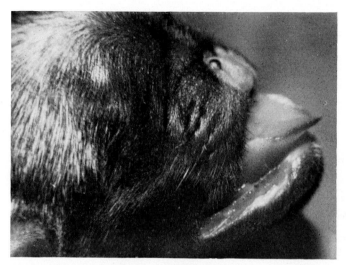

Fig. 114. *Anophthalmos.*

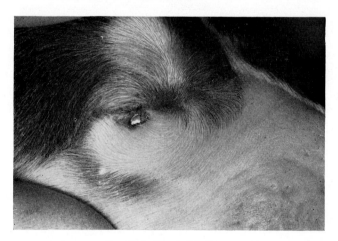

Fig. 115. *Microphthalmos.*

unilateral or bilateral, usually the former, and may be associated with strabismus, aniridia or nystagmus. It is a relatively common abnormality, seen most often in the Pekingese. Some cases may be hereditary in origin, and others may be associated with albinism or heterochromia. Possible hereditary types occur in the Collie, Great Dane and Shetland Sheepdog, usually homozygous merles and harlequins, and in dappled Dachshunds.

Buphthalmos, in which there is excess fluid in the anterior chamber, and bulging of the eyeball, is caused by errors at the filtration angle and excessive thinness of the cornea or sclera.

Megalophthalmos, a rare condition, is one in which the eye is excessively large, without the presence of excess fluid.

Exophthalmos, or protrusion of the eyeball, is normal, to a degree, in such breeds as the Pekingese, Japanese Spaniel, Pug and the King Charles Spaniel.

Enophthalmos, or sinking of the eyeball, is usually found with microphthalmos.

Strabismus, or squint, is seen particularly in the Pekingese and Boston Terrier, and may be convergent or divergent (Fig. 116).

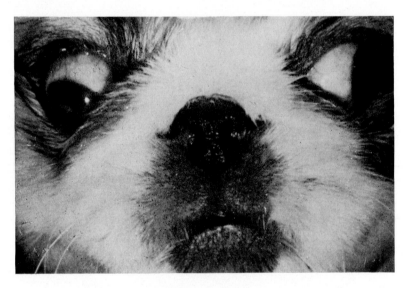

FIG. 116. *Strabismus.*

EXOPHTHALMOS

Acquired anterior displacement of the eyeball may be due to fracture of the orbital ring, to postorbital abscess or haematoma formation, to orbital neoplasia, to tumours involving the oculomotor muscles, or to strangulation, and will be exhibited in the early stages of eosinophilic myositis and some cases of lymphatic leucosis.

A case of anteriovenous fistula in the orbit has been described, probably congenital in origin, in which exophthalmos was a prominent feature. In this case, the chief diagnostic sign proved to be a continuous murmur over the site of the fistula.

Blastomycosis affecting the bones of the orbit, and cryptococcosis of the optic nerve, have been reported as causes of exophthalmos.

Endocrine exophthalmos, associated with hyperthyroidism, may occur in a slight degree in some dogs, but never to that extent associated with Grave's disease in the human. Mild hyperthyroidism may occur in those breeds which normally present some degree of exophthalmos, such as the Pekingese and French Bulldog, where thyroid hyperplasia may be regarded as normal.

ENOPHTHALMOS

Any debilitating disease, resulting in absorption of the postorbital fat, will produce an acquired enophthalmos. Other possible causes are eosinophilic myositis, in the later stages, when the muscles have atrophied; atrophic myositis; irritation of the cornea causing reflex contraction of the retractor bulbi muscle; or trauma to cranial nerves resulting in atrophy of the temporal, masseter or pterygoid muscles.

Enophthalmos, associated with unilateral miosis, narrowing of the palpebral orifice, relaxation of the membrana and ptosis, together with vasomotor and trophic disturbances, has been reported in the dog. Such a syndrome—the Claude Bernard-Horner syndrome—is a cervical hypo-sympathicotonia, caused by lesions paralysing the cervical sympathetic portion of the autonomic nervous system and lesions of the hypothalamus.

Such lesions may be produced by infections, neoplasia or trauma, either affecting the pupillo-dilating centre in the hypothalamus, or interfering with the neuron pathways. It has been suggested that the use of 4% cocaine chlorhydrate and 1:1000 adrenaline as collyria, applied two or three times at 2-minute intervals and observed three times at 15-minute intervals is a useful diagnostic aid. Mydriasis with cocaine indicates a lesion of the first neuron (central neuron); no reaction to either cocaine or adrenaline indicates a lesion of the second neuron (medullo-ganglionic neuron); mydriasis with adrenaline and not cocaine indicates a lesion of the third neuron (peripheral neuron).

The Claude Bernard-Horner syndrome has been noted in cases of tumours affecting the anterior mediastinum, cervical cord lesions, and tumours of the hypothalamus. Similarly, the syndrome has been reported as occurring in cases of hemifacial spasm (Roberts & Vainisi), associated with irritative lesions of the facial nerve in the area of the middle ear, affecting the sympathetic enervation to the eye.

STRABISMUS

Strabismus or squint denotes a deviation of the globe from its proper axis, due either to excessive slackness or excessive tension in opposing extraocular muscles (Fig. 116). Squint in the dog is usually congenital but other cases may be seen associated with virus infections, perforation of the ear tympanum, cerebral disorders, morphine and alkaloid poisoning, and rabies. Strabismus may be either vertical, horizontal or oblique, the commonest type in the dog being horizontal. Most commonly, this is convergent, although the Pekingese and the Pug will more often exhibit a divergent squint. It may be either unilateral or bilateral. Congenital convergent strabismus, affecting one or both eyes, has been reported in the Collie, often associated with other ocular defects.

Congenital strabismus may be treated surgically, but the results are often disappointing. In this operation, the conjunctiva and Tenon's capsule are incised, a strabismus hook is inserted beneath the appropriate muscle, and the muscle is divided close to its sclerotic insertion. In convergent strabismus, the internal rectus muscle is severed, whereas in divergent strabismus, the external rectus muscle is divided.

THE DISEASED OR INJURED EYEBALL

Endophthalmitis and panophthalmitis

Suppuration of the contents of the eyeball (endophthalmitis), or suppuration involving all the coats of the eyeball as well as the contents (panophthalmitis) (Plate III, Fig. 10, facing p. 104) may be endogenous in origin, the infection entering via the blood stream; or exogenous, due to penetrating wounds of the eye, corneal ulceration, shotgun wounds, burns, neoplasia, or intraocular foreign bodies. It may, on rare occasions, follow intraocular surgery.

A possible sequel to infection within the eyeball is meningitis as an extension of the infection through the ophthalmic veins. One case has been reported (Rogers & Elder) of a panophthalmitis and purulent leptomeningitis, associated with an aerogenic *Pasteurella multocida*; in this case, spread was thought to be from the orbital cavity to the meninges via the optic nerve.

On rare occasions, panophthalmitis may be associated with spontaneous rupture of the eyeball. Treatment is by excision of the eyeball and the control of infection with antibiotics.

Trauma of the eyeball

Injury to the eyeball is not common, due to its protection within the orbit, but may at times be seen associated with shotgun wounds, blows and kicks. The eyeball may be injured by compression or fracture of the orbital ring. Subconjunctival haemorrhage may be caused by contusion. Rupture of the eyeball will occasionally occur from direct blows.

Simple wounds are treated by saline cleansing and antibiotic dressings. Extensive injury may lead to panophthalmitis. Burns and scalds are occasionally seen from boiling fat and water, lime, acids and disinfectants.

Prolapse of the eyeball

Prolapse of the eyeball is most commonly seen in the brachycephalic breeds, due to pressure on the supraorbital fossa during fights or street accidents, but may be seen in other breeds when the orbital ligament is ruptured. The condition is usually unilateral, and the prolapsed eye will quickly become inflamed and congested as the eyelids close behind it. Desiccation of the cornea follows, together with oedema of the conjunctiva, and sometimes haematoma formation. In some cases, the eyeball may be perforated or ruptured.

Replacement of the eye must be performed immediately, for the dry cornea soon becomes ulcerated and the prolapse of the eyeball may cause damage to the optic nerve.

An attempt must be made to replace the eye, firstly through the palpebral orifice and then into the orbit, lubricating it well first, and then drawing the eyelids over the prolapse. A canthotomy may have to be performed, or sutures may be inserted through the eyelids to apply traction. Once replaced, any tendency to prolapse again can be counteracted by suturing the lids together over a gauze pad; by suturing the membrana nictitans to the skin above the upper lid; by forming a conjunctival flap; or by a temporary lateral tarsorrhaphy. The retrobulbar injection of a corticosteroid preparation will reduce oedema in the orbital tissues and assist in the maintenance of the globe in its correct position. Intraocular tension changes may be prevented by the administration of a carbonic anhydrase inhibitor.

In any case in which, for one reason or another, it is not possible to replace the eye immediately, the cornea must be kept constantly moist using saline or, preferably, artificial tears; and further self-mutilation by the patient must be avoided.

Nystagmus

An involuntary to-and-fro oscillation of the eyes—nystagmus—is invariably bilateral and is normally regular, although very occasionally, irregular nystagmus may be presented. In most cases, the rhythmical movement is horizontal, very rarely vertical. Nystagmus may be either ocular or labyrinthine. The ocular form usually exhibits a pendular, regular and equal movement of the eyes, whereas labyrinthine nystagmus displays jerky, slow and fast, movements.

Ocular nystagmus, which may be congenital in origin, or may result from disease conditions where fixation is difficult or impossible, is essentially an exaggeration of the normal fixation movements. In some cases, even when the exciting cause is eliminated, the condition may persist as an established habit.

Labyrinthine nystagmus normally follows lesions or stimulation of the labyrinth, cerebellum or associated areas of the brain-stem. It may be seen in cases of brain tumour, apoplexy, otitis media or encephalitis.

Spontaneous nystagmus, following vestibular nerve damage, is horizontal, and tends to be controlled within a relatively short time, by central compensation. Positional nystagmus, which may be elicited by inclining the head backwards or laterally, is associated with lesions of the eighth nerve and posterior fossa. Fixating nystagmus, associated with cerebellar lesions, is exhibited with a quick phase towards the periphery when the eyes are deviated laterally and fixed on an object; this is most marked on deviation towards the side where the lesion is situated.

A horizontal nystagmus, of very fine amplitude and great frequency, may occur as a congenital defect in the Collie. It is exhibited at the age of three to four weeks and tends to disappear with age.

EXCISION OF THE EYEBALL

Removal of the eyeball is indicated in the following cases:
(1) Large ocular wounds, particularly if the lens is displaced.
(2) Excessive loss of vitreous or extensive prolapse of the uveal tract.
(3) The presence of a large foreign body within the eye.
(4) Panophthalmitis.
(5) Hydrophthalmos that cannot be corrected surgically.
(6) Some cases of ocular or orbital neoplasia.
(7) Some cases of prolapse of the eye.

The eye may be removed by evisceration enucleation, or extirpation.

Evisceration of the eyeball

This is undertaken usually when an artificial eye is contemplated. In this operation, the cornea and the whole contents of the eyeball are removed, leaving the sclera, conjunctiva and musculature intact. This operation should not be performed when any intraocular tumour is present, where the sclera may be involved. It may be indicated in cases of panophthalmitis, where division of the optic nerve sheath may result in a fatal meningitis. Following evisceration, the remaining tissues partly fill the orbital cavity after healing has taken place.

Operation. An incision is made at the limbus and the cornea removed, allowing the intraocular fluids to escape. The uvea is then removed by a curette, taking care that all uveal tissue is cleansed from the inner scleral surface and the cavity packed with adrenaline-soaked gauze. If no artificial eye is to be inserted later, the eyelids are then trimmed and sutured together leaving a gap at the nasal canthus through which the gauze strip is brought out. The gauze is removed after 24 hours, and irrigation of the cavity can be carried out through the opening if required. If an artificial eye is to be used later, the eyelids are sutured together without the preliminary trimming.

Enucleation

This is carried out when it is desired to remove the conjunctiva and the eyeball, but leave intact most of the oculomotor muscles and the whole of both eyelids. It is indicated for eyes which are blind and painful, or for any intraocular tumours.

Operation. The bulbar conjunctiva is incised at the limbus for the whole of the circumference of the eyeball, the connective tissue between sclera and conjunctiva broken down, Tenon's capsule is incised, and the extrinsic muscles divided close to their insertions. The eyeball is then withdrawn as far as possible, and the retractor bulbi and optic nerve severed as far back as may be, using curved enucleation scissors. The globe is lifted from the socket and any remaining muscular and vascular attachments are incised. Haemorrhage from the central artery of the nerve, which is usually severe, is controlled by forceps pressure and packing, and the lids are trimmed and sutured.

Subconjunctival ablation

A method that may be preferred is that in which the conjunctiva is left intact to form a partition directly behind the sutured lids, to help in preventing a sunken socket. In this technique, the incision is made at the limbus, and the conjunctiva reflected from the sclera. The muscles are severed at their scleral insertions, and the optic nerve exposed and severed. The eyeball is then removed and the edges of the conjunctiva are drawn together with Lembert catgut sutures. The third eyelid is removed, the conjunctiva repaired and the lids trimmed and sutured.

Extirpation

Otherwise known as exenteration, this is the operation of choice where there is suppuration within the eyeball, for in this case the eyeball is removed in one piece together with the entire orbital contents. Both eyelids are removed completely and the whole of the orbital contents extirpated, including all of the conjunctiva and the oculomotor muscles.

Operation. The eyelids are first sutured together. The skin surrounding the eyelids is then incised between the insertion of the eyelids and the orbital ring. The eyelids are dissected away, leaving the conjunctiva intact. A spatula is then passed round the orbital cavity to break down any connections. The eyeball is drawn forward, the optic nerve and the muscles are severed with long curved scissors, and the eye is removed. When possible, the optic nerve is clamped with curved artery forceps before it is cut, and plugging is not usually necessary. Lastly, the skin is sutured and a pressure pad of gauze sutured to the skin over the wound. A disadvantage of this technique is the subsequent sinking, which leaves a large and rather noticeable cavity.

ARTIFICIAL EYES

Artificial globes, made either of glass, vulcanite or plastic, either solid or with a hollow posterior surface, can be used in the dog, but may be resented, and may be increasingly difficult to remove and replace.

Insertion must not be attempted for at least 3 or 4 months after excision of the eye, to allow the cavity to reach its maximum contraction. At first, they should be left in position for only an hour or so, gradually increasing the time until they are worn permanently. They must be removed for cleansing, however, at regular intervals.

INTRASCLERAL PLASTIC PROSTHESIS

The use of an intrascleral prosthesis (which has been described by H. D. Simpson) is suitable in cases of panophthalmitis, hydrophthalmos and in most cases of traumatic loss of eye. It is not suitable where the blood supply to the globe is severed, where the extraocular muscles are ruptured deep in the orbit or where infection is coexistent with excessive scleral trauma.

The prosthesis, which has a standard corneal diameter of 15 mm is covered in its posterior part with a tantalum mesh, moulded into the plastic at its free borders. It is sterilized chemically.

Operation. A canthotomy is performed and the eyeball is eviscerated, taking care that all uveal tissue is removed. The bulbar conjunctiva is then separated from the sclera at the limbus to allow these two structures to be sutured to the prosthesis separately. The sclera is incised posteriorly, to allow the insertion of the prosthesis, which is placed in an introducer and orientated. The blades of the introducer are placed within the sclera and the prosthesis is deposited in the cavity. Fixation is maintained by interrupted catgut sutures, approximating first the sclera to the tantalum mesh, and then the conjunctiva.

The operation is followed by extensive oedema for 7 to 10 days, and by a marked conjunctivitis for 21 to 28 days. Following this operation, there is an increased susceptibility to conjunctivitis which needs constant supervision. Neglect of the conjunctivitis will lead to separation of the conjunctiva from the tantalum, and the prosthesis may be extruded if this separation is not dealt with promptly and adequately.

The same operation has also been described by D. G. Lewis, who advises that the operation be done in two stages and suggests that this will avoid most of the undesirable reactions and discomfort. An optically clear methyl methacrylate lens is used, moulded over a painted iris and pupil. The prosthesis, which is made of the same plastic, has tantalum type 50 mesh drawn over it and secured by a tantalum wire circlip.

The first operation consists of the removal of the cornea and uveal tract, following which the cavity is treated with antibiotics and the lids are sutured. At the second operation, which is performed 6 to 10 days later, the sutures are removed, the conjunctiva is dissected from the sclera at the limbus and the prosthesis is inserted. The conjunctival edge is then sutured to the edge of the mesh at the rim of the prosthesis, and the outer canthus is sutured for one week.

INTRAOCULAR FOREIGN BODIES

Foreign bodies within the eye of the dog are rare, the most commonly encountered being airgun pellets.

Many foreign materials, such as glass, wood and metallic alloys, are normally well tolerated by the eye, and are best left in situ. On the other hand, iron particles may cause siderosis and later degenerative changes within the eye.

Foreign material within the eye may often be localized by using a loupe or an ophthalmoscope. Radio-opaque objects may be located by orbital X-ray examination. The exact location of such bodies, however, may prove difficult, although accurate positioning of a guide post and geometric calculation may allow the position of the object to be plotted, enabling an assessment to be made of the position of the object within or outside the eyeball.

Foreign bodies anterior to the lens may be removed through a limbal incision into the anterior chamber. The extraction of a foreign body from the posterior segment of the eye is hazardous, and in nearly all cases it would prove preferable to leave the object in position.

11

THE LACRIMAL APPARATUS

ANATOMY

The lacrimal apparatus consists of a lacrimal gland, the ducts of which open into the dorso-lateral fornix (the secretory portion); and a drainage system, from the conjunctiva to the nasal cavity (the excretory portion),

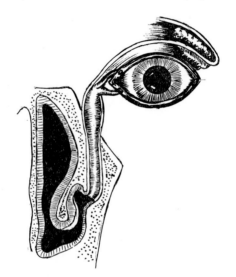

Fig. 117. *The lacrimal apparatus. (After Magrane)*

comprising two canaliculi, a lacrimal sac and a nasolacrimal duct (Fig. 117). Only a small part of the tear fluid produced finds its way to the nasolacrimal duct, most being evaporated from the surface of the cornea.

The lacrimal gland is situated on the dorso-lateral aspect of the eyeball, within the periorbital tissues, in the region of the orbital ligament. It is light red in colour, with rounded edges, and slightly lobulated, shaped to blend with the surrounding tissues.

This gland is normally approximately 12·5 mm wide and 15·0 mm deep (Prince), and is flat. It is a tubuloracemose gland, composed of serous and mucus acini and a connective tissue network forming lobules. Fifteen to twenty lacrimal ducts open from the gland into the conjunctival sac at the outer part of the upper fornix.

The lacrimal puncta form the two openings into the canaliculi. Two puncta are present, one in each lid, and are situated near the medial commisure of the eyelids. They are set away from the lid margin, and are directed slightly backwards towards the eyeball. Each punctum is normally slit-like, but occasionally appears circular or oval. The two puncta may be of different size, and may be pigmented.

The lacrimal canaliculi run from the puncta, away from the lid margin, converging upon one another to join on entering the lacrimal sac.

The lacrimal sac lies in the lacrimal fossa in the medial orbital wall. It is very underdeveloped in the dog and represents merely a slight dilatation of the junction of the two canaliculi and the nasolacrimal duct.

The nasolacrimal duct lies in the bony nasolacrimal canal, between the maxilla and lacrimal bone, and normally opens into the nasal cavity. It may be interrupted along its length.

LACRIMATION

The eye is bathed in a fluid that is the composite product of many glands —tears from the lacrimal gland, mucus from the conjunctival glands, oil from the tarsal glands, and mucus and serum from the nictitans gland. The exact composition of this film—the precorneal film—is unknown, but it serves to moisten, lubricate, clean, protect and disinfect the cornea. The cornea and conjunctiva are dependent for their normality on the adequate production, distribution and drainage of the tears.

In composition, tears are similar to blood plasma, but contain enough protein to lower the surface tension sufficiently to allow thorough wetting of the epithelial surfaces. This results in an even film being spread over the tissues. The secretion of tears is a continuous process except during sleep. In addition, tears have a bactericidal effect from the contained enzyme, lysozyme. This specific enzyme is mucolytic, and in physiological concentration is capable of dissolving many common airborne bacteria. The level of lysozyme in the tears of the dog would appear to be considerably lower than that in man.

The tears flow over the cornea to the lower fornix, helped by the movements of the eyelids and nictitating membrane, towards the lacrimal puncta. Overflow over the lower lid margin is prevented by the meibomian secretion. The entrance of the tears into the puncta is probably effected by capillary action, and their flow through the canaliculi into the nasolacrimal duct is probably brought about by negative pressure. The siphoning action of the lacrimal sac and nasolacrimal duct is controlled by contraction of the orbicularis muscle, which in turn forces the tears along the nasolacrimal duct into the nasal cavity. Gravity and capillary action are also probably involved in the flow of tears from eye to nose.

The rate of secretion

The rate of lacrimation may be measured by Schirmer's test in which a strip of sterile filter paper, normally measuring 4×30 mm (Schirmer's papers), is bent and inserted under the lower lid so that approximately 5 mm is in direct contact with the conjunctiva, the remainder of the strip protruding forward from the eye.

The rate at which the paper becomes moistened is measured. A normal reading would be between 5 and 35 mm/min, with an average of 20 mm/min (Rubin), less than 9 mm/min probably indicating a deficient tear secretion. As each unit of paper absorbs a given amount of fluid, the rate of secretion may be calculated by noting the total amount of paper wetted in a given time. This figure may be recorded in μl/min, and a range of 2·8 to 40·0 μl/min, with an average figure of 10·5 would be considered normal (Roberts & Erickson). Under-secretion might give figures between 2·4 and 7·0 μl/min, average 4·4.

The tears that are obtained in a Schirmer test are those produced by irritation of the conjunctiva, and may not be the same as normal tears. The wide variation that may be expected in normal eyes shows that, in the first place, small amounts are capable of efficient lubrication and, in the second, that large amounts are removable by evaporation when required. In any case, a reading of less than 2·5 μl/min may be taken as indicative of a deficiency, but readings are of little value unless correlated with the clinical condition, or unless a pair of eyes is compared.

Excessive secretion produces tears with a low protein content; in under-secretion the protein content is greatly increased.

DISEASES OF THE LACRIMAL APPARATUS

LACRIMAL GLAND

Over-secretion

Excessive production of tears—*excessive lacrimation*—results from trigeminal stimulation by inflammatory conditions. Possible causes, therefore, are allergies, irritative conditions such as trichiasis, distichiasis, entropion, ectropion, nasal fold stimulation, or nictitans gland adenitis. The correction of these various conditions is dealt with in other chapters.

Chronic *epiphora*, or overflow of tears, in the dog, is most commonly associated with disturbances in the drainage system, rather than to over-secretion.

An excessive secretion of tears or epiphora does not appear to affect vision, but does cause unsightly staining on the face in the tear streak (Fig. 101). This, in turn, may lead to excoriation, depilation and eczematous conditions.

Under-secretion

A lacrimal deficiency may follow motor lesions of the facial nerve, sensory lesions of the trigeminal nerve, diseases of the lacrimal gland, or mechanical obstruction of the ductules resulting from conjunctival infection or scarring.

A lacrimal deficiency may produce a degenerative keratoconjunctivitis —keratitis sicca; or, in other circumstances, chronic undersecretion may follow a chronic keratoconjunctivitis, where there is scarring of the conjunctival openings of the various glands concerned in the production of the precorneal film. In either case, the result may be blindness from pannus formation, corneal keratinization and pigment migration.

In cases of chronic under-secretion occlusion of the lacrimal puncta helps to conserve the limited tear supply. Such occlusion, of all four puncta if both eyes are affected, may be accomplished by diathermy.

Dacryo-adenitis

Inflammation of the lacrimal gland is uncommon in the dog.

Acute dacryo-adenitis will occasionally be seen, sometimes with abscess formation, associated with infection of other glands in the head region with pyogenic bacteria. Such cases exhibit pain and tenderness, with a yellow discoloration over the gland. Treatment is by hot compresses, antibiotics and the evacuation of any abscess.

Chronic dacryo-adenitis is rare but may, very occasionally, be associated with granuloma formation. It can be felt as a hard mass in the area of the lacrimal gland. Lacrimal gland tumours are rare, but adenoma and adeno-carcinoma are the types most likely to be found.

Mikulicz's syndrome—enlargement of the lacrimal and salivary glands, due to replacement of tissue with lymph cells—has been described in the dog, in a case of leukaemic lymphosarcomatosis.

Xerophthalmia. Dryness of the cornea that results from failure of the lacrimal gland to secrete tears is relatively common in the dog. The condition may be temporary or permanent, and possible causes are virus infections, injuries to the lacrimal gland, senile changes in the gland, damage to the fifth or seventh cranial nerves, cerebral disorders, or, most commonly, chronic keratoconjunctivitis. In such cases the cornea is lustreless, later being dry, shrunken and insensitive, with pigment migration and vascularization. The conjunctiva is thickened, granular and shrunken, and a tenacious conjunctival secretion is apparent. This is the condition of keratitis sicca.

Early cases of desiccation may sometimes be detected by the installation of 1% Rose bengal, when the affected areas are dyed bright red. Treatment depends on the removal of the cause where possible, the frequent use of saline lotions and artificial tears, stimulation of the lacrimal gland where this is still functional, by parasympathomimetic drugs, and occlusion of the puncta to conserve any remaining secretions. Transplantation of the parotid salivary duct into the conjunctival sac promises to be a useful technique in the treatment of xerophthalmia.

LACRIMAL PUNCTA AND CANALICULI

Congenital closure

Congenital closure of the puncta—agenesis—is most commonly observed in the Toy and Miniature Poodle and the Cocker Spaniel, although cases

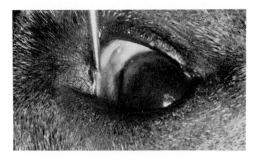

FIG. 119. *Location of punctum using a dilator.*

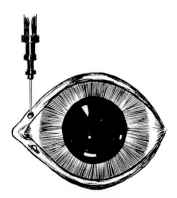

FIG. 120. *Ballooning of occluded punctum by irrigation.*

may be seen in many other breeds. One or both eyes may be affected, and either the upper or lower or both puncta may be closed, although the condition is most likely to be found in the upper punctum.

In some cases, the punctum and canaliculus are absent; in others, the punctum is covered by a membrane, the canaliculus being patent. The presenting signs will be those of epiphora and the presence of a tear streak, although, in many cases, compensatory mechanisms resulting in a lowered tear production mean that no epiphora is evident. Closure of the upper punctum only is unlikely to result in any overflow of tears.

The patency of the punctum can be investigated by the insertion of a Nettleship's canaliculus dilator (Fig. 118), followed by a probe or cannula. Recognition of the punctum although sometimes easy, particularly when

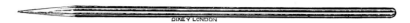

FIG. 118. *Nettleship's canaliculus dilator.*

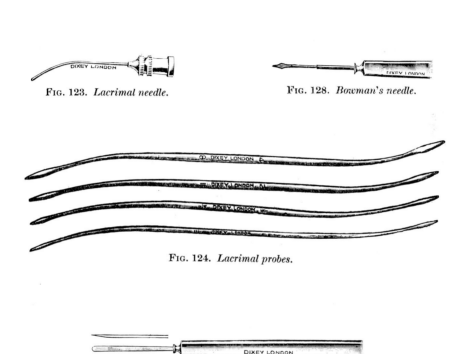

FIG. 123. *Lacrimal needle.*

FIG. 128. *Bowman's needle.*

FIG. 124. *Lacrimal probes.*

FIG. 127. *Eye spud.*

the edge is pigmented, may prove difficult if there is a tendency for it to be enveloped in a small fold of conjunctiva. Location of the punctum, in difficult cases, is best accomplished with a dilator (Fig. 119). When only one punctum is covered by a membrane this may be demonstrated by inserting a cannula into the patent punctum and the injection of a little saline, with the resultant ballooning of the membrane over the opposite punctum (Fig. 120).

If the lacrimal punctum and canaliculus is absent, no treatment is possible. If one only is covered by a membrane, this may be cut away after ballooning as described above. Such a procedure should be followed by enlargement of the punctum with a dilator, and daily irrigation until the patency is ensured.

Acquired closure

Occlusion may occur as the result of damage to the puncta due to trauma, foreign bodies, scarring due to burns or caustics, catarrhal thickening due to infections, or scarring resulting from chronic infections.

Imperfect drainage may also be caused by eversion of the punctum in cases of congenital or acquired entropion or ectropion, or by senility causing relaxation of the lower lid. In the Toy and Miniature Poodle, in which chronic epiphora is often a problem, the cause may be found either in malpositioning of the puncta or in pressure from the nictitans gland upon the puncta or canaliculi.

All cases of puncta occlusion will be accompanied by some degree of epiphora, sometimes combined with a discharge resulting from a canaliculitis or secondary conjunctivitis. The patency of the puncta can be investigated by the use of fluorescein, or by the use of a dilator and subsequent irrigation. The installation of fluorescein is not entirely reliable as a test for patency; in a small proportion of dogs the nasal portion of the nasolacrimal canal is interrupted, so that fluids enter the pharynx instead of appearing at the nostril. Cases will be seen of dogs without epiphora, where dyes fail to pass down the nostril—in such cases, irrigation can be used to demonstrate patency, unless some obstruction is present.

Treatment. Where the punctum is too small or narrow, it may be enlarged with a dilator, or the canaliculus may be opened with a knife for a few

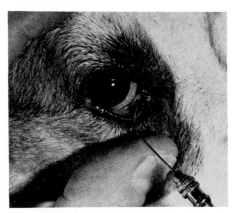

FIG. 121. *Irrigation of the canaliculus with saline.*

millimetres from the punctum. Such openings will usually remain patent. Simple blockage can be cleared by passing a fine strand of nylon through the punctum and down the canaliculus; or the canal may be irrigated with normal saline introduced through a lacrimal needle (Fig. 121).

Where eversion of the punctum results from ectropion, an operation to correct the latter may be sufficient to correct the epiphora. If the ectropion operation fails to produce adequate apposition of globe to punctum, or if the punctum is malpositioned, the 'three-snip operation' may be employed (Fig. 122). In this, the first cut with scissors opens the canaliculus, the second cuts vertically downwards between punctum and conjunctiva, and the third is placed obliquely, to remove a triangular flap. Any thickened conjunctiva around the punctum may be removed by electrocautery.

Dogs having occlusion of the canaliculi resulting from inflammatory or catarrhal thickening may be treated by enlargement of the puncta and subsequent repeated irrigation with antibiotic-corticosteroid solutions.

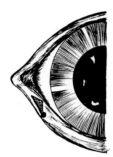

FIG. 122. *The three-snip operation.*

In the Poodle, cases associated with malpositioning of the puncta may be improved by careful surgical eversion of the nasal edge of the lid; cases associated with pressure on the canaliculus from the nictitans gland will improve following the surgical removal of the gland.

Epiphora

Epiphora, or 'weeping', is caused by impaired outflow of tears, rather than over-production of tears, or 'lacrimation'.

Possible causes are congenital or acquired occlusion of the puncta or canaliculi; canaliculitis; congenital or acquired malpositioning of the puncta; orbital tumours invading the lacrimal duct; tumours of the lacrimal sac; foreign bodies in the lacrimal sac; stenosis of the naso-lacrimal canal; or dacryocystitis.

LACRIMAL SAC AND NASOLACRIMAL DUCT

Occlusion

Occlusion of the lacrimal sac and nasolacrimal duct is common, and results in epiphora. A few cases may be due to congenital imperfections, but the majority result from inflammatory fibrosis. Such cases are frequently associated with chronic conjunctivitis.

Inflammation of the lacrimal sac—dacryocystitis—is usually chronic, associated with epiphora and chronic conjunctival infection. Acute, local-ized, pyogenic infections are uncommon. Other cases, where there is stenosis of the nasolacrimal duct, will be associated only with persistent epiphora.

The cause of a dacryocystitis may be a primary infection, associated with oedema of the mucous membrane, or a secondary infection arising from the conjunctiva, nasopharynx or sinuses. A very few cases may be due to neoplasia, and melanosarcoma of the orbit and fibroma and sarcoma of the lacrimal sac have been reported.

Diagnosis of chronic cases is established by demonstration of the patency or otherwise of the duct by dye tests and syringing. The puncta should first be dilated with a dilator, and a slightly curved lacrimal needle (Fig. 123) or cannula is then inserted into the punctum. Such a procedure must be carried out under anaesthesia, the instruments should be lubricated, and great care must be taken, when inserting the cannula, that the direction of the canaliculus is followed carefully and that no damage is done to the lining membrane. Saline is normally used for irrigation, and, if a little fluorescein is added, its presence at the nostrils can be easily seen. Radiographically, the lacrimal passages may be visualized by inserting an opaque dye such as lipiodol, and a dose of 0·3 to 0·4 ml is suggested.

Treatment of chronic dacryocystitis depends on syringing and probing of the duct. Syringing with saline is often sufficient in mild cases, by washing away mucous obstruction and breaking down adhesions of the mucosa. A trypsin or fibrolysin solution may be used to control cicatrization, and a combined antibiotic-corticosteroid preparation may be used to control infection and inflammatory changes. Such irrigation may need to be repeated daily, or at frequent intervals, before success is achieved.

Probes (Fig. 124) may be used prior to irrigation with antibiotic-corti-costeroid solutions, but their use without these drugs is likely to lead to further irritation of the inflamed mucosa and further stenosis. Probes must be well lubricated and their negotiation through the canal must be accom-plished atraumatically with great care.

Operations commonly employed in man, to provide a new passage from lacrimal sac to nasopharynx—dacryocystorrhinostomy—have not been employed, to date, in the dog.

12

THE CORNEA AND SCLERA

ANATOMY AND PHYSIOLOGY

The cornea

The cornea, or anterior transparent coat of the eyeball, is continuous with the sclera, and occupies the anterior sixth of the globe. The radius of curvature is slightly greater than the remainder of the globe, and, although roughly circular, the transverse measurement is usually about 1 mm greater than the vertical measurement. The diameter varies, in different species of dog, from about 12 mm to 17 mm, and the radius of curvature is approximately 8 mm. As the cornea of the dog is slightly thicker in its central portion, the anterior and posterior surface radii differ slightly. The central thickness is recorded by Prince as being from 0·73 to 0·95 mm.

The junction of cornea and sclera is marked by a circumferential depression, the scleral sulcus. The transitional zone, known as the limbus, is approximately 1 mm in width, and has a different histological structure to the cornea.

Although the cornea has dense nerve fibre plexuses, it is entirely devoid of blood vessels. The nerve plexuses render it more sensitive to pain than other parts of the eye. Histologically, it is made up of five layers (Fig. 125).

(1) *Corneal epithelium*. The anterior coat of the cornea is a continuation of the conjunctiva, and is approximately 0·08 mm in thickness. It is composed of stratified squamous epithelium, the deepest layer of which—the basal cells—is composed of columnar cells, with their flat surface towards the next layer of the cornea, Bowman's membrane. Anterior to the basal cells is a zone of polyhedral cells—the wing cells—which are convex anteriorly and concave posteriorly. The wing cells form some 2 to 4 layers, and processes pass from the inner surface of these cells between the basal cells. Between the wing cells are lymph spaces and lymphoid cells. The remaining 4 to 10 layers of cells, in the anterior part of the cornea, are composed of flattened polyhedral cells, the degree of flattening increasing towards the surface of the cornea, thus giving the cornea a perfectly flat anterior surface. The corneal

epithelium, which has great powers of regeneration, is innervated by many free nerve endings. The cells, even on the surface, retain their nuclei, and never, under normal circumstances, show keratinization.

(2) *Bowman's membrane*. The epithelium is separated from the substantia propria by a thin, structureless, homogeneous, non-elastic membrane,

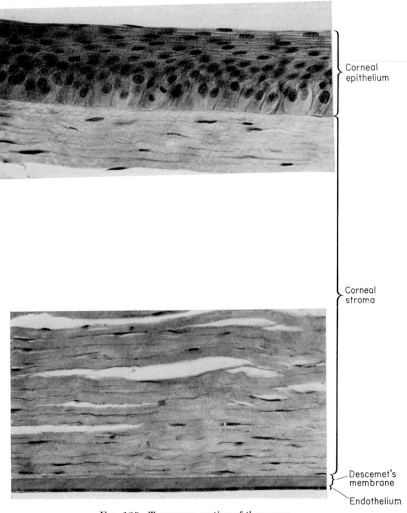

FIG. 125. *Transverse section of the cornea.*

approximately 1·5 μ thick (1 μ = 1 micron = 0·001 mm). Although the anterior border is sharply defined, the posterior border merges into the superficial cells of the substantia propria. Although a fairly tough membrane, Bowman's membrane does not possess any power of regeneration. Although some authors (Oda & Fukuda) have been unable to demonstrate the existence of Bowman's membrane in the dog, others (Prince *et al.*; Spreull) maintain that it does, in fact, exist.

(3) *Substantia propria.* The stroma constitutes about 90% of the thickness of the cornea, and has an average thickness of 0·5 to 0·6 mm, being rather greater in the central part of the cornea. It is composed of connective tissue cells and fibres. The fibres consist of thin, straight, transparent collagen fibrils, which cross and interlace, and form lamellae parallel to the surface of the cornea. Fixed cells are interposed between the lamellae and their branching processes unite with one another. Between the lamellae are fine nerve fibres and lymph spaces, and leucocytes migrating from the neighbouring capillaries.

(4) *Descemet's membrane.* A thick (14 μ), structureless, elastic membrane forms the inner limitation of the stroma, from which it is sharply differentiated. It is continuous at the limbus, where it covers the trabeculae at the angle of the iris and cornea, whereas Bowman's membrane ends abruptly at the limbus. Descemet's membrane, which is normally in a state of tension, is able to regenerate.

(5) *Endothelium.* The inner layer of the cornea is composed of a single layer of rectangular cells, approximately 4 μ thick, which are continuous with the cells on the anterior surface of the iris. This layer acts as a barrier, preventing contact of the cornea with aqueous humour.

The sensory nerve supply of the cornea is derived from the ophthalmic branch of the trigeminal nerve, small branches of which enter the cornea at its periphery and branch extensively in the stroma and pass both towards Bowman's membrane and to the centre of the cornea. Fibres penetrate Bowman's membrane and terminate between the epithelial cells. There are many nerve endings and, therefore, corneal lesions will cause pain and photophobia; this pain may be increased by the movements of the eyelids and of the nictitating membrane. In many Pekingese and other breeds with protruding eyes, the sensitivity of the cornea is often considerably reduced.

In order that no shadows should be thrown upon the retina, the cornea is entirely devoid of blood vessels. This avascularity reduces the surface temperature of the cornea $\frac{1}{2}$ to 1°C (1 to 2°F) below that of the body. Those breeds which show a large area of cornea are likely to be less resistant to corneal infection and ulceration because of the lower sensitivity and the lower temperature.

The cornea is nourished by diffusion from the superficial marginal plexus of vessels, from the aqueous and from the tears. During waking hours, oxygen is absorbed from the air. Lubrication and cleansing are provided by the movements of the nictitating membrane.

The first essential of the cornea is to transmit light freely, and this is dependent on its transparency. The transparency of the cornea is in turn due to its avascularity, uniform structure and deturgescent state. Any force that breaks the regularity of structure will cause cloudiness—such as distortion of the cornea in glaucoma, or the swelling of the stroma by absorption of fluid.

Water can pass freely, by diffusion, into the cornea from both endothelium and epithelium, these layers acting as semipermeable membranes. Under normal conditions, the stroma is not fully hydrated, the corneal tissue fluids being hypotonic to both tears and aqueous. Water that enters the cornea tends to be drawn out, with the result that the cornea contains far less water than it is capable of imbibing. The dehydration of the cornea results from constant metabolic activity, centred in the limiting membranes, although the exact mechanism involved is still obscure.

The maintenance of the correct intraocular pressure is essential for the proper functioning of the cornea. Any lowering of the tension results in a rapid opacity, indicating that the pressure of the aqueous on the posterior surface of the cornea influences the intake and loss of fluid by osmosis.

The limbus

Histological changes take place in the transitional zone between the cornea and the sclera and conjunctiva. There is an increase in thickness of the corneal epithelium as it passes into the limbus, the basal cells becoming smaller, but the surface cells retain their corneal characteristics. The lamellae of the stroma become more irregular and assume more of the characteristics of the scleral cell arrangement.

The blood vessels which nourish the cornea—the marginal vascular plexus—are found at the limbus, in the superficial stroma, extending as far as Bowman's membrane. Descemet's membrane and the endothelial cells continue onto the scleral trabecular meshwork and pectinate ligament.

In the coarser part of the trabecular network, at the limbal iris angle, the fibres are arranged to form channels. Similar channels are to be found in the area of finer trabeculae, close to the angle and the cornea, and these channels drain the aqueous from the anterior chamber to the vessels of the scleral venous plexus. There is no definite canal of Schlemm as in man. The spaces formed by the trabecular network are known as the spaces of Fontana. The large vessels in this area are normal veins, but the smaller ones contain no blood.

Drugs will penetrate the corneal epithelium if they are fat-soluble, whereas penetration of the stroma will only be possible if they are water-soluble. In order to penetrate the entire cornea, therefore, a drug must be both fat and water soluble.

The sclera

The outer layer of the wall of the eyeball, the tunica fibrosa, comprises the cornea and sclera. The sclera forms the opaque posterior five-sixths of the tunica fibrosa, and is composed of dense fibrous connective tissue. There is considerable variation in thickness, the thicker parts (0·8 to 1·0 mm) being at the insertions of the extraocular muscles and the penetrations of vessels. Over the remainder of the globe, the thickness varies from 0·3 to 0·4 mm. The sclera is pierced by three sets of apertures, through which pass nerves, blood vessels and lymphatics. The largest structure to enter —the optic nerve—is situated in the posterior wall, usually lateral and inferior to the posterior pole. At this point, the sclera forms a sieve-like membrane, the lamina cribrosa, through which the nerve enters the eye. The lamina cribrosa, however, is poorly developed in the dog, in comparison with man. The ciliary nerves travel in the substance of the sclera.

The sclera is composed of three layers of tissue, which are not sharply defined. The outer layer—the episclera—is composed of loose elastic and collagen fibres, is vascular in nature although not coloured and unites with the conjunctiva. The sclera proper, the central layer, is composed of dense collagen fibre bundles, parallel to the surface, between which are small elastic fibres and fixed cells, forming a syncytium. The inner layer—the lamina fusca—is the transitional zone between sclera and choroid, and exhibits smaller collagen bundles, increased elastic fibres and pigment cells. This transitional zone is the suprachoroidal space, a lymph space continuous with those contained within the cribriform ligament. This loose connective tissue area permits the passage of aqueous into the venous plexus. The greatest areas of pigmentation within the sclera appear at the limbus. The sclera contains no large blood vessels, but only a capillary network.

The sclera and cornea are continuous with one another, through the transitional zone of the limbus. On the inner surface of the sclera, at the junction, a slight inward projection—the scleral spur—forms the point of attachment of the ciliary body.

The functions of the sclera are twofold—first, to maintain the shape of the eye, and afford protection to the deeper structures; secondly, by its rigidity, to maintain a constant length of the eyeball, despite the pressures exerted by the action of the eyelids and the extraocular muscles.

AESTHESIOMETRY OF THE CORNEA

The sensitivity of the cornea would appear to vary from one individual to another, and particularly from one breed of dog to another. This factor may have particular significance in the development of socalled neurotrophic ulcers. The degree of sensitivity will also vary with age and with the development of various pathological corneal lesions.

The sensitivity of the cornea may be determined accurately by means of an aesthesiometer, such as that of Cochet and Bonnet, by which pressure is transmitted axially on the cornea by a nylon monofilament, of known diameter but of variable length. The instrument consists of a nylon mono-filament, of 0·12 mm diameter, held within a sleeve within which it may be retracted (Fig. 126). Changes in length of the filament are made by a rack and pinion, the length protruding from the sleeve being measured on a scale incorporated in the instrument. The length of the filament may be varied from 60 down to 5 mm, and, as the length is decreased, so the pressure transmitted to the cornea will vary from 0·96 to 17·68 g/mm^2.

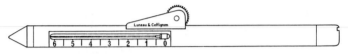

Fig. 126. *Aesthesiometer.*

In use, the dog is seated on a table, and the head steadied. Measurements are started with the nylon monofilament fully extended and the tip is applied perpendicularly to the corneal surface. Slight pressure is exerted until a bending of the filament is just visible. The procedure is repeated with decreasing lengths until a reaction is obtained, consisting of retraction of the globe and blinking. A note is made of the length of filament at which reaction is first obtained.

Congenital anomalies

Microcornea may be encountered on rare occasions, but will normally be seen only as part of a generalized microphthalmos.

Corneal opacities may occur as the result of congenital anterior synechiae, or may be due to defects in Descemet's membrane.

Megalocornea, in which the cornea is excessively large, although otherwise normal, is rarely encountered. It must be distinguished from buphthalmos, in which there is a large cornea associated with glaucoma.

CORNEAL WOUNDS

The eyelids, the bony orbit, the retraction of the eyeball into the orbit, and the cushioning effect of the retrobulbar fat all help to protect the eye from injury. Nevertheless, corneal injuries are common in the dog, and may result from foreign bodies, thorns, grass seeds, motor accidents or injuries received in fights or scratches from cats.

Corneal injuries are likely to be painful, and examination of the cornea may prove difficult, particularly if blepharospasm is produced by the pain. In such cases, it may be necessary to instil a topical anaesthetic solution to facilitate examination; refractory cases may necessitate the use of thiopentone.

Examination should be carried out in good light, with the aid of a magnifying loupe, and the corneal surface should be checked for foreign bodies and wounds. In cases of doubt, fluorescein should be used to demonstrate small abrasions, foreign bodies or lacerations that may not be noticeable otherwise. Small particles of foreign matter may often be more easily demonstrated by oblique illumination. The regularity and lustre of the cornea should be noted, as well as the depth of the anterior chamber.

The healing of the cornea

Epithelium. Following loss of epithelium, epithelialization commences immediately and proceeds rapidly, so that even large defects will be covered in a few days. Columnar epithelial cells rearrange themselves, spreading and migrating over the surface of the defect, in addition to the normal proliferation of these cells.

Substantia. Injuries to the deeper layers of the cornea heal by proliferation of connective tissue cells. No granulative tissue is formed, but some fibrous scar formation is likely to result in all but young animals.

Endothelium. The inner layers heal by migration of endothelial cells.

Nonpenetrating wounds

Most corneal injuries that are encountered will be of the nonperforating variety.

Abrasions should be cleansed and all foreign matter removed by irrigation with saline. Topical anaesthetic agents may be required, both for examination and to prevent the animal inflicting further self-damage through pain or irritation. An antibiotic or sulphonamide preparation may be used to prevent bacterial infection of the wound, which should be inspected regularly for evidence of such infection or of ulceration.

Foreign bodies on or in the cornea are not common, but, on occasion, metallic bodies, splinters or thorns may be encountered. Fluorescein may be necessary to demonstrate small particles of foreign matter. Rust from metallic foreign bodies that have remained in the cornea for some period of time may cause further penetration of the cornea.

Small foreign bodies, if not embedded in the cornea, may be removed gently with a piece of moistened cotton wool, taking care not to inflict further damage upon the cornea.

Foreign bodies embedded in the superficial layers of the cornea may usually be removed satisfactorily with the aid of a magnifying loupe, although a slit-lamp and binocular microscope will prove more satisfactory.

11

General anaesthesia will usually be required and absolute asepsis is essential. The most useful instrument is an eye spud (Fig. 127), the tip of which may be passed beneath the edge of the foreign body, which is then levered forward.

Those foreign bodies embedded more deeply, in the superficial layers of the stroma, are best removed with a sharp curved needle. The needle is used to cut through the epithelium and Bowman's membrane, along the edge of the foreign body; the point of the needle is passed behind the body which is levered forward. A Bowman's needle (Fig. 128) may also be used for the same purpose.

Although tough, the cornea is very thin and it is important that it is not penetrated in the process of removing a foreign body. Following the removal, an antibiotic ointment should be used to prevent infection, combined with anaesthetic preparations in cases showing pain or irritation. The eye should be inspected regularly to detect any complications.

Foreign bodies lying deep in the cornea are, if non-metallic, often best left alone, provided there is no irritation or inflammatory reaction. At a later stage, it is sometimes found that they will approach nearer to the surface where they can be more easily removed. Metallic foreign bodies, on the other hand, may cause considerable staining of the surrounding tissue, and are best removed. This is often difficult, but may usually be accomplished by incising the cornea over the foreign body with the point of a cataract knife, undermining the edges of the incision, and thus gaining access to the foreign body. If the foreign body is near Descemet's membrane, it is possible that these manipulations may cause it to enter the anterior chamber. Should this happen, it will be necessary to make a keratome incision into the anterior chamber, and remove the foreign body, either with a pair of capsule forceps or a blunt iris hook.

Burns affecting the cornea are not common, and are more likely to be encountered affecting the protective eyelids. Cases will occasionally be met where the cornea is burned by acids or alkalis splashed into the eye; alkali burns from soap will be the most common type seen.

Mild cases will require nothing more than irrigation of the conjunctival sac with sterile normal saline, to remove debris, followed by a mydriatic and an antibiotic cream. In cases where the damage is more severe, the area should be cleansed as far as is possible, and all devitalized tissue removed, and covered with a conjunctival flap. If the damage to the cornea is sufficient to cause sloughing of corneal tissue the eye may have to be removed, or at best will exhibit extensive scarring. It may be possible, however, in such cases to perform a superficial keratectomy, or even a corneal graft, at a later stage.

Acid burns will cause precipitation of the tissues and penetration will thus be limited. No such precipitation will occur with alkali burns, in which the degree of penetration is likely to be greater.

Penetrating wounds

Simple perforating wounds are usually caused by penetration of the cornea with a sharp instrument, such as scissors whilst trimming, or by car accidents or cat scratches (Fig. 129). They may be detected in the same way as non-perforating wounds and, in addition, the anterior chamber may be found to be shallow due to loss of aqueous humour.

Unless heavily contaminated, such wounds usually heal quickly. If there is no evidence of prolapse of the intraocular structures, and if the wound is clean or free from gross contamination, simple perforating wounds may often be repaired by a direct suturing technique. Under general anaesthesia,

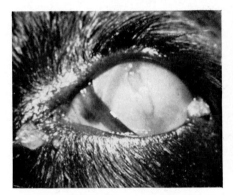

FIG. 129. *Corneal wound.*

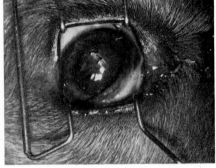

FIG. 130. *Suturing of corneal wound.*

and with magnification and good illumination, the wound is sutured using a corneal needle, with interrupted sutures of 6/0 silk. The lip of the wound is grasped with fine corneal forceps, and each suture is inserted through the cornea, about 1 to 2 mm from the wound edge, to a depth of half the corneal thickness. The corneal edge opposite is then grasped, and the needle is passed through the middle thickness of the cornea to emerge on the surface about 1 to 2 mm from the edge. The edges of the wound must be accurately apposed to avoid buckling, and the sutures must be tied firmly but not so tightly as to cause sloughing of tissue. As many sutures as are required to make the wound watertight are placed in position (Fig. 130).

Care must be taken that the sutures do not penetrate the thickness of the cornea, and thus act as a filtering wick, or cause epithelialization of the anterior chamber. Following suturing, the anterior chamber should be entered with a paracentesis knife and any blood clots removed by irrigation. Air is injected into the anterior chamber to prevent the formation of anterior synechiae. The pupil should then be dilated with atropine, an antibiotic ointment applied to the cornea, and systemic antibiotics given to prevent infection.

Small perforating wounds that do not warrant suturing, or those wounds in which there is so much loss of tissue as to make suturing impossible, should be covered with a conjunctival flap.

Complicated perforating wounds will be associated with loss of aqueous and prolapse or entanglement of the iris in the wound. Large wounds may involve the loss of iris, lens or even vitreous humour. Deep wounds, passing farther into the eye, may produce injury to the anterior lens capsule and subsequent traumatic cataract. Wounds at the corneoscleral junction may produce prolapse of the ciliary body and iris (Fig. 131).

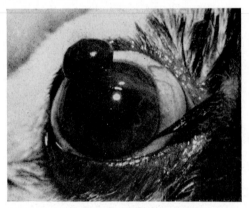

Fig. 131. *Prolapse of iris through a limbal wound.*

Successful treatment of corneal wounds with iris prolapse depends on early diagnosis, to prevent massive contamination and to prevent the iris from becoming adherent to the lips of the wound. In cases where the iris is entangled in the deep lips of the wound, the use of miotics is indicated to constrict the pupil, free the iris and draw it back into the anterior chamber. Where the pupil margin is similarly involved the use of mydriatics may be effective. Cases of iris prolapse should be treated by the replacement of the iris within the anterior chamber, or excision of the prolapsed part with control of the inevitable haemorrhage. The wound should then be closed in the same manner as a wound without prolapse. Antibiotic therapy is recommended in all cases, with atropine to prevent spasm of the iris and the formation of synechiae. Severe wounds, or cases where complete closure cannot be maintained, should be covered with a conjunctival flap.

Prolapse of the ciliary body is likely to be followed by extensive fibrous tissue formation within the eye and consequent obstruction to the entry of light.

The eye should be enucleated if there is extensive trauma with injury to the lens, much loss of vitreous or extensive prolapse of the ciliary body, large foreign bodies within the eye that cannot be removed, endophthalmitis or panophthalmitis.

Perforation of the cornea, and the ensuing complications or the resulting scar formation, is a major cause of blindness in the dog. Many cases can be treated successfully with the minimum of scar formation, but visual impairment can be avoided only if appropriate treatment is started promptly.

CONJUNCTIVAL FLAPS

In the case of corneal wounds to which the direct suturing technique is unnecessary or not applicable, the use of a conjunctival flap is recommended. The flap is designed to protect the wound mechanically, to seal the defect and prevent further loss of aqueous, to prevent infection from the conjunctival sac, and to bring an immediate blood supply to the injured, avascular cornea.

General principles. The wound should be cleansed with saline, and any dirt or debris removed as completely as is possible. Prolapsed tissue, which has become contaminated, should be cut away. Structures adjacent to the wound are replaced into their normal position, and the defect is then covered by the conjunctival flap. In certain cases, a combination of direct suturing and a conjunctival flap may be considered necessary.

Types of flap

Many methods of forming conjunctival flaps have been described. Each is of value under certain conditions, and the type chosen will depend on the condition under treatment, the area of cornea which it is proposed to cover, and the length of time necessary for the flap to stay in position. Flaps may be fashioned so that the conjunctiva covers either the upper or lower half of the cornea (hood flap), or so that it covers the whole of the corneal surface (full flap, or two hood flaps joined together). Alternatively, a strip of conjunctiva may be placed to cover the corneal lesion (strip flap or pedicle flap); or the membrana nictitans may be drawn over the cornea and fixed in position (membrana flap).

Hood flap. This technique is suitable for wounds in the upper third of the cornea. A hood flap may also be used in the lower quadrant, but the approach to the formation of a lower hood flap is not easy in the dog. The conjunctiva is incised, just posterior to the limbus as far as, and sometimes beyond, the horizontal meridian. It is undermined for 6 to 8 mm, drawn over the cornea, and secured by mattress sutures inserted 2 mm behind the free edge of the flap and 3 to 4 mm from the ends of the incision, on the nasal and temporal sides. The sutures are then carried through the episcleral tissues and conjunctiva, just behind the limbus, beyond the limit of the incision on each side (Fig. 132).

If required, two hood flaps may be formed, one in the upper quadrant, and one in the lower. These two flaps may then be sutured together across the centre of the cornea (Fig. 133).

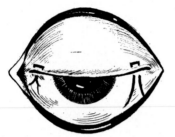

FIG. 132. *Conjunctival hood flap.*

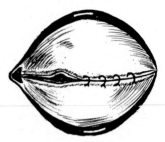

FIG. 133. *Double hood flap.*

Full flap. An incision is made through the bulbar conjunctiva, immediately above and parallel with the limbus. The position and length of the incision are determined so that the flap, when fashioned, will cover the corneal defect. Two incisions are then made, at right angles to the original, one at each extremity, and carried upwards for approximately 1·5 mm. The flap is then undermined and dissected away from the eyeball, making it as thick as

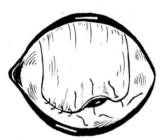

FIG. 134. *Full conjunctival flap.*

possible. The edge of the flap nearest the cornea is drawn over the defect, and sutured, with fine catgut or cotton, to the bulbar conjunctiva of the lower lid (Fig. 134).

The flap must be of sufficient length to fit over the cornea without undue pressure. Any pressure exerted on the cornea will tend to increase the loss of aqueous if the cornea is perforated; a flap that is too long is to be preferred. Haemorrhage experienced at the time of cutting the flap may be controlled by the subconjunctival injection of adrenaline.

As an alternative, the edge of the flap may be secured by two mattress sutures carried through the substance of the lower lid, and tied off on the outer side of the lid.

Strip flap. A strip flap is fashioned approximately twice the width of the corneal lesion. The conjunctiva is dissected from the cornea at the limbus for about half the corneal circumference. It is freed from the sclera so that it may be drawn over the lesion, and a second incision is then made, parallel to the first, fashioning a strip of suitable width that will cover the defect. This flap is secured at either end, passing the suture from the limbal border into the conjunctival fold. Such a flap becomes atrophic, and is severed and trimmed after about 9 days (Fig. 135).

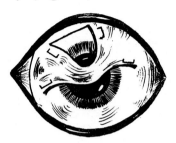

FIG. 135. *Conjunctival strip flap.*

Pedicle flap. This type of flap is recommended for large wounds that will not heal in 6 to 8 days, after which time other flaps often become detached and regain their normal position spontaneously.

The pedicle is brought down from the upper fornix and secured by passing beneath bridges of conjunctiva, 4 mm wide, cut at the limbus on either side

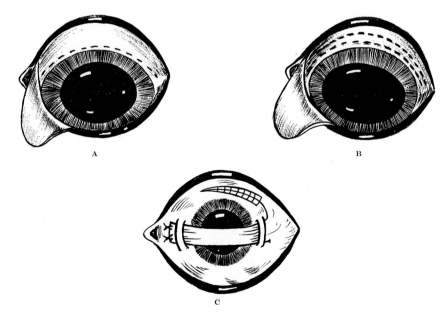

FIG. 136. *Conjunctival pedicle flap.* A *stage 1,* B *stage 2,* C *stage 3.*

in the horizontal plane. The free end of the pedicle is sutured to the conjunctiva after passing beneath a bridge on the opposite side of the cornea to the base of the pedicle (Fig. 136).

Preparation of the pedicle may be facilitated by the subconjunctival injection of saline. The pedicle is based about 4 mm from the limbus, on the temporal side, in the 3/9 o'clock meridian. The incision passes upwards towards the upper fornix in a curve concentric with the limbus. The edges of the conjunctival incision are reflected and a pedicle, containing episclera and Tenon's capsule if necessary to conserve tissue, 5 mm wide, is cut and reflected towards its base. At the limbus, a conjunctival bridge and a conjunctival pocket, each 4 mm wide, are fashioned on either side of the transverse meridian. The pedicle flap is now threaded through between the temporal bridge, carried into the nasal pocket, and secured under the conjunctiva by two mattress sutures of fine silk passing through the overlying conjunctiva.

Membrana flap. The membrana nictitans may be used to cover corneal defects; a full flap is to be preferred if the injury is extensive, or if a marked blood supply is required.

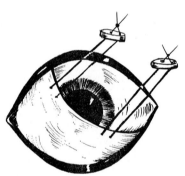

Fig. 137. *Membrana flap.*

Two mattress sutures are inserted through the membrana, about 4 to 5 mm from the free edge, one at either end, using a round-bodied needle. Then, using a cutting needle, the sutures are passed into the upper conjunctival fornix, so that they emerge in the skin, approximately 13 to 19 mm above the upper eyelid. Tension on the sutures draws the membrane completely across the eye, and the sutures are fastened over a small button to prevent them pulling through the skin (Fig. 137). In cases where an additional blood supply is desirable, the inner surface of the membrane may be scarified before the sutures are tied.

This technique may not prove suitable in those animals with markedly protruding eyes, when it may be found impossible to draw the membrane over the cornea.

Postoperative treatment

The site should receive daily cleansing with saline, and a suitable antibiotic preparation should be applied regularly. The time for removal of a conjunctival flap will depend on the severity of the condition, but in most cases 7 to 10 days is sufficient. In some cases there is spontaneous extrusion of the sutures, and the flap may have to be replaced if the time interval is not adequate; this is less likely to happen with the pedicle and membrana flaps. Once the sutures are removed, the conjunctival flap quickly heals in its original position. On rare occasions, the flap will become adhered to the corneal wound; in such cases the flap will have to be severed and trimmed. That part of the flap adhering to the wound will eventually slough and the surface of the cornea will be reconstituted.

Contraindications

The use of a conjunctival flap is contraindicated when the wound is small and sutures alone will make a suitable closure. Although also used in the treatment of corneal ulceration, it is not advocated for extensive ulceration to which the flap might adhere, particularly in the case of superficial pseudomonas ulceration where massive antibiotic therapy will be required.

KERATITIS

Keratitis signifies any inflammation of the cornea. The cornea is exposed and more liable to injury and infection than other parts of the eye. Certain protective mechanisms and reflexes protect the eye to a large extent—the long mobile neck allows rapid head movements and the protective eyelid reflex, and the rapid movement of the membrana nictitans across the eye, accompanied by retraction of the eye into the orbit, all play their part in preventing injuries.

Most animals are extremely 'eye conscious', but this is less noticeable in some of the brachycephalic breeds. In these animals the eyes tend to be very prominent and more prone to injury and drying; there is also reduced corneal sensitivity which diminishes the effectiveness of the protective reflexes. These factors mean that breeds such as the Pekingese are particularly likely to suffer from the effects of corneal damage, and it is possible also that some of these animals have a hereditary defect of the sensory root of the trigeminal nerve, predisposing them to keratitis and corneal ulceration.

Of the many breeds of dog, it would seem that some are extremely susceptible to various forms of keratitis, whilst others appear to be comparatively immune. The brachycephalic types with prominent eyes are particularly susceptible to corneal injuries and ulceration, often with perforation. Corneal erosion is common in the Boxer, but this breed rarely exhibits ulceration of other types, melanosis or interstitial vascularization. Similar superficial erosions are encountered in the Corgi. Keratitis with deep vascularization, and also pannus, are extremely common in the Alsatian, while keratitis with melanosis is most frequently encountered in the Toy breeds, Cocker Spaniel, Boston Terrier, and the small Terriers such as the Cairn and West Highland White.

Keratitis may be either superficial, affecting the surface layers of the cornea only, or interstitial, affecting the deeper layers, together with the uveal tract. It may be accompanied with one or more of the following conditions—loss of transparency, ciliary injection, vascularization of the cornea, cellular deposits in the anterior chamber and ulceration of the cornea.

Loss of transparency may be partial or complete, and is due either to oedema of the corneal epithelium, oedema of the substantia propria or infiltration of the cornea by inflammatory cells.

Oedema of the epithelium is found in cases of acute glaucoma, interstitial keratitis and iritis. It is due to an interference with the drainage of fluid from the cornea and produces a diffuse haziness together with diminished power of reflection from the corneal surface. Oedema of the substantia propria is due to excessive amounts of fluid in the corneal substance and produces faint grey lines in the depth of the cornea, which may be detected with the aid of an ophthalmoscope.

Infiltration of the cornea is either by leucocytes or lymphocytes which migrate either from the normal blood vessels at the corneoscleral junction or from newly formed vessels in the substance of the cornea. This infiltration is seen as a grey-white localized haze, which may be of a yellowish colour in infected wounds or ulcers. Such infiltrations may be followed by complete absorption, or an incomplete absorption leaving either a residual opacity or cicatricial tissue.

Ciliary injection signifies engorgement of the circumcorneal vessels, coming from the anterior ciliary blood supply. At the same time, the conjunctival vessels are often congested.

Vascularization of the cornea may be either superficial or deep, the vessels being derived, in the superficial type, from the conjunctival vessels at the limbus, or, in the deep type, from the anterior ciliary vessels. The new blood vessels invade the cornea from the limbus. *Superficial vessels* (Fig. 138A), from the conjunctiva, extend over the limbus, are continuous with the conjunctival vessels, are bright red in colour, and branch widely in a tree-like fashion. A group of vessels, superficial and sinuous and with many fine branches, lying between the epithelium and Bowman's membrane and associated with some degree of grey or white opacity, is known as a pannus. *Deep vessels* (Fig. 138B), appear at the margin of the cornea, and from under the limbus. They are dull red in colour, and appear as long, straight lines or in the form of brush-like groups; these often coalesce to form a vascular ring.

Vascularization may arise from injury, infection, nutritional disturbances or allergic reactions. Adventitious vascularization of the dog's cornea normally proceeds at a relatively slow rate. In most cases, a period of around 17 or 18 days will elapse before new vessels, arising at the limbus, have reached a central corneal lesion. This relatively long period often allows perforation to take place before the defence mechanism can become fully operative.

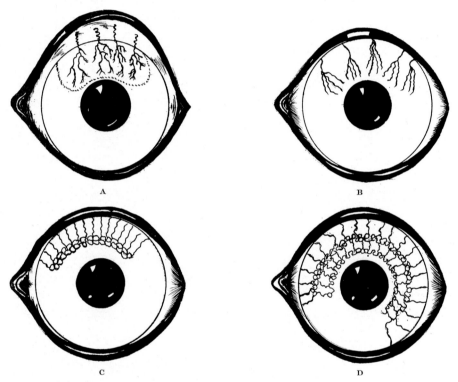

FIG. 138. *Vascular changes in keratitis.* A *superficial vessels*, B *deep vessels*, C *and* D *vascular ring formation.*

Cellular deposits in the anterior chamber are an indication of involvement of the uveal tract. In some cases, only a slight turbidity may be found, but any wound involving Descemet's membrane may lead to the formation of a hypopyon—deposits of exudate and leucocytes in the anterior chamber —at the lower edge of the iris, forming a grey or yellow deposit in the aqueous humour. A hypopyon may clear spontaneously, and will rarely lead to a panophthalmitis.

Ulceration of the cornea may be either superficial or deep, ranging from mild erosion of the surface epithelium to destruction of the substantia.

Deep ulceration may or may not be associated with rupture of Descemet's membrane. Superficial ulceration may be difficult to detect with the naked eye, but may be easily demonstrated with the use of fluorescein.

Keratitis is likely to be accompanied by pain, photophobia, blepharospasm and lacrimation, the severity of these signs depending on the type and severity of the keratitis.

Aetiology of keratitis

As with conjunctivitis, many factors may operate in the production of a keratitis, and, in many cases, both conditions will be present at the same time; a keratitis will often be secondary to an infection of the conjunctiva.

Virus infections, bacterial infections and fungal infections may be involved, and the infection may be self-inflicted by persistent rubbing at some periorbital lesion. In other cases, the infection may be introduced by trauma, as from wounds of the cornea, lids or conjunctiva, burns, foreign bodies, contusions or irritating drugs or chemicals; or the injury may be produced by such conditions as entropion, blepharospasm, trichiasis or dermoids.

Intraocular infections, either from viruses or from penetrating wounds or ulcers, are likely to produce a deep keratitis. Glaucoma will produce a keratitis due to interference in the water metabolism of the cornea from the increased intraocular pressure. Deficient tear production, or exophthalmos, and subsequent drying of the cornea, trophic changes and nutritional deficiency lesions may lead to infection.

Malignant lymphoma may produce changes in the cornea, as well as the uvea and retina. Tumour cells enter the eye by passive infiltration from the blood stream, and may result in a variety of secondary inflammatory and degenerative lesions, including vascularization, ulceration and opacities of the cornea, and, on occasion, keratic precipitates.

Corneal opacity has been noted in some cases of trypanosomiasis in India.

Keratitis may be classified as superficial, interstitial, pigmentary or ulcerative, but many clinical cases cannot be allocated to one group only and may present features from more than one type. The classification of the types of keratitis produces many difficulties, for the term virtually covers all forms of corneal pathology. The reactions of the cornea to various stimuli are many, and the resulting clinical picture will depend on the areas of the cornea that are involved in pathological changes; these may vary and change as the disease process continues.

The superficial layer of the cornea—corneal epithelium—may be regarded as an extension of the conjunctival epithelium and, therefore, will show the pathological changes that might be expected in the conjunctiva or even the skin. The substantia is continuous with the sclera, differing from that structure in its cellular arrangement, allowing transparency, and reactions in this part will affect the transparency of the cornea. The deep layers— Descement's membrane and endothelium—are related to the anterior uvea and will reflect pathological changes in that part of the eye.

Although these three layers may exhibit individual changes, disease processes in one are likely to lead to changes in the others so that eventually the whole of the cornea may become involved.

From this, it will be apparent that cases of superficial disease processes of the cornea are invariably associated with conjunctival involvement, whereas deep lesions of the cornea are invariably associated with an anterior uveitis. As an example of the gradual involvement of all layers of the cornea in a keratopathy, one might consider an ulcer, caused initially by a corneal wound and subsequent infection. Initially the corneal epithelium only is involved with, perhaps, superficial vascularization and ultimately melanosis. Deepening of the ulcer leads to involvement of the substantia, with altera- tion in the fluid balance and loss of transparency. Further deepening of the ulcer may result in intraocular infection, hypopyon formation or anterior uveitis, with subsequent interstitial neovascularization.

SUPERFICIAL KERATITIS

Acute superficial keratitis

This, as the name signifies, is an acute condition, limited to the corneal epithelium and, sometimes, the superficial part of the substantia. A co- existent conjunctivitis is usually present and, although there is no true ulceration, the epithelium may be denuded in places.

The cause might be injury or infection, such as might occur with foreign bodies, trichiasis, entropion, or neoplasia of the lid; nutritional deficiencies, particularly of riboflavine; an extension of a conjunctival infection; or allergy.

The patient will usually exhibit pain, lacrimation and photophobia, and sometimes, blepharospasm and impairment of vision. Superficial lesions of the cornea are likely to involve the superficial nerve plexus and these mani- festations are, thus, likely to be more marked than with deeper involvement of the cornea. In some cases, reflex contraction of the pupil may be noted.

Physical signs. Epithelial oedema will be present, producing a general haziness of the cornea and loss of the natural reflective surface. This will be followed by infiltration, superficial vascularization and circumcorneal congestion. The haziness of the cornea will increase as the infiltration of cells continues, and some loss of transparency may occur. The infiltration of cells—polymorphonuclear leucocytes and lymphocytes—will produce an overall opacity if the infection is generalized or may, in other cases, be limited to small areas of the cornea.

Vascularization will occur in most instances of acute superficial keratitis, the vessels invading the cornea being derived from the conjunctival vessels. The newly formed vessels pass into the cornea from the limbus, where they may be seen to be continuous with the conjunctival vessels. These vessels are superficial, slightly raising the corneal epithelium, are bright red in colour, and form convolutions or loops at the limbus or may branch, in a tree-like fashion, over the cornea (Plate III, Fig. 11, facing p. 104).

Treatment. The neovascularization will regress as soon as the underlying cause is removed, and this must form the basis of treatment. Where the primary cause is injury to the cornea from foreign bodies, entropion, trichiasis or lid tumours, correction of these disorders will often resolve the keratitis without further treatment.

Infections, coexistent with a conjunctivitis, are best treated with antibiotics, after culture of the causal organism and sensitivity tests. Corticosteroids and β-ray irradiation are useful to limit and resolve neovascularization, provided that infection has been controlled.

Vascularization due to riboflavine deficiency will respond dramatically to the administration of this vitamin. It is probable that true cases of riboflavine deficiency are uncommon or even rare, in the dog, but the administration of this vitamin in daily doses of 10 to 25 mg is indicated in all cases of acute corneal vascularization.

Antihistaminics, in ointment or drop form, are indicated in cases of acute keratitis associated with allergy. They are most likely to be associated with an acute conjunctivitis, and be caused by pollen allergy. Corticosteroids are also of value and may be combined with antihistaminics if required.

Superficial punctate keratitis

Keratitis of this type usually affects the central part of the cornea, is usually bilateral and is not usually associated with other corneal or conjunctival disease. The cause is unknown, but thought to be of viral origin. The opacities may be due to an antibody-antigen reaction in the cells of the substantia propria (Fig. 139).

The condition usually commences with signs of pain, photophobia and lacrimation, but sometimes only mild irritation may be shown. In the former cases, the third eyelid may be drawn over the eye, and blepharospasm and spastic entropion may be present. Fluorescein staining reveals small punctate ulcers in the corneal epithelium followed by diffuse opacity, more marked in the upper nasal and temporal quadrants. The cornea is somewhat oedematous and a superficial vascularization may appear, the vessels invading the corneal epithelium for only a short distance. Later, this vascularization may invade the deeper structures and produce an interstitial keratitis. This may be followed by anterior uveitis, pigment migration and later still, by retinal degeneration and xerosis of the cornea. A mass of fine vessels forming a bulbar hyperaemia may be found at the limbus. In other cases, the disease appears to be self-limiting, the ulcerated areas forming opacities which may be permanent, or may resolve within months or even years. The ultimate prognosis, despite the protracted course, is usually favourable.

Treatment is of little avail, but should be directed towards the prevention of secondary infection and the relief of pain. The use of corticosteroids, riboflavine and vitamin A in full doses is suggested.

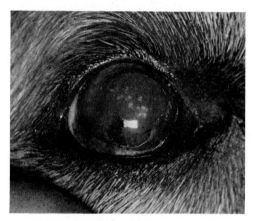

Fig. 139. *Superficial punctate keratitis.*

Pannus

Pannus is a subepithelial vascular or fibrovascular infiltration of the cornea. Part of the substantia is replaced by vascularized connective tissue, and the overlying epithelium becomes conjunctival in nature (Plate III, Fig. 12, facing p. 104). Although the cause is unknown, and it may be seen in any breed, it is most commonly met in the Alsatian and Boxer.

Signs are usually first seen in the lower quadrant on the temporal side, where a greyish haziness develops at the limbus. This area subsequently becomes vascularized, and sometimes pigmented, and gradually extends onto the cornea. Many cases appear to be self-limiting, affecting only quarter to a third of the corneal surface, but in other cases the condition spreads over the whole cornea and may result in total blindness.

Treatment in some cases, particularly those that extend rapidly, is often most unsatisfactory. Beta-ray therapy has given consistently poor results, and early improvement is often followed by recurrence. Similarly, cauterization with phenol, to destroy the superficial epithelium and connective tissue, may be followed by a return of the pannus.

In the milder type of case, repeated subconjunctival injections of corticosteroids, combined with the parenteral and topical application of the same drugs, have given good results in many cases. In more advanced cases, success may follow a superficial keratectomy, vascularization of the regenerated epithelium being controlled by corticosteroids, or β-ray treatment.

DEEP KERATITIS

Deep keratitis includes two clinical entities—interstitial keratitis, in which there is a severe inflammation of the deep structures of the cornea, with ingrowth of deep corneal vessels; and keratitis profunda, a more mild, diffuse inflammation of the corneal parenchyma.

Interstitial keratitis

In interstitial keratitis, the usual irritative signs of photophobia, pain and lacrimation are present, and vascularization takes place in the deep layers of the parenchyma. In the early stages, short vessels radiate in an even fashion, from the limbus towards the centre of the cornea, sometimes over the whole circumference of the cornea. These vessels originate from the limbal loops of the ciliary vessels, where they pass over and into the corneal substance; they tend to be arranged in close, parallel, straight lines (Plate IV, Fig. 1, facing p. 168). The vessels concerned in deep keratitis are not bright red in colour and wavy as are superficial vessels from the conjunctiva, but tend to show a slate-coloured appearance and, at their terminations, form minute arcs which join to an arc or circle (Plate IV, Fig. 2, facing p. 168). Later, these vessels assume a brush-like pattern and are more prominent. There is thickening of the cornea, a gradually increasing haze of the parenchyma leading to a variable degree of corneal opacity, and folding of Descemet's membrane. In addition, there may be some superficial vascularization and, sometimes, a greyish-pink appearance of the cornea at the limbus, due to the oedema and vascularization.

The aetiology of interstitial keratitis is obscure, but in all cases the uveal tract is involved forming the basic lesion of the acute interstitial keratitis. Some cases arise as a complication of ulcerative keratitis, traumatic or operational wounds. Primary causes may be focal infections in tonsils, teeth or prostate gland; virus infections such as distemper, or leptospirosis or toxoplasmosis. The condition, which may be either unilateral or bilateral, is most commonly seen in the Alsatian.

Treatment must be directed to the primary cause if known, and to the anterior uveitis that is present. Atropine, in the form of drops or ointment should be applied several times daily, to lessen congestion of the iris, reduce spasm and pain, and to prevent synechiae.

Corticosteroids are of value in the treatment of interstitial keratitis, and may be used locally as a suspension or an ointment. As drops they

PLATE IV

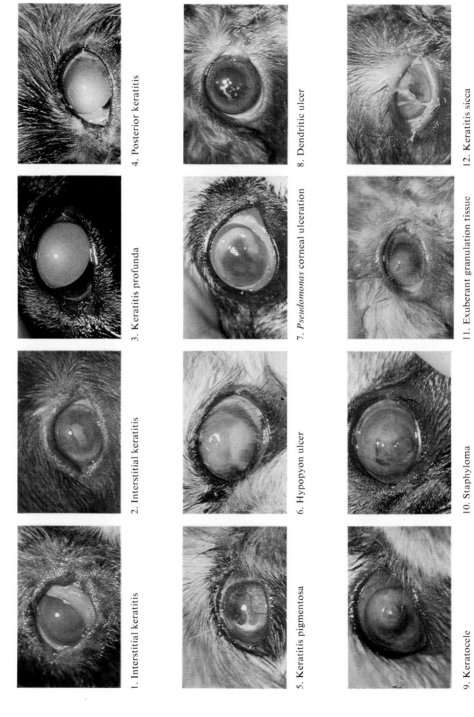

1. Interstitial keratitis

2. Interstitial keratitis

3. Keratitis profunda

4. Posterior keratitis

5. Keratitis pigmentosa

6. Hypopyon ulcer

7. *Pseudomonas* corneal ulceration

8. Dendritic ulcer

9. Keratocele

10. Staphyloma

11. Exuberant granulation tissue

12. Keratitis sicca

should be applied frequently—every hour for the first 24 hours, and then five or six times daily; as ointment, application three times daily is adequate. In view of the involvement of the deeper ocular structures, these drugs should also be administered systemically and by subconjunctival injection; the latter should be repeated every 2 to 4 days, or repository injections may be used.

The use of foreign proteins, given by injection, has been recommended and irradiation with β-rays has a palliative effect and also limits vascularization. Chronic cases of interstitial keratitis, seen particularly in the older Spaniel, and associated with a chronic mucopurulent conjunctivitis, may benefit from the use of silver nitrate, used as a 1 to 2% solution, neutralized by saline.

Keratitis profunda

This condition, which is usually associated with or, more often, follows infection with canine virus hepatitis, is usually unilateral and sudden in onset. Occasional cases have been reported following the use of live hepatitis vaccine.

The affected eye is usually not painful, and photophobia and lacrimation are invariably absent. The cornea, which is thickened and oedematous, exhibits a dense, diffuse bluish appearance, affecting the deeper layers of the parenchyma (Plate IV, Fig. 3, facing p. 168). The iris is sometimes involved and, on rare occasions, a secondary glaucoma or a keratoconus may result. Vascularization of the cornea is uncommon, and the condition will usually resolve spontaneously in 7 to 10 days. The use of chloramphenicol, in ointment form, is recommended, in an effort to prevent secondary complications. In a few cases the opacity may be permanent and in these extensive corticosteroid therapy is suggested.

Keratitis pigmentosa

Pigmentation of the cornea by the deposition of melanin is a common condition in the dog and is responsible for many cases of impaired vision. Pigmentation is usually secondary to some other corneal or uveal disease where vascularization has already occurred; the deposition of melanin frequently follows inflammatory reaction in the dog. Those breeds in which conjunctival pigmentation is normal are naturally more prone to corneal pigmentation. The pigmentation is usually superficial (although it may on occasion, affect the deeper layers), insidious in onset and progressive (Plate IV, Fig. 5, facing p. 168). Only rarely will blindness occur, except in cases with deep deposits, and dogs with advanced melanosis of the cornea will often retain some vision. The breeds most often affected are the Pekingese,

12

Cocker Spaniel, Pug and small Terriers; and the condition is usually bilateral.

The main endogenous pigments concerned in keratitis pigmentosa are melanin and haemoglobin derivatives. Melanosis normally involves the epithelial layer, although some involvement of the substantia propria may also occur, even extending to the basal cells. Haemoglobin derivatives—haematoidin and haemosiderin—cause pigment formation of the cornea, also, extending as far as the endothelium. Haematoidin appears as yellow granules and tends to disappear rapidly; haemosiderin, the iron-containing pigment, produces the condition of siderosis—the presence of particles of iron, giving a rusty brown or greenish discoloration.

The normal cornea contains no pigment cells. Melanosis occurs by migration of melanin from either a pigmented conjunctiva or, in cases of corneal perforation and subsequent anterior synechia formation, from the uveal tract. In cases in which the cornea becomes pigmented, melanocytes are found in the corneal epithelium, superficial stroma and around the superficial vessels. It would appear that, in most cases, corneal vascularization precedes the migration of melanocytes from the limbus, although it is possible that in other cases the basal cells of the epithelium also produce melanin.

Keratitis pigmentosa is not a specific entity but represents a complication of chronic keratitis and subsequent vascularization of the cornea. The conditions under which corneal pigmentation may occur are as follows:

(1) From the bulbar conjunctiva in cases of trichiasis, entropion, chronic conjunctivitis and pannus formation. In the Pekingese, it commonly arises on the inner aspect due to irritation from nasal hairs on a protruding eye.

(2) Following any keratitis involving vascularization, particularly interstitial varieties. Some pigmentation will also be caused by the deposition of haemosiderin following the breakdown of blood vessels.

(3) Following corneal ulceration and penetration, resulting in anterior synechiae or prolapse of the iris. In these cases, uveal pigment migrates from the ciliary vessels and is deposited in the stroma as well as on the surface.

(4) From melanotic tumours involving the limbus.

(5) In cases of senile degeneration of the cornea.

The primary changes are usually seen at the limbus, more often on the nasal side, as brown or brownish-black patches in the epithelium. The initial lesions are usually small and irregular. Spread occurs onto the surface of the cornea in irregular areas, which may later coalesce and obscure vision. In advanced severe cases showing deep pigmentation the cornea may appear dry and irregular, and the dog may exhibit some conjunctival discharge and discomfort. The pigmentation is preceded by vascularization. Blood vessels may be seen in the corneal epithelium and, on occasions, in the stroma as well. In many cases, particularly those arising from irritation of the cornea by hairs or eyelashes, the area of pigmentation remains localized at the periphery of the cornea.

Treatment of corneal pigmentation must primarily be directed against the cause if possible, involving the correction of any entropion, treatment of conjunctivitis and the removal of lashes in cases of trichiasis. Cases of melanosis associated with superficial keratitis and vascularization will resolve when the vascularization is treated. Little attention need then be paid to the pigmented areas, provided that they do not obscure the pupillary opening. Pekingese, with their prominent nasal folds, are best treated by excision of the folds, thus eliminating contact between hairs and cornea.

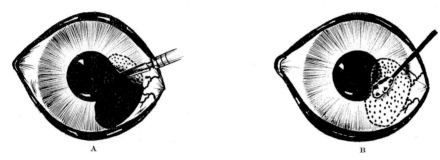

A   B

FIG. 140. *Surgical removal of superficial pigment.* A *stage 1*, B *stage 2.*

Treatment with corticosteroids, applied locally, systemically and, particularly, subconjunctivally is of great value, although prolonged courses of treatment may be required.

Superficial pigment may be removed surgically under general anaesthesia (Fig. 140A). The eyeball is immobilized with fixation forceps and the pigment then scraped using a no. 15 scalpel blade, following which the underlying vascular bed is destroyed by swabbing with phenol (Fig. 140B). At the same time, the larger vessels at the limbus supplying the pigmented area should be destroyed by either peritomy or diathermocoagulation. Postoperative care consists of protecting the eye from self-damage and the installation of a suitable antibiotic-corticosteroid ointment.

Good results in the treatment of pigmentary keratitis have been reported following the use of β-ray therapy. Radioactive strontium applicators are used as the source of β-radiation, the limited penetration of which allows treatment of superficial conditions without danger to the deeper structures. The endothelium of blood vessels is particularly sensitive to radiation, and the use of this type of therapy will allow the destruction of the vessels concerned in the neovascularization, thus discouraging the deposition of pigment. Suggested doses are 5000 to 15,000 rep, repeated at intervals of 7 to 21 days, depending on the degree of vascularization. Favourable results may follow in early cases of pigmentation, although there is, on the other hand, some evidence that radiation may activate the formation of melanin in potential melanoblastic cells. Following β-ray therapy, it may be possible to still see the pigmented areas and some very small blood vessels after several months.

Uveal pigment deposited in and on the cornea cannot be treated surgically, and treatment with corticosteroids, directed towards the elimination of any interstitial keratitis, is recommended. The use of corneal grafts is not advised, for, even if successful, the graft will invariably become pigmented in the same way as the surrounding host cornea. In some cases, however, where treatment fails to produce any improvement, the use of a corneal graft, and attempted subsequent control of neovascularization by means of β-rays, might be considered worthwhile.

The use of factors containing melatonin from the pineal body has recently been suggested as a treatment for canine melanosis. It would appear that such treatment has no effect on established corneal melanosis but may prevent the deposition of melanin.

CORNEAL ULCERATION

Scarring of the cornea as the result of corneal ulceration or penetration is a major cause of blindness in the dog. With certain exceptions, most cases of ulceration, even of penetration, will be followed by reasonable healing and the restoration of vision if suitable treatment is instituted promptly.

Corneal ulceration is associated with loss of corneal substance. It may or may not be associated with corneal oedema, vascularization, pain or photophobia. The latter signs are more often associated with superficial ulceration than with deep involvement.

The classification of corneal ulcers has taken many forms in the past, most systems being concerned with the type or shape of ulcer rather than the cause. In many cases, however, the precise cause can be determined, and an aetiological classification is probably more satisfactory.

(1) *Bacterial causes*
  Haemolytic *Streptococcus*
  Staphylococcus
  Pseudomonas pyocyanea
  Moraxella
  Proteus vulgaris
  Micrococci
  E. coli

(2) *Viral causes*
  Distemper virus
  Hepatitis virus (rarely)
  ? other unidentified viruses

(3) *Fungal causes*
  Candida
  Nocardia

(4) *Hypersensitivity reactions*
   To unknown allergens or
      toxins
   To bacterioproteins

(5) *Vitamin A deficiency*

(6) *Neurotrophic ulceration*

(7) *Exposure*

(8) *Unknown causes*
   Chronic serpiginous ulcer
   Chronic epithelial ulcer

The pathogenesis of ulceration

The stages in the formation and regression of a corneal ulcer have been described by **R. J. Beamer** as follows:

(1) Progressive stage

(a) The ulcer begins as an infiltrate shown clinically as a cloudy spot on the cornea.

(b) The epithelial cells swell, the nuclei undergo cloudy swelling and then break down.

(c) Albuminous fluid collects between the lamellae.

(d) The lamellae swell and become hazy through a dust-like deposit, and eventually break down into a granular mass.

(*e*) The most infiltrated portion becomes necrotic and forms an ulcer.

(2) Regressive stage

(*a*) A line of demarcation forms and dead tissue is shed.

(*b*) The size of the ulcer increases but its floor and edges become smooth and transparent, and the cloudiness disappears.

(3) Cicatrization stage

(*a*) Vessels extend from the nearest portion of the limbus towards the ulcer.

(*b*) The neighbouring epithelium grows over this.

(*c*) Nuclei and vessels disappear and are replaced by a mass of fibrous tissue, forming a scar.

Bacterial corneal ulcers

Streptococcal ulcer. The streptococcus is a common bacterial cause of ulceration, usually following trauma to the cornea, but occasionally associated with a chronic streptococcal conjunctivitis or nictitans gland infection. In the case of conjunctivitis, the organism may enter the corneal substance and multiply after the corneal epithelium has been damaged by the infection.

Traumatic ulcers infected with the streptococcus are usually superficial, show little tendency to spread and will heal rapidly. When associated with coexistent conjunctival infection, a well-circumscribed ulcer is produced, again with little tendency to spread, but with some tendency to deepen (Fig. 141). This may result in the production of a hypopyon (Plate IV, Fig. 6, facing p. 168)—an accumulation of pus in the anterior chamber—due either to the passage of bacteriotoxin through Descemet's membrane, or, sometimes, to perforation of the cornea.

Local treatment is usually effective, using sulphonamides or antibiotics.

Staphylococcal ulcer. Corneal ulcers produced by the staphylococcus are very uncommon, although the reason for the lack of affinity of this organism for the corneal tissues is not understood (Fig. 142).

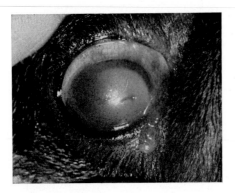
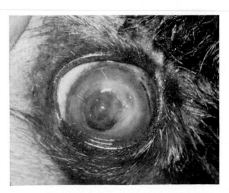

FIG. 141. *Streptococcal corneal ulceration.*   FIG. 142. *Staphylococcal corneal ulceration.*

The ulcer produced by the staphylococcus is similar to the streptococcal ulcer, but shows more tendency to spread, shows a necrotic centre, a diffuse keratitis and some infiltration of the substantia propria. The creeping effect over the cornea is similar to that of the acute serpiginous ulcer in man, although the cause in that instance is usually the pneumococcus.

Pseudomonas ulcer. Pseudomonas pyocyaneus, although not a common cause of ulceration in the dog, can cause destruction of the cornea overnight. This particular organism has a great affinity for corneal tissue, on which it flourishes, thus early diagnosis and rigorous treatment are absolutely essential. Entry of the organism into the cornea usually takes place through traumatic wounds. Attention should be drawn to the fact, however, that *Pseudomonas* thrives in fluorescein solutions and to a lesser extent in physostigmine solution. As there is no suitable antibacterial preservative that can be used in these solutions, they should be autoclaved at frequent intervals, or individual sterile packs should be used.

Ulcers of this type usually start in the centre of the cornea and spread rapidly, showing large areas of necrosis, a diffuse keratitis and infiltration of the substantia. The epithelium is undermined and raised, but there is little tendency to penetrate the cornea (Plate IV, Fig. 7, facing p. 168). Large areas of the cornea may be badly damaged, and healing may be followed by marked scar formation.

The most consistently effective antibiotic against *Pseudomonas* is poly-mixin, although some strains are also susceptible to streptomycin. Both these antibiotics should be used in treatment. Polymixin is best adminis-tered by subconjunctival injection ($\frac{1}{3}$ ml of a solution containing 30,000 units/ml) and also as a solution instilled into the conjunctival sac every hour. Before each application, the conjunctival sac should be irrigated with saline solution, and a polymixin-bacitracin ointment applied every 4 hours. In addition, streptomycin should be given by intramuscular injection and as an ointment (5 mg/g) at the same time as the polymixin ointment. Provided the conjunctiva does not show undue reaction, the subconjunctival injections should be repeated daily.

Moraxella ulcer. Ulcers produced by this organism may occasionally be seen associated with a conjunctivitis produced by the same cause. Usually, the ulcers are only slowly progressive, superficial and central on the cornea. Perforation is unlikely. Treatment with sodium sulphacetamide or with antibiotics is usually effective.

Viral ulcers

Ulcers may occasionally be seen in cases of infection with canine distemper virus, more often in those cases in which an acute purulent conjunctivitis or keratitis is present. Ulceration may be due either to a direct effect of the virus on the corneal tissue or to the effect of secondary bacterial infection.

Ulceration may, on rare occasions, be noted in association with the keratitis profunda produced by the canine hepatitis virus.

Fungal ulcers

Fungal corneal ulcers are usually slowly progressive, grey and indolent, and usually result from damage to the corneal epithelium by either trauma or infection. The use of long-term antibiotics and corticosteroids may allow a fungal overgrowth to take place. Various fungistatic preparations, such as nystatin and amphoterycin, may be used in treatment.

Ulcers due to hypersensitivity reactions

Catarrhal ulceration in old and debilitated dogs, often as an extension of a chronic conjunctivitis, may be due to exotoxins from the bacteria present in the conjunctiva, or to an allergic reaction from the bacterial infection (Fig. 143).

Pain, photophobia and lacrimation are present, and small, punctate ulcers are seen, usually towards the limbus. These ulcers have a tendency to coalesce. There is usually some coexistent vascularization of the super-ficial layers of the cornea around the ulcerated area.

Treatment must be directed towards the chronic conjunctivitis if present. Vitamin A therapy is often beneficial, applied both locally and systemically. Desensitization with staphylococcal toxoid may be of value.

Ulcers due to vitamin A deficiency

These ulcers are extremely rare in the dog, but, when they do occur, mostly in undernourished puppies, they are associated with a dry conjunctiva—xerophthalmia—and with a desiccation and necrosis of the cornea —keratomalacia. The ulcers are usually situated in the centre of the cornea and are bilateral; they appear grey and indolent and corneal perforation is common. Keratinization of the conjunctiva may be present.

Treatment consists of the administration of large doses of vitamin A, both intramuscularly and orally, together with local antibiotic treatment to prevent secondary infection.

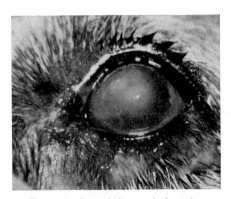

Fig. 143. *Catarrhal corneal ulceration.*

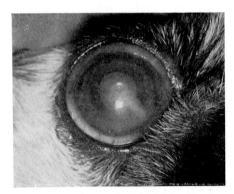

Fig. 144. *Neurotrophic corneal ulceration.*

Neurotrophic ulcers

Ulceration, due to a loss of sensation in the ophthalmic branch of the fifth cranial (trigeminal) nerve which supplies the cornea, caused by trauma, surgery, inflammation or other agents, is most commonly seen in the brachycephalic breeds; in these animals there is possibly a deficiency of the Gasserian ganglion. The sensitivity of the cornea is lost, thus its defence against degeneration, infection and ulceration, and the reflexes that control the disposal of toxins and metabolites, are diminished in power.

In the early stages of neurotrophic ulceration, widespread superficial ulceration of the epithelium occurs, which may be demonstrated by the use of fluorescein. These ulcerated areas tend to coalesce at a later stage producing irregular areas denuded of epithelium, often in the central portion of the cornea. The ulcers remain superficial and show no tendency to perforate, neither do they show any tendency to heal with the usual forms of therapy (Fig. 144).

If untreated, there is a likelihood of the ulcerated areas becoming infected. Provided the corneal surface can be kept moist with artificial tears, the continuity of the corneal epithelium can be maintained. Healing of large areas of superficial ulceration will usually take place under the protection of a conjunctival flap; in some cases, however, it will be found necessary to perform a tarsorrhaphy along two-fifths of the lid margins, leaving openings at either end for the escape of tears and the installation of drops, and to leave this union in place over a prolonged period.

Ulcers due to exposure

Any condition in which the surface of the cornea is not properly moistened and covered by the eyelids may lead to ulceration due to exposure. Such conditions include ectropion, exophthalmos, deficiencies in the structure of the lid margin as the result of injury, or any inability to close the lids properly. Breeds with protruding eyes are particularly susceptible to corneal

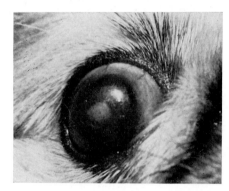

FIG. 145. *Corneal ulceration due to exposure.*   FIG. 146. *Chronic epithelial erosion in the Boxer.*

drying or injury and it is these two factors which are responsible for ulceration. In addition, these dogs very often show a poorly developed corneal reflex and appear to be far less 'eye conscious' than other animals. Vascular and nervous disturbances of the lacrimal glands may also result in excessive drying of the corneal surface (Fig. 145).

Unless secondarily infected, this type of ulcer will be sterile, and treatment must be aimed at providing protection and moistening of the corneal surface. In some cases surgical manipulations on the lids will correct the underlying cause. With breeds having normally proptosed eyes, resort may have to be made to the use of artificial tears composed of $\frac{1}{2}$ to 1% methylcellulose.

Ulcers of unknown cause

Dendritic ulcer. Ulceration of the dendritic type occasionally occurs in the dog, giving an appearance very similar to that of *Herpes simplex* ulceration in man. Although no causal organism has been isolated, a virus is probably responsible.

In the early stages, a catarrhal conjunctivitis is often present, followed by the appearance of minute punctate opacities in the superficial layers of the cornea, giving a picture very similar to superficial punctate keratitis. The opacities vesicate and rupture and coalesce, forming a serpent-like pattern on the cornea (Plate IV, Fig. 8, facing p. 168). Fresh foci may appear later isolated from the main ulceration, or the irregular pattern of ulceration may spread over the cornea. Erosion of the corneal epithelium and secondary infection may follow at a later stage. Relapses are frequent and, despite treatment, the ulceration may continue for several weeks. Eventually, the ulceration is self-limiting, but corneal scarring is likely to remain, particularly when secondary infection has occurred.

Treatment often appears ineffective, and antibiotic and chemotherapeutic agents are of little value except to control secondary infection. Cauterization of the entire corneal surface with phenol or iodine may prove helpful, but may need to be repeated several times. Covering the ulcer with a conjunctival flap will sometimes limit the spread, and the use of vitamin A, locally or orally, is suggested. Subsequently, if scarring is excessive, a lamellar keratoplasty may be needed.

Chronic epithelial ulcer. Chronic superficial epithelial erosion of the cornea is most often seen in the Boxer and Corgi, of any age group. It is not associated with any drying or exposure of the cornea, and its aetiology remains obscure. Neither is it associated with any systemic disease, nor have any causal organisms been isolated (Fig. 146).

The area most often affected is in the lower lateral segment, 2 to 3 mm from the limbus, although this may spread at a later date to involve a considerable proportion of the corneal surface. Extensive areas of ulceration, 10 to 14 mm in diameter, are not uncommon. In the early stages, the ulceration is very superficial, with no evidence of corneal oedema or cellular infiltration, and is often only detected after the application of fluorescein. A mild conjunctivitis is sometimes present. Pain and photophobia are exhibited, often to a marked degree, and, sometimes, lacrimation and blepharospasm, particularly in the early stages. There is no associated iridocyclitis or hypopyon.

In most cases, one eye only is affected; it is not uncommon, however, to find both eyes involved, occasionally concurrently, but more often, consecutively.

Most cases show little tendency to heal spontaneously, and the ulcerated area becomes indolent. At this stage, the ulcer is clearly defined in depth and area and stains vividly with fluorescein, suggesting that in some cases the superficial layers of the substantia are involved. The margin of the ulcer appears ragged and fluorescein tends to undermine the margin, suggesting that new epithelial cells are being produced, but are incapable of adhering to the underlying stroma. After the ulcer has been in existence for some time, vascularization of the cornea may take place, commencing at the edge of the ulcer nearest to the limbus. This may result in resolution of the ulcer, leaving a persistent haziness, or exuberant granulation tissue may be formed.

Ulceration of this type is usually resistant to medical treatment, and the most favourable results are obtained by stripping the epithelial edge from the ulcer and covering the cornea with a conjunctival flap. In some cases, a superficial keratectomy may have to be performed and, at a later date, the vascularization may have to be controlled by the use of subconjunctival corticosteroids. In other cases phenol cauterization will often prove effective. Corticosteroids should be avoided in the active stages, for they will delay healing. In all cases, however, there is a tendency to recur at some future date.

Chronic epithelial erosion, as seen in the Boxer, presents two interesting features; firstly, the failure of the corneal epithelium to become re-established, secondly, the delayed onset of neovascularization. Epithelial defects defects normally become filled rapidly, abrasions of up to 5 mm in diameter being covered by new cells within 24 hours. Repair is normally accomplished by a combination of cell migration and mitosis. In this particular corneal disease, cell migration does not appear to occur, and the mitosis of cells at the periphery of the lesions fails to repair the defect because of a lack of cohesion.

Lesions of the cornea adjacent to the limbus might be expected to initiate neovascularization within 48 to 72 hours. The delayed onset of vascularization in this particular condition might be explained by lack of infection and of corneal oedema, which is normally regarded as a prerequisite for vascular invasion.

THE GENERAL TREATMENT OF CORNEAL ULCERATION

Certain general principles apply to the treatment of corneal ulceration of any type, whatever the cause. It must first be appreciated that small, punctate, or superficial ulcers are not always easily detected on examination, even under good lighting conditions, and the value of the use of fluorescein in the detection of such ulcers must be borne in mind. The use of fluorescein will also help to differentiate active ulceration from these cases in which epithelialization of the defect has occurred before the loss of corneal tissue has been replaced, leaving a shallow circular or oval depression on the corneal surface.

Cleanliness of the ulcerated area and conjunctival sac is important, and should be maintained by irrigation with normal saline. The use of cotton-wool swabs to cleanse the eye and the infliction of further damage on the corneal epithelium, must be avoided. Self-inflicted damage is an ever-present danger in the dog, particularly where either irritation or pain is present; in such cases, the use of topical anaesthetic agents is of value in preventing further injury to the eye. In all cases of threatened or actual penetration of the cornea, painful spasm of the iris may be controlled by the use of atrophine, which also helps to prevent synechia formation.

In those cases in which bacteria are present, either as primary or secondary agents, antibiotic therapy is indicated. The value of cultural examinations and sensitivity tests must be considered. Infected ulcers of a superficial type may be treated with topical applications, but in those cases in which the deeper structures of the cornea or anterior chamber are affected, these agents should be administered by the subconjunctival route. At the same time, it may prove beneficial to administer these drugs orally or parenterally as well.

Superficial ulcers, particularly those situated on the periphery of the cornea, may sometimes be treated by cauterization with iodine (tinct. iod. fort.). Cauterization with more drastic agents such as phenol, is of value in cases of chronic epithelial ulceration.

The use of vitamins in the treatment of corneal ulceration is usually of value. It is normally accepted that, as a general rule, the dog cannot make its own vitamins. Vitamin D may be manufactured, provided that there is sufficient irradiation of the skin with summer sunshine, and it is probable that the healthy dog can produce its own vitamin C. Fat-soluble vitamins can of course be stored for long periods in the body, mainly in the liver. Vitamins of the B complex are likely to occur in sufficient quantities in the diet, provided this contains sufficient protein in the form of natural foods. Vitamin A is obtained by the conversion of carotene, found in fresh green vegetables; it may also be obtained from liver, provided that the animal from which the liver was obtained had access to regular supplies of carotene of vitamin A. The requirements of working dogs are likely to be considerably higher than those of non-working pets, particularly in respect of the vitamin B complex.

However, it is possible that sub-optimal levels of vitamins occur in many of the diets given to dogs, and this relative insufficiency may at least hinder the healing of ulcerated tissue. The vitamins most intimately concerned with the cornea will be vitamin A and riboflavin, and it would seem prudent to assure an adequate intake of these two factors in any case of corneal ulceration.

Due to their effect of suppression of the natural inflammatory response, and their delaying effect on the regeneration of epithelium, corticosteroids are normally contraindicated in the treatment of corneal ulceration. Use of these agents may allow a superimposed infection with various fungi and, on occasion, a mycotic keratitis.

Irradiation with β-rays is occasionally successful in the treatment of indolent ulcers, particularly those of metabolic origin.

Paracentesis of the anterior chamber may be indicated to evacuate a hypopyon, to relieve any secondary ocular hypertension, and to allow the aqueous to escape and be replaced by fresh aqueous, rich in antibodies.

Complications of ulcerative keratitis

Uveitis. Deep ulceration may allow the passage of toxins through Descemet's membrane, producing an anterior uveitis. Under these conditions, leucocytes may collect in the anterior chamber, either as small clumps, adherent to swollen endothelial cells (keratic precipitates or K.P.s) or as a copious exudate, gravitating as a fluid level of sterile pus (hypopyon) (Plate IV, Fig. 6, facing p. 168). The formation of K.P.s is uncommon in the dog.

Panophthalmitis. A purulent infection of all coats of the eyeball, as well as its contents, with pus filling the anterior chamber, may occur without actual perforation. In such cases, removal of the eye by evisceration will be necessary.

Perforation. Corneal penetration will follow deep ulceration whether the ulcer be large or small. The whole thickness of the substantia propria may be lost, so that only Descemet's membrane remains. The normal intraocular pressure causes bulging of this elastic membrane, which will project as a clear vesicle, known as a keratocele or descemetocele, above the corneal surface (Plate IV, Fig. 9, facing p. 168 and Fig. 175, p. 214). This may or may not burst, but if it should do so through a large opening, the aqueous will flow out carrying with it the iris and possibly the lens or even the vitreous. In such cases a panophthalmitis is likely to follow.

If the herniation should burst through only a small aperture, the aqueous will trickle out slowly, and a clot will be formed by the membrane and by fibrin from the aqueous. The iris will often be entangled in the wound, or may herniate through the opening becoming engorged and forming, with collected exudates and lymphocytes, an anterior staphyloma (Plate IV, Fig. 10, facing p. 168). This will result in anterior synechia formation, and occasionally, in fistula formation. In other cases, an anterior uveitis or even panophthalmitis will result. Perforations with prolapse and incarceration of the iris result, when the ulcer is healed and the aqueous reformed, in anterior synechiaë leading up to the base of the scar; this is then known as a leucoma adherens (Fig. 147).

Occasionally, the corneal epithelium around the perforation proliferates very rapidly, covering the edges of the corneal wound; in other cases the scar formed with an adherent leucoma degenerates, forming a cystoid cicatrex which breaks through the epithelium. Either way, a corneal fistula may be formed. In the case of a cystoid cicatrex, the fistular normally closes after the aqueous has escaped and the intraocular pressure is lowered, only to form again when the wound has healed and pressure restored.

Impending perforation may be demonstrated by the intravenous injection of 0·5 to 1 ml of 2% fluorescein solution, producing a fluorescent aqueous flare.

The treatment of corneal perforation

In the early stages of threatened perforation, the ulcer may be cauterized with iodine. Deeper ulcers, in the early stages, may sometimes be treated with phenol cautery. Antibiotics should always be used, but the use of corticosteroids should be avoided, at least until the repair process has started.

In all cases in which there is a tendency to penetrate, paracentesis of the anterior chamber should be performed immediately through a healthy part of the cornea, and repeated every 24 to 48 hours if necessary. This releases aqueous and reduces intraocular pressure.

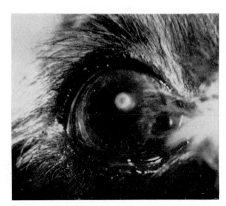

Fig. 147. *Leucoma adherens.*

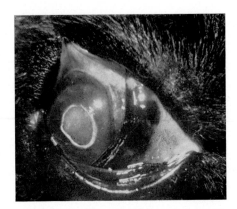

Fig. 148. *Cauterization of corneal ulcer with phenol.*

Perforation in a peripheral ulcer, with incarceration of the iris, may be treated, in addition, with frequent applications of eserine sulphate, to draw the iris back into position. Mydriatics should be used in all other cases.

Where perforation has occurred, or is threatened, a conjunctival keratoplasty should be performed.

Cauterization. The use of phenol is indicated in some cases where the ulcer is indolent and resistant to treatment, particularly in those cases caused by pathogens resistant to antibiotic and chemotherapeutic agents. It is of particular value in indolent epithelial ulceration. The operation should be performed under general anaesthesia. A thin wisp of cotton wool is wound around a carrier, ear probe or mosquito forceps, tightly wrapped and dipped in phenol. Any excess is removed by squeezing against the side of the containing dish or bottle. The eye is fixed in position with forceps so that the ulcerated area is accessible, and the surface dried with filter paper. The ulcer is then gently touched with the phenol swab, paying particular attention to the edges of the ulcerated area. The treated area will immediately turn grey-white. In the case of deep ulcers, the bottom of the crater is left untreated, to avoid the risk of perforation. The ulcer is then dried again with filter paper, to remove any excess phenol, or may be flushed with saline. An ophthalmic ointment is applied, but no after-treatment is normally required. Healing of superficial ulcers is normally complete in a few days, but the procedure may be repeated if necessary (Fig. 148).

Iodine in alcoholic solution may be used, but is less easily transferred to the eye; and as it does not, like phenol, whiten the corneal epithelium, the area treated is less easy to judge accurately. Iodine cauterization should be followed by cocaine drops, thus fixing the iodine as cocaine iodate.

Paracentesis. Paracentesis of the anterior chamber (Fig. 149) should be performed under general anaesthesia. A speculum is inserted and fixation

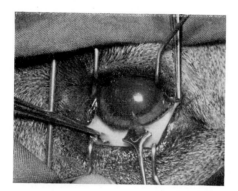

FIG. 149. *Paracentesis of the anterior chamber.*

forceps applied to the lower nasal quadrant. Full aseptic conditions must be applied, and a broad paracentesis knife (Fig. 150) is passed obliquely through the cornea, close to the limbus in the lower temporal quadrant, if possible through a healthy part of the cornea. An oblique incision allows for a safer closing action of the wound which, for the evacuation of aqueous, need only be approximately 3 mm long; larger incisions may be required for the removal of a blood clot or soft lens material in other circumstances.

Great care must be taken to avoid damage to the iris, and, on removal of the knife, the aqueous should be allowed to escape slowly. It may be necessary to remove pus, which has formed a coagulum, by grasping it with capsule forceps and gently delivering it through the wound; irrigation of the anterior chamber, using an irrigator and normal saline may on occasion be necessary. No sutures are required following this procedure, but sometimes it may be necessary to cover the wound with a conjunctival flap.

Conjunctival keratoplasty. The technique used for the application of conjunctival flaps has already been discussed in connection with corneal wounds. The employment of this technique in cases of threatened or actual corneal perforation due to ulceration, will allow a successful conclusion in a

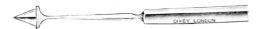

Fig. 150. *Paracentesis knife.*

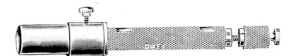

Fig. 158. *Franceschetti's trephine.*

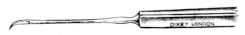

Fig. 165. *Cystitome.*

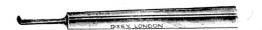

Fig. 167. *Paufique's angled knife.*

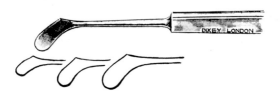

Fig. 168. *Desmarre's scarifier.*

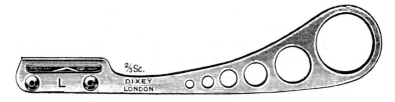

Fig. 170. *Franceschetti and Bock lamellar knife.*

high percentage of cases. Healing of the defect is often rapid and the resultant scar formation is minimal.

Exuberant granulation tissue

As a result of corneal injury, ulceration or pannus formation, granulation tissue will sometimes form on the cornea and reach the point where it is no longer of value, producing an area of red, raised tissue, over and around the corneal scar (Plate IV, Fig. 11, facing p. 168). If such vascularization is, in fact, an obstructing mechanism rather than a defensive one, then peritomy —the division of the new vessels as they enter the cornea—is of value. The granulation will often disappear within 48 hours allowing the cornea to

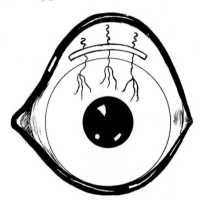

Fig. 151. *Excisional peritomy.*

regain its transparency. This division may be accomplished by either coagulating diathermy or electrocautery, or by the excision of a strip of conjunctiva at the limbus containing the blood vessels.

Thermocautery. The vessels arising in the bulbar conjunctiva are touched with the hot tip of the instrument and severed. Only those vessels in the conjunctiva, just posterior to the limbus, are divided, the corneal continuations being left untouched. Care should be taken that no heat is applied to the cornea, or opacity may result.

Surgical division. In some cases, thermocoagulation will be found to be inadequate, as the collateral circulation quickly bridges the gap; in these cases, excisional peritomy is indicated (Fig. 151). Under general anaesthesia, and using a speculum and fixation forceps to control the globe, the conjunctiva is incised with a diathermy needle, 3 mm posterior to and concentric with the limbus, over the area containing the vessels to be destroyed. The incision is carried down to the sclera and then a second incision is completed, equal in length, parallel to, and 3 mm from, the first. One end of this strip is then lifted with forceps and cut away from the underlying sclera with sharp-pointed scissors. Any bleeding points are controlled by diathermy and the eye is cleansed and dressed with sterile liquid paraffin. Subsequent treatment consists of daily cleansing and liquid paraffin installations until healing is complete. Corticosteroids may be used to check any further neovascularization, although the formation of scar tissue at the limbus will usually prevent any further extension of capillary loops into the cornea.

Posterior keratitis

This will result from anterior luxation of the crystalline lens, resulting in damage to the corneal endothelium and oedema of the deeper structures of the cornea. A marked, diffuse and evenly-spread milkiness of the cornea is produced (Plate IV, Fig. 4, facing p. 168). If in existence for any length of time, some opacity will remain even after the successful extraction of the dislocated lens.

Corneal opacity, produced by the deposition of a precipitate on the posterior surface of the cornea, has recently been reported by J. H. Wilkins and his co-workers, associated with the disease termed tropical canine pancytopaenia.

Keratitis sicca

An insufficiency of lacrimal secretion, which may be either congenital or acquired, may affect one or both eyes. Possible causes of acquired types include injuries to the lacrimal gland or chronic inflammatory conditions of the conjunctiva. The condition is seen particularly in the Boston Terrier, Miniature Poodle and Cocker Spaniel.

The conjunctiva becomes red and thickened, with a ropy secretion, and the cornea becomes dry, with numerous defects, taking a light fluorescein staining over the whole surface (Plate IV, Fig. 12, facing p. 168). The condition is similar to xerophthalmia resulting from avitaminosis.

No improvement can be expected in the condition, although it might be possible to control the effects upon the cornea by the use of artificial tears, consisting of $\frac{1}{2}$ to 1% methylcellulose, for the rest of the animal's life.

In those cases where a minimal lacrimal secretion is still present, some benefit may result from the occlusion of the lacrimal puncta by diathermy, in order to preserve in the conjunctival sac any tears that may be present.

Permanent lubrication of the eye can be achieved in cases of keratitis sicca by the transplantation of the parotid duct into the conjunctival sac at the lateral canthus. The lacrimal and parotid secretions would appear to be similar enough to allow this technique to be successful, and the preliminary reports are encouraging. Some epiphora is present postoperatively, especially in association with feeding, but it would seem that, in time, some regulation of the parotid secretion takes place, allowing the eye to be regularly moistened without excessive overflow.

Keratomalacia

Keratomalacia, resulting from a lack of vitamin A, is rare in the dog. It is characterized by desiccation and subsequent necrosis of the cornea and conjunctiva, the conjunctiva at first becoming dry—xerophthalmia— followed by drying of the cornea and subsequent ulceration and necrosis (Fig. 152). Perforation is likely to occur. The epithelium becomes keratinized and stained conjunctival scrapings will show saprophytic bacilli and keratinized epithelial cells.

Treatment consists of the administration of vitamin A, in a daily dose of 25,000 units, and the use of vitamin A drops as a topical dressing, together with any routine ulcer therapy.

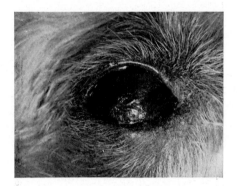
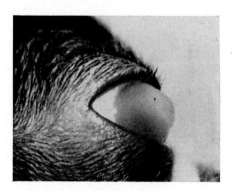

Fig. 152. *Keratomalacia.*   Fig. 153. *Keratoconus.*

Keratoconus

A bulging of the cornea into a cone shape may be due to a weakening of the cornea from trauma, ulceration or nutritional deficiency, or may have genetic origins. Cases have occasionally been seen associated with the keratitis profunda of canine virus hepatitis (Fig. 153). The condition is usually unilateral, not associated with any rise of intraocular pressure, and perforation is rare. Opacity and astigmatism are likely to result, and consideration might be given to the use of a penetrating corneal graft to correct the deformity.

Corneal opacities

Opacities of the cornea are the result of loss of substance, either from epithelium or substantia propria. Permanent scars are associated with the production of fibrous tissue, during the natural process of healing of an ulcer or wound; other opacities may be due to leucocytic or lymphocytic infiltration.

Corneal opacities are classified according to the degree of density as: *nebula*, a faint clouding of the cornea; *macula*, a definite grey opacity; and *leucoma*, a dense white opacity (Fig. 154). If a leucoma should form, with a dark spot in the centre due to attachment of the iris, this is then known as *leucoma adherens*.

The effect of an opacity will, of course, depend on its density and position on the cornea. Many scars appear to have little effect on the visual acuity of the dog. Others, where the cornea is extensively affected, may cause blindness. This is particularly true of the leucoma that may follow chemical injury of the cornea.

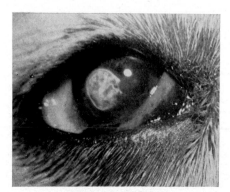
FIG. 154. *Leucoma.*

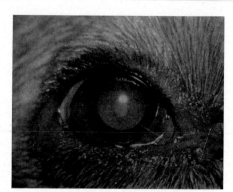
FIG. 155. *Corneal dystrophy.*

For aesthetic reasons, scars may be stained with platinum. The epithelium covering the area to be stained is first removed. This is marked by means of a trephine, cutting through the epithelium, and then outlined by placing a drop of sterile rose bengal on the cornea and washing off with saline. The epithelium inside the trephine cut is then scraped away using a small curette. Finally, the cornea is washed with saline, and the denuded area dried with filter paper. The platinum is applied as a 2% solution of platinum chloride, transferred to the cornea by means of a disc of filter paper, the same size as the trephine, dipped in the solution and placed upon the denuded area of cornea. The platinum is left in place for two minutes, following which it is reduced by means of a freshly prepared 2% solution of hydrazine hydrate, applied at the rate of one drop (0·05 ml) every 3 seconds for 24 seconds. The eye is then washed with distilled water, followed by normal saline, and a dark grey-black colour immediately appears. The staining tends to fade in a year or two and may have to be repeated.

In other cases, it may be possible to remove the defect by employing a corneal graft.

Corneal dystrophy

The corneal dystrophies are rare degenerative disorders of the cornea normally seen in older animals. They are usually bilateral, non-inflammatory and slowly progressive. They result in impairment or loss of vision. Some are hereditary in origin, some follow inflammatory diseases and some are of unknown aetiology (Fig. 155).

In human ophthalmology, several types are recognized—fatty degeneration, marginal dystrophy, zonular dystrophy, familial and hereditary dystrophy, epithelial dystrophy and so on. The various degenerative changes taking place in the cornea of the dog have not been categorized, but cases will be encountered, from time to time, corresponding to types seen in the human subject.

In fatty degeneration, there is a generalized deposition of lipoid material within the stroma and a thickening of the epithelium with some infiltration. Secondary fatty degeneration may result from the transformation of scar

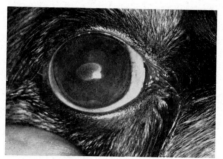

FIG. 156. *Corneal lipidosis.*

tissue. Primary fatty degeneration—corneal lipidosis—has been described in the dog (Fig. 156). Of unknown aetiology, seen most often in the Alsatian, it is exhibited as opacities in the centre of the substantia, 1 to 8 mm in diameter. These opacities, composed of neutral fats and cholesterol, are normally bilateral, although often unilateral in the initial stages, and appear as needle-shaped crystals on biomicroscopy. There is no inflammatory reaction, and in some cases, spontaneous resorption takes place over a number of years.

Marginal dystrophy exhibits a replacement of the corneal stroma by loose connective tissue. In the limbal area the cornea becomes thinner, and there is a bulging of Descemet's membrane. Some irritative signs may be shown.

Zonular dystrophy is often associated with chronic uveitis, and shows a deposition of calcium salts in the superficial layers of the cornea, frequently extending over a considerable proportion of the cornea. Corneal infection and ulceration may occur as a complication.

Familial and hereditary dystrophy is slowly progressive throughout life, and is characterized by the deposition of hyaline material in the superficial lamellae, degeneration of the lamellae, and thickening of the epithelium. Different forms may appear as a diffuse opacity, or as particles or nodules.

Epithelial dystrophy is again slowly progressive and shows hyaline deposits on Descemet's membrane, corneal oedema, epithelial degeneration and defects. Complete opacity of the cornea may follow, and the epithelial defects may lead to secondary infection and ulceration.

KERATOPLASTY

Corneal transplantation or keratoplasty has been practised in human ophthalmology, in some form or other, for nearly 200 years and great advances in the technique have been made in the last two decades. The procedure entails the replacement of an unhealthy area of cornea by a homograft of healthy cornea; the donor graft may be obtained from a cadaver or an enucleated eye.

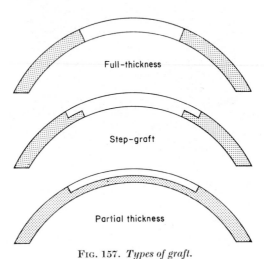

FIG. 157. *Types of graft.*

A true graft is possible with the cornea, for a transparent graft retains the normal structure of the cornea and, with the exception of the nerves, most of the tissue constituents probably survive. Some degeneration of the elements of the graft takes place in the early stages, giving rise to a characteristic opacity, but later, new cells from the host invade the donor tissue and in many cases the graft will clear. Failure of a graft is manifested by opacity and not rejection by the host. The reason for this is not understood, but it may be due to an antigen-antibody reaction.

The types of graft that may be used are either penetrating, full-thickness grafts, or lamellar, non-penetrating, partial-thickness grafts, or a combination of the two, the so-called 'mushroom' grafts (Fig. 157). Lamellar keratoplasty carries a considerably lower operative risk than full-thickness keratoplasty where, in the dog, the graft is more liable to be dislodged. The size of the graft will depend on the area of diseased cornea that is to be removed. Generally, however, penetrating grafts in the centre of the cornea, will rarely exceed 5 to 7 mm diameter, whereas lamellar grafts will vary from 5 to 10 mm in diameter. Total grafts of the entire cornea are rarely successful.

Indications. Optical indications for corneal grafting would appear to be absent in the dog, except possibly in rare cases of bilateral keratoconus, and cosmetic grafts will rarely be utilized. The main indications would appear to be corneal dystrophies, leucoma formation, thermal and chemical burns, certain types of keratitis and ulceration, and certain neoplasms.

A lamellar graft is normally used to replace superficial scars, but a penetrating graft will be required if the scarring reaches Descemet's membrane. Lamellar grafts may be used to hasten the healing of corneal burns, and in cases of recalcitrant ulcers. They may also be used as a preliminary to a penetrating graft, to improve the nutrition of the cornea and to have a trophic effect on the adjacent recipient cornea.

The guiding factor in corneal grafting is the presence of corneal vascularization and its extent, depth and age. In the absence of any vascularization the prognosis is favourable, whereas in its presence, particularly if it affects the deeper tissues, the chance of a successful outcome is greatly diminished. Unfortunately, the condition of keratitis pigmentosa is not suitable for grafting operations, for the graft will certainly become vascularized and pigmented itself.

Other contraindications include xerosis, active infections and the presence of any anterior uveitis, which may be aggravated by the operation, and glaucoma, where grafting may cause a rise in tension. Factors which favour success are a surround of normal corneal tissue, no anterior synechiae, and no vascularization.

Donor eyes. Either cadaver eyes, or eyes enucleated for some other disease not involving the cornea, may be used as donors. Cadaver eyes should be removed within 10 hours of death, and may be stored in a refrigerator at 4°C (39°F), placed in sterile liquid paraffin in a sterile, wide-mouthed stoppered jar. The donor graft should be taken from the centre of the cornea. Whenever possible, the donor graft should be used as soon after the death of the donor as the circumstances permit.

FULL-THICKNESS GRAFTS

General anaesthesia is essential for all keratoplasty operations in the dog, and this, together with a consideration of sedation, asepsis, operating conditions, illumination and instruments, is discussed in chapter 4 which deals with operative technique.

If possible, miosis should be maintained during penetrating keratoplasty operations. It is, as a general rule, easier to obtain and maintain than mydriasis, it allows for better vision of the anterior chamber, and the closed iris affords some protection to the lens. Retraction of the eyelids must be maintained without pressure on the eyeball, and suitable retractors for this purpose are discussed elsewhere. Movements of the eyeball while trephining is in progress may be prevented by the use of suitable fixation forceps, such as those of Barraquer-Llovera.

Type and size of graft. A penetrating graft may be either round or square, although the cylindrical graft is usually used. In addition, it may be made in the form of a step-graft, in order to obtain a more secure closure of the anterior chamber. The graft should always be placed in the centre of the cornea and whenever possible adjacent to normal corneal tissue. The thicknesses of both donor and recipient corneas should be as nearly equal as is possible. The maximum diameter of full-thickness graft likely to be successful is 7 mm and sometimes, 5 or 6 mm will suffice.

Centering the graft. The graft is most accurately centred by measuring the diameter of the cornea with Castroviejo's calipers (Fig. 66, p. 67). The horizontal and vertical measurements divided into two, after the subtraction of the trephine diameter, allow the marking of four points on the cornea to indicate accurately the trephining area. For marking, the points are dipped in dye.

Cylindrical grafts

Many models of corneal trephines are available, that most commonly used being Franceschetti's, available in diameters from 2 to 12 mm (Fig. 158). The cutting depth may be varied by amounts of 0·1 mm. Pairs of trephines, with 0·1 mm difference in diameter are also available, although under normal conditions the same dimensions are kept for both receptor and donor. In human ophthalmology, grafts slightly smaller than the receptor trephine are used when it is intended to increase hypermetropia, and slightly larger when myopia is desirable. All trephines must have a perfect cutting edge, thus ensuring a clean cut which will seal rapidly in a water-tight union.

Preparation of the receptor. Fixation of the globe is maintained with fixation forceps, ensuring that there is no deformity in the globe that might produce irregularities of the section. The trephine is held between the index and middle finger on one side and the thumb on the other. The cutting edge is placed in contact with the corneal epithelium, making sure that the trephine is in the exact vertical position, and the trephining is continued with a rotary movement (Fig. 159A). The trephining is continued until aqueous begins to escape, great care being taken that the incision is not continued too far and risk damage to the iris or lens. In most cases only a small incision will be made in the cornea, and the section will never be completed with the trephine only (Fig 159B).

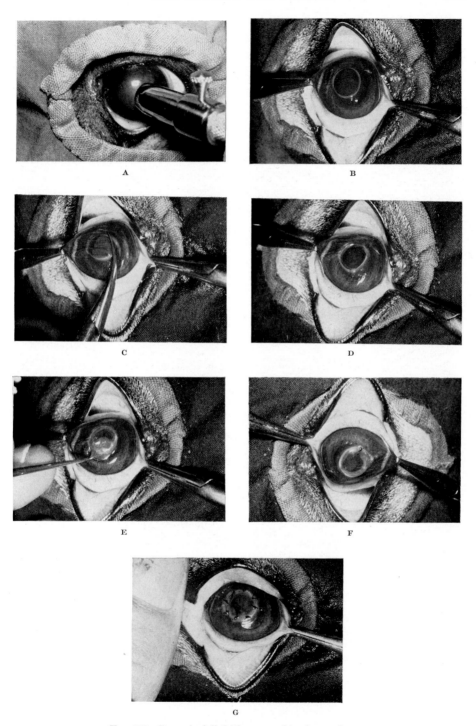

FIG. 159. *Stages in full-thickness trephine keratoplasty.*

Completion of the section is accomplished with either scissors or knife, whilst slightly lifting the disc with forceps (Fig. 159c). Excessive traction on the disc must be avoided or irregularities will result. More accurate sections are obtained by using a knife, and the models of Arruga (Fig. 160) or Barraquer may be used for this purpose. The excised disc is then left in position until the graft is prepared (Fig. 159d).

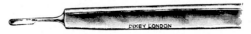

FIG. 160. *Arruga's corneal knife.*

Preparation of the graft. The graft is normally obtained with the same trephine that has been used for the receptor. It is taken from the centre of the donor cornea, the eye being held in the hand whilst the trephine is applied. The trephine is used to complete the whole section, for damage to the iris or lens is of no importance.

The graft should be handled, either by holding the epithelial border with fine forceps, or by using a spatula. It should be washed in saline to remove any particles of aqueous humour, iris pigment or lens material, and then placed in a watch glass, resting on its epithelial surface.

Positioning the graft. The receptor disc is removed and the graft is placed in position, holding the anterior border in fine forceps (Fig. 159e). A perfect fit should be obtained. Before placing the graft in position, the receptor area may be cleaned gently with a small brush.

Suturing. Needles used for graft suturing are normally 4 to 7 mm long and, to avoid unnecessary trauma, must have fine points, perfect edges and be highly polished so that they run smoothly. The curvature of the needle must be such that will enable the cornea to be entered close to the wound margin and yet avoid penetration of the parenchyma. Needles with the cutting edge only on the convexity, such as those of Vogt-Barraquer, are generally preferable to those with both edges sharp, such as those of Castroviejo. In the latter case, any tilting of the needle whilst it is penetrating the cornea is likely to cause the suture to cut-out.

When using such small needles, it is essential that suitable needle holders and suturing forceps be used as well. Fine needle holders (Barraquer) (Fig. 53) and fine forceps (Barraquer) (Fig. 46) are best used with needles of 4 or 5 mm. More robust needle holders (Castroviejo) (Fig. 52) and forceps (St. Martin) (Fig. 45) may be used where needles of 7 mm are employed.

The suturing materials must be fine. Those most commonly employed are Kalt silk (0·09 to 0·1 mm) or Barraquer pure silk (0·04 mm). The latter is probably better tolerated by the tissues.

The sutures are regularly oriented around the graft, great care being taken that none of the sutures enters the anterior chamber, and that there is no resulting deformity of either graft or receptor cornea. The first one is placed in the 12 o'clock position (Fig. 159F), followed by those in the 6, 3 and 9 o'clock positions. When these four sutures are positioned, the remaining sutures are placed regularly between them. The number of sutures employed will depend to a certain extent on the size of the graft, but, bearing in mind the possibility of postoperative interference by the patient, the number of sutures required will always be large. Using Kalt silk, a minimum of 12 sutures may be employed; using Barraquer silk, up to 24 may be required (Fig. 159G).

The epithelial surface of the graft is held with forceps in the 12 o'clock position where the first suture is to be applied, and the needle is held at right angles to the needle holder, and as close to its eye as possible. The needle is introduced into the epithelial surface of the graft, near to the holding forceps, and approximately 1 mm from the edge of the graft. It emerges in the centre of the cut surface of the graft, and is then introduced into the centre of the sectioned corneal edge. After travelling through the corneal tissue, it emerges approximately 1 mm beyond the section in the corneal epithelial surface. Before penetrating the receptor cornea, the forceps are moved from the graft edge to the corneal epithelial edge. The sutures are tied only sufficiently tightly to close the wound accurately, avoiding any distortion.

The ends of the sutures are cut to approximately 2 mm long. Care must be taken that none of the cut ends enter the wound and so delay healing.

Wound protection. Following the completion of the suturing, the eye is irrigated with warm saline to remove any debris and may, if necessary, be cleaned with a small brush. Atropine may be applied to dilate the pupil and so help to prevent synechia formation. Antibiotic drops are used and, if there is any inflammatory reaction, a subconjunctival injection of cortisone may be given.

The value of bandages in the dog is doubtful, because of the difficulty of application in this species, and the increased interference that they will often evoke in the dog. The most satisfactory protection may be obtained by using a conjunctival flap.

Step grafts

A step graft allows a more perfect closure of the anterior chamber and is probably a safer technique for application to the dog.

The details of general technique are identical to those used with a cylindrical graft, but a special trephine is required, such as Appolonio's (Fig. 161), which has an external guide concentric with the trephine and of the same diameter as the trephine used for the section of the anterior layers. The two trephines used will normally differ in diameter by 1 to $1\frac{1}{2}$ mm.

Preparation of the graft (Fig. 162). The trephine used for the section of the anterior layers (normally of 7 mm diameter) is regulated so that the piston depth is 0·3 mm and the anterior layers of the cornea are incised to this depth. A wing, approximately 1 mm in width, is then dissected around the whole of

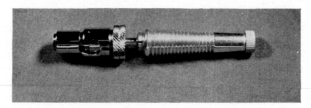

FIG. 161. *Appolonio's trephine for step grafts.*

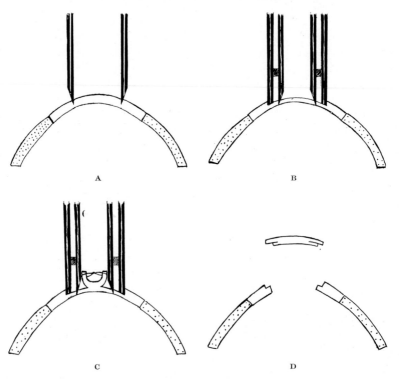

A   B

C   D

FIG. 162. *Step keratoplasty. (After Rycroft)*

the perimeter of the trephine incision, and at a uniform depth of 0·3 mm using a pyriform spatula as in lamellar keratoplasty.

A continuous suture is then placed in the free edge of the dissected wing so that, when it is tied, the edge folds upwards. The smaller trephine (usually 5·5 mm) is then placed on the eye, with the folded portion inside the barrel, and rotated so that a disc is cut. The disc is removed, washed, and placed in a dish.

Preparation of the recipient eye. Using the same trephine, with the piston in the same position, the superficial layers of the cornea are incised to a depth of 0·3 mm, and this part is dissected away using the pyriform spatula.

The guide is then placed on the eye so that it coincides exactly with the bed of the previous resection, the inner trephine is regulated so that approximately 0·3 mm project over the border of the guide, and the posterior layers of the cornea are sectioned. The disc is removed with the aid of a small knife as in cylindrical grafting.

The graft is placed in the recipient cornea, and should fit the prepared bed well. Using small (4 mm) needles, the graft is secured with a minimum of 8 sutures.

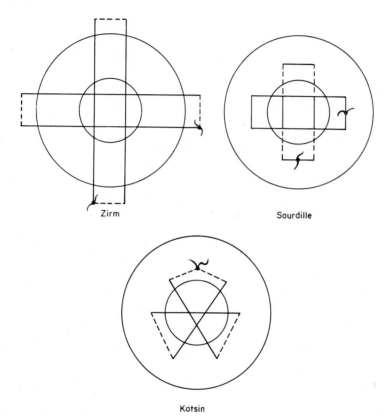

FIG. 163. *Types of bridge sutures.*

Alternative techniques for fixing the graft

Edge to edge techniques will normally be employed in the dog, because of the greater security offered. However, the instrumentation involved, and the handling of the tissues necessary, may cause damage to the edge of the graft and consequent faulty healing. For these reasons, some authors have recommended other techniques for the fixation of the graft by means of bridge sutures.

Bridge sutures may be either continuous or interrupted, inserted in the limbus or close to the graft. Interrupted sutures are easier to apply, and the consequences of breakage at one point are not necessarily serious. On the other hand, continuous sutures exert a more even pressure. For the application of bridge sutures, curved needles with about 10 mm of curvature are used, together with 6/0 silk or cotton.

Zirm's suture utilizes two perpendicular U-sutures, inserted parallel to the limbus, whereas Sourdille's suture is similar but inserted as near as is possible to the graft. Katzin's clover-leaf method is a continuous method allowing firm fixation of the graft. Many other modifications of bridge sutures will be found (Fig. 163).

To protect the edges of the graft from erosion by the threads and to spread the pressure more evenly, egg membrane may be interposed between the graft and the sutures. The egg membrane may be prepared by boiling a fresh egg for one hour, cooling, and peeling the membrane from the shell. Using sterile instruments, discs of membrane are cut with a trephine, of a size slightly larger than the graft. These discs may be kept indefinitely in absolute alcohol. Before use, the disc is washed in saline and a few small cuts are made around the periphery to ensure a good fit to the cornea.

Postoperative treatment

If a conjunctival flap has been used, this may begin to recede about six to eight days after the operation. It should be released by about this time if it has not receded. Daily cleansing of the lids should be carried out, and steps taken to prevent any self-mutilation by the patient. Antibiotic drops should be used routinely, and cortisone ointment 1·5% should be applied at each dressing; in this dosage it does not interfere with healing. If there are signs of excessive irritation, corticosteroids may be given systemically.

The corneal sutures are removed only when the wound is well healed. This will depend on the size of the graft, but will usually be around 15 to 20 days in small grafts and up to 30 days in larger grafts, provided there is no irritation from the sutures. Many of the sutures will be extruded spontaneously.

To avoid any possible opening of the wound, suture removal should always be carried out under general anaesthesia and with full asectic precautions. Great care should be taken, using very fine forceps to hold each suture, and special small spring scissors to cut the silk (Fig. 164). Pure silk can be visualized by staining it with a drop (0·05 ml) of a solution of methylene blue, 0·06%, or sulpha green 1%. If there is any evidence of conjunctival or iris irritation at this stage, a subconjunctival injection of cortisone may be given. Installations of cortisone may be maintained for days or months after the operation, according to the degree of the resultant reaction, and should continue well beyond the time of apparent absolute normality.

Operative complications

Most complications will arise from faulty trephining—off-centre or oblique sections—and this will result in bad coaptation of the wound edges. Damage to the iris will inevitably result in haemorrhage, which may necessitate the abandonment of the operation. Damage to the lens, if slight, may not be noticed, but any appreciable damage should be followed by irrigation

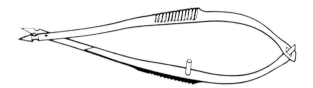

FIG. 164. *Suture removing scissors.*

to remove as much soft lens tissue as possible, and the injection of sterile air. Loss of vitreous may follow in aphakic eyes or in cases of lens luxation. Penetrating sutures should be removed and replaced.

Postoperative complications

Most postoperative complications result from faulty coaptation of the graft, or faulty suturing. Penetrating sutures may lead to fistula formation and delay in the reformation of the anterior chamber. Faulty sutures or fistulas may often be demonstrated with the use of fluorescein.

Anterior synechia formation, more common with step grafts, may respond to the alternate use of miotics and mydriatics, or may need separation using a Bowman's needle. Postoperative hypertension may follow anterior synechiae. Iris herniation will necessitate the incision being opened well beyond the area of prolapse, replacement of the iris and resuturing. Displacement of the graft, due to defective fixation, may require its replacement with a new graft; ectasia of part or the whole of the perimeter of the graft is more common and will require resuturing.

Infection is a rare complication, but keratitis may result in some cases, rendering the graft opaque, caused by the disease which was responsible for the original opacity of the cornea.

Biological complications, due to an immune response in the recipient to the transplanted cornea, are characterized by vasodilatation in the limbal area, oedema of the cornea, corneal vascularization and opacity of the graft. Early necrosis of the graft may be seen in some cases. Such complications are more likely to follow the insertion of a large graft, or if the host cornea is vascularized. Provided treatment is started at an early stage, corticosteroid therapy may save the graft; other cases will require a new transplant.

LAMELLAR KERATOPLASTY

Non-penetrating lamellar keratoplasty, although a more difficult operation to perform than a penetrating graft, is safer and even if the visual results are not so marked vision will rarely be worsened by the operation. Complications arising during and after the operation are not so frequent, and it is possible to repeat the operation, or follow it with a penetrating graft at a later stage.

This operation is indicated particularly in superficial lesions of the cornea, where the deeper layers of the cornea are clear, such as traumatic superficial keratitis or chemical burns, superficial leucoma following corneal ulceration, and corneal dystrophy.

In most cases, a central lamellar keratoplasty will be indicated, varying in size from 4 to 9 mm, usually 6 to 7 mm. The graft must be cut of equal thickness throughout and great care must be taken not to penetrate the anterior chamber.

Preparation of the graft site. The details of general technique, anaesthesia and conservation of the donor eye are the same as with a penetrating graft. As a preliminary step, the centre of the cornea is marked using a cystitome (Fig. 165), the tip of which has been dipped in gentian violet (Fig. 166A). The size of the graft required is measured with calipers and a suitable trephine is chosen.

Preparation of the graft bed. The piston of the trephine is adjusted to give the desired depth of incision, the eye fixed with forceps and the trephine applied vertically to the cornea. Quick complete turns of the trephine are made and the depth of the incision is checked with a fine cyclodialysis spatula (Fig. 166B). The incision is repeated until the required depth is reached, carefully avoiding penetration of Descemet's membrane. Direct sutures are usually indicated in canine surgery, but if indirect sutures are to be used, these are now inserted.

Using a Paufique's knife (Fig. 167), the splitting of the posterior corneal layers is begun by sliding the knife into the trephine incision and cutting the corneal substance with small lateral movements (Fig. 166c). The segment that is thus freed is then held by fine forceps and lifted, allowing the remaining corneal layers to be split with a small Desmarre's scarifier (Fig. 168). Small movements of the instrument are required and the cornea will split along the natural lines of cleavage (Fig. 166D).

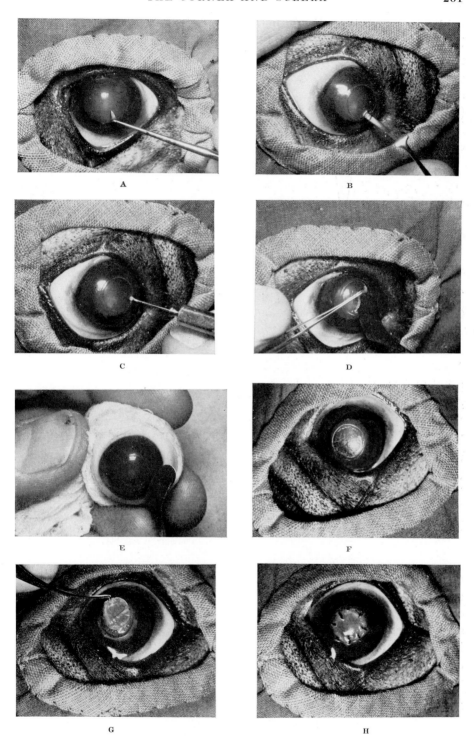

FIG. 166. *Stages in lamellar keratoplasty.*

If a deep graft is required, the Desmarre's knife is used to cut obliquely into the corneal substance, until the level of Descemet's membrane is reached. A small amount of aqueous is then evacuated from the anterior chamber by puncture at the limbus, thus allowing the cornea to become slightly flattened and preventing the bulging of the thin posterior layers (Fig. 169). Any haemorrhage from small vessels in the graft bed is best controlled by cauterization with a heated spatula point, or small electro-cautery.

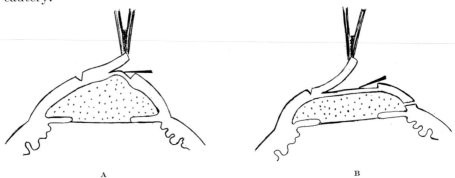

A   B

FIG. 169. *Puncture of the anterior chamber to reduce the risk of penetration.* (*After Rycroft*)

Preparation of the graft. The donor eye is held by hand, in a swab, and is trephined in the same way as the recipient cornea, using the same trephine adjusted to the required depth.

Using a large Desmarre's scarifier, the cornea is incised obliquely 1 mm beyond the trephine incision (Fig. 166E). The oblique incision is continued until the blade enters the desired depth at the bottom of the trephine incision, the blade is then turned horizontally, and the cutting is continued, by small to-and-fro movements, until the opposite edge of the trephine incision is reached. Alternatively, an accurate incision may be made by using the knife of Franceschetti and Bock (Fig. 170).

The graft is placed, lying on its epithelial surface, on moistened gauze.

Fixation of the graft. The bed of the graft is first washed to remove debris or small blood clots (Fig. 166F). The graft is then placed into the bed and smoothed with a spatula to remove any air bubbles (Fig. 166G). Edge-to-edge sutures, 6 to 8 in number, are used to fix the graft, using 6/0 silk on suitable needles (Fig. 166H). It is probably easier and less traumatic, to insert the sutures in the graft before it is completely detached from the donor eye. Alternatively, indirect sutures, applied over an egg membrane, may be employed. A conjunctival flap may be used to give added security. Antibiotic drops and atropine complete the operation.

Postoperative treatment. The details of postoperative management closely follow those advocated for penetrating grafts. Sutures are removed on the seventh day.

Operative complications. The anterior chamber may be opened, either by the trephine incision, or during the splitting of the cornea. If the opening is only very small, it may be possible to continue cautiously. If the opening is large, the operation must be abandoned until a later date, replacing the corneal disc, or a penetrating keratoplasty must be performed.

Postoperative complications. Complications less commonly follow lamellar keratoplasty than penetrating grafts. Infection is unlikely to occur in the dog, and cases of keratitis or corneal vascularization should be treated immediately with corticosteroids or β-rays. Openings in the anterior chamber may lead to delayed reformation of the chamber or synechia formation. Displacement of the graft will require resuturing or replacement. Haemorrhage in the graft bed may occasionally occur, and the use of heparin drops in such cases is recommended. Local areas of necrosis are usually absorbed, and biological complications are less likely to be exhibited.

KERATECTOMY

Small, very superficial lesions of the cornea, not warranting a corneal graft, may often be treated successfully by means of a keratectomy (Fig. 171).

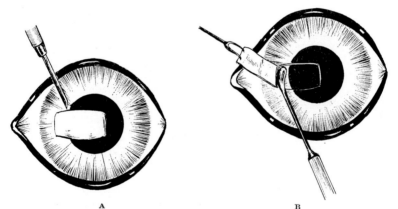

FIG. 171. *Partial superficial keratectomy.* A *stage 1,* B *stage 2.*

A partial superficial keratectomy is carried out by first outlining the area of cornea to be incised with the point of a cataract knife or, in the case of a circular lesion, with a trephine. The outline is marked by installing a drop of dye.

Cleavage of the cornea, in the desired plane, is commenced with a cataract knife, and continued with a Desmarre's scarifier. The edge of the excised area may be held, and lifted as the dissection proceeds, with a fine hook (Fig. 57, p. 65). Following the keratectomy, the eye is covered with the membrana and this is left in place for 10 to 14 days. No adhesions between cornea and membrana are likely to occur.

Removal of corneal epithelium

The corneal epithelium may be removed in cases of recurrent corneal erosion or where there are multiple small foreign bodies in the epithelium.

The epithelium, which is loosely attached to Bowman's membrane, may be easily stripped off by grasping with fine forceps, over the affected area, as far as the limit of normal, well-attached epithelium. Regeneration of the epithelium is rapid under normal conditions, and a membrana flap may be used to prevent self-inflicted damage.

Fixation of globe in corneal surgery

The performance of surgical procedures upon the cornea is sometimes rendered difficult by virtue of the limited access available in many dogs. The tendency for the eyeball to rotate under anaesthesia, retraction of the globe, the protrusion of the nictitating membrane, and the loose nature of the bulbar conjunctiva, are all factors which hinder the approach.

W. G. Magrane has described the production of artificial proptosis, using a strabismus hook (Fig. 59, p. 65), and this method, in addition to making the cornea more accessible, also tightens the bulbar conjunctiva and reduces haemorrhage from the vascular limbal area. The procedure is easy to perform in the Pekingese, Pug, Boston Terrier, Cocker Spaniel and Alsatian, but, in other breeds, a preliminary canthotomy will probably be required.

To proptose the eye, the hook is inserted underneath the nictitating membrane, in the area of the inferior rectus muscle. The eylids are spread with the fingers, and the eye proptosed by exerting pressure on the hook in a lifting manner. Once proptosed, the eye may be held in this position by the application of clip-on rat-toothed forceps. There is no danger to the eye in this procedure, the extraocular muscles allowing this degree of movement.

The strabismus hook, applied in the same manner, may also be used to rotate the eyeball in any direction, so that the limbus at any point, or the inferior aspect of the globe, may be made accessible.

Once the eye is correctly positioned for the procedure in-hand, it may be maintained, without movement, by the application of fixation forceps, or by the use of stay sutures placed in the body of either the superior or inferior rectus muscle. Stay sutures may be maintained in position by clipping them to the drapes with bulldog forceps.

Proptosis performed in this manner should never be used where intra-ocular operations are to be performed. In such instances, prolapse of the intraocular structures would be likely and accurate corneal sectioning and apposition would become difficult.

Tumours of the cornea

Tumours of the cornea are rare and invariably secondary to primary tumours of the uvea. A primary epithelioma of the cornea of the dog has been described, however, affecting the upper layers of the cornea only (Fig. 172). In such cases, surgical excision might prove possible, or the tumour might be removed by a penetrating corneal graft.

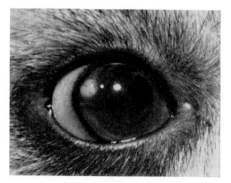

FIG. 172. *Epithelioma of the cornea.*

OCULAR NODULAR FASCIITIS

A recent report (Bellhorn & Henkind) describes a subconjunctival nodular growth, arising at the limbus, composed of bundles of connective tissue, with capillaries, fibroblasts and strands of collagen. The tissues involved were the corneal stroma and sclera but not the overlying conjunctiva. This lesion, which has been termed ocular nodular fasciitis, was successfully excised, and it is suggested that it must be differentiated from neurofibroma and fibrosarcoma.

DISORDERS OF THE SCLERA

Scleral injuries

The sclera is seldom involved in infections or inflammatory processes, and even injuries are not common. Trauma, causing injury to or fracture of the orbital ring, may result in bruising of the sclera. Other causes of injury may include bites, shotgun wounds, pellets from air-guns or balls thrown towards the eye. Rupture of the sclera, usually at the corneoscleral junction, may be associated with prolapse of the eyeball, usually in the Pekingese. Posterior staphylomata are rare in animals, but have been reported in young animals suffering from calcium deficiency.

Perforating wounds of the sclera require similar treatment to wounds of the cornea, but suturing is difficult in the posterior areas. Rupture of the eyeball, with ciliary prolapse, will usually necessitate the removal of the eyeball. This course will prove necessary if the injury is extensive, if there is damage to the lens, if there is much loss of vitreous or prolapse of uveal tissue, if there is a large retained foreign body, or if an endophthalmitis develops. In those cases in which the injuries are not too serious, treatment will consist of wound toilet, the removal of contaminated tissue, suturing where possible, the use of conjunctival flaps and of antibiotic therapy.

Scleritis

Inflammation of the sclera—usually of the superficial layers, an *episcleritis*—is most often associated with a uveitis. In the course of uveal infection, a hyperaemic condition of the sclera in the perilimbal area may sometimes be exhibited.

Local inflammatory lesions of the episcleral tissues, nodular in character, with a full overlying conjunctiva, have been occasionally noted in the dog. Although the aetiology of such lesions is not understood, they probably represent a collagen degeneration. A favourable response, in such cases, is often obtained with corticosteroid therapy, but relapses are common.

Ectasia of the sclera

Ectasia of the sclera will occur in cases of buphthalmos and hydrophthalmos. In such instances, the sclera appears thinned, and the underlying uveal tissue gives it a blue appearance over the area of the ciliary body. On occasion, the sclera may bulge in areas that are particularly weakened.

Congenital posterior ectasia of the sclera in the Collie has been described. Further consideration is given to this under the ectasia syndrome (page 341).

13

THE UVEAL TRACT

ANATOMY AND PHYSIOLOGY

The intermediate coat of the eye, known as the uvea, uveal tract or tunica vasculosa, consists of the choroid, ciliary body and iris, and is characterized by the presence of numerous blood vessels and pigment cells. The iris is separated from the cornea by the anterior chamber, whereas the choroid and ciliary body are adherent to the sclera.

The choroid forms the posterior part of the uveal tract, separating the sclera from the retina. It is a vascular, pigmented membrane, which absorbs any light that passes through the retina and which is not reflected by the tapetum. It is approximately 0·1 mm thick around the optic nerve and around the ora ciliaris, and approximately 0·2 mm thick where it is associated with the tapetum.

The choroid is attached loosely to the overlying sclera, and is separated from the sclera by a potential space, the perichoroidal space. The two layers are connected by delicate strands from the superficial layers of the choroid blending with the lamina fusca of the sclera. The lacunae between the strands form the perichoroidal lymphatic spaces. Posteriorly, around the optic nerve, and anteriorly, where the ciliary muscle fibres are inserted into the scleral spur, the choroid is attached more firmly to the sclera.

Histologically, four layers of the choroid are usually described. The superficial layer—the suprachoroid—is composed of delicate fibres passing from choroid to sclera. These lamellae consist of structureless endothelial membranes, supported by a reticulum of elastic fibres, containing many large pigment cells filled with black-brown granules of melanin pigment.

The vessel layer consists of an outer layer of large vessels, which is prominent in the dog, and an inner layer of small vessels. Arteries and veins are present, but the majority of vessels present are veins, the arteries breaking up into capillaries. The veins are arranged in whorls—the vortices—and pass out through the sclera as the vortex veins.

Between the two layers is a layer of medium vessels in which is situated the elastic reticulum containing the tapetum. This is a reflecting layer which serves to reflect light that has passed through the retina back to the receptor cells in that structure, so that a double stimulus is received. This tapetum —the tapetum lucidum—is composed of a number of layers of flattened, irregular cells, with doubly refractile crystals, and is responsible for the brilliant luminosity that is seen when the animal faces a light at night. In the central areas, 9 or 10 rows of cells may be present, but towards the optic nerve and the periphery of the choroid the number of layers gradually decreases.

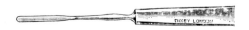

Fig. 173. *Iris repositor.*

The tapetum, which develops soon after birth, varies greatly in colour, even within a single breed, and even within an individual's two eyes. Normally, the colour is within the range of gold to pale green, shading off towards the periphery into browns and mauves. The shape, also, varies in different breeds and in different individuals, but is normally triangular or almost semicircular, with the base straight and lying horizontally at the level of the optic disc. The apex is situated at the upper outer posterior quadrant of the eye, and the tapetum normally extends to a little more than half-way to the periphery of the choroid. In some cases, an area free of tapetum will be found around the optic nerve head. The capillaries joining the two vascular layers pass through the tapetum.

The lower part of the tapetum—the tapetum nigrum—lies in the lower part of the fundus, and is normally distinctly separated from the tapetum lucidum by a difference in coloration. Normally it is of a chocolate colour but may contain large masses of black pigment.

The capillary layer of the choroid, which is not well differentiated in the dog, consists of a network of capillaries connected with a stroma, and serves as the nutritional layer for the retina.

The innermost layer of the choroid—Bruch's membrane—is a structureless, noncellular layer, not easily demonstrable, approximately 1 μ thick, bordering on the pigment layer of the retina.

The ciliary body is wedge-shaped in section, lying between the iris and the choroid, attached to the internal surface of the sclera. The inner surface is in contact with the vitreous, and it projects to form a barrier between this body and the posterior chamber. The anterior part of the ciliary body forms the root of the iris and, laterally, helps to form the angle of the anterior chamber. The junction of the ciliary body and choroid forms the ora serrata,

or ora ciliaris retinae. The posterior two-thirds is smooth, and is known as
the pars plana. The anterior third—the pars plicata—forms the surface of
attachment of the zonular ligaments, and shows an irregular surface bearing
the ciliary processes.

The ciliary body is a highly vascular, highly muscular structure, innervated, via the parasympathetic, by the third nerve. It provides the contraction necessary to alter the shape of the lens, and so provides accommodation. Relaxation of the ciliary muscle tightens the suspensory ligaments, and so reduces accommodation. Contraction of the ciliary muscle
relaxes the suspensory ligaments, thus allowing the lens to assume the
shape dictated by its elastic capsule and so increase its curvature. The
degree of accommodation in the dog is limited.

The structure of the ciliary body is similar to that of the iris. The outer
part contains the ciliary muscle, composed of unstriped fibres, which
encircles the eye within the ciliary body, forming a sphincter. The inner,
vascular region, extends into the ciliary processes, composed mainly of veins,
continuous with those of the choroid. Each ciliary process, of which there are
70 to 80 in the dog, is from 1·5 to 2·5 mm in length. Between the veins is a
network of connective tissue, and the ciliary processes have an overlying
Bruch's membrane. Covering this is an epithelial layer, continuous with the
retinal pigment layer.

The hyaloid membrane ramifies between the ciliary processes and is
reinforced, over the ciliary body, by the addition of some radial fibres. The
union of hyaloid membrane and fibres from the ciliary body—the ciliary
zonule—divides into two parts, the posterior of which remains as the hyaloid
membrane, the anterior of which forms the suspensory ligaments.

The iris forms the anterior part of the uveal tract, arising from the anterior
portion of the ciliary body, and is the disc perforated by the pupil. The
pupil, which is circular in the dog, varies in size according to the amount
of light entering the eye, adjustments in the size being made by the contraction of its sphincter or dilator muscles. Separating the iris from the cornea
is a mushroom-shaped space—the anterior chamber; between the iris and
the lens, against which the iris rests lightly, is a very shallow space—the
posterior chamber. By virtue of the convexity of the lens, the iris is pressed
very slightly forward.

The iris may be divided into two distinct zones: the narrow inner ring
—the pupillary zone; and the main outer ring—the ciliary zone. The inner
edge, forming the pupil, is known as the collarette. At its outer edge, the iris
is continuous with the ciliary body and the cornea, via the pectinate ligaments. The thickness of the iris varies from approximately 0·5 mm at the root
to 0·01 mm at the collarette.

The iris is highly vascular and in most dogs pigmented, the colour varying
in the majority from yellow to brown, often with more heavily pigmented

areas. The posterior surface is more irregular in appearance, and is heavily pigmented.

Two muscles are present in the iris structure, the sphincter muscle and the dilator muscle. The sphincter muscle encircles the pupil, extending almost to the tip of the pupillary edge. It reduces the size of the pupil by contraction and is innervated by a branch of the motor root of the third nerve. The dilator muscle, which is well developed in the dog, extends from near the root of the iris towards the pupillary edge but without encroaching upon it. This muscle dilates the pupil and is innervated by the sympathetic nerves.

The arterial blood supply of the iris is derived from the posterior ciliary arteries, the upper and lower branches of which lie in the horizontal meridian of the iris. These proceed to the ciliary portion of the iris in a ring-like manner at about the height of the margin of the lens, where they send numerous strong branches posteriorly towards the ciliary body, and only weaker vessels to the region of the sphincter. The arterial 'ring' formed in the iris by the circulus iridis arteries, following a circular course within the iris, is extremely well-developed in the dog. The terminal branches, however, do not anastomose and a complete ring does not exist in the dog. The veins of the iris are comparatively weak and are unevenly distributed.

Histologically, the iris may be divided into four layers. The anterior endothelium consists of a single layer, continuous with the posterior endothelium of the cornea, composed of flattened cells, which are largely absent over the numerous crypts. The stroma, consisting of loose connective tissue, contains the sphincter, vessels, nerves, pigment cells, plasma cells and wandering cells; in addition, some collagen fibres are present, and small cells with oval nuclei and branching processes—the chromatophores. These latter cells tend to cover over the vessels and nerves, particularly in the anterior parts of the iris, giving the iris its characteristic coloration. The vessels, having a thick adventitia, tend to stand out on the surface of the iris as ridges; between the ridges, where the stroma is less thick and where the chromatophores are less numerous, the relative absence of pigment gives the iris its characteristic furrowed appearance. Tissue fluid occurs in the stroma, entering the stroma, through pores, from the aqueous humour. This transfer of fluid, from aqueous to iris, is concerned with the function of the iris, and not with the disposal of aqueous. Entry of the fluid occurs through semipermeable membranes, and not by any open connections. The presence of tissue fluid within the iris stroma allows rapid displacements of different parts of the iris as changes in the size of the pupil take place. The posterior stroma (Bruch's membrane) is the dilator muscle which originates in the ciliary muscle and the pectinate ligament. The posterior epithelium, composed of two layers of cells, is heavily pigmented.

THE FUNCTION OF THE IRIS

The two muscles controlling the movements of the iris—the sphincter muscle and the dilator muscle—are innervated reciprocally; one contracts as the other relaxes, although, of the two, the sphincter would appear to be the stronger. Both cholinergic and adrenergic (inhibitory) fibres innervate the sphincter, through the parasympathetic system, and it is probable that reflex dilatation of the pupil is due to inhibition of the sphincter as well as to circulating sympathetic agents.

The purpose of pupillary contraction is to regulate the amount of light entering the eye, dependent upon the retinal adaptation that is present; to increase the depth of focus for near objects; and, to a lesser extent in animals, to reduce optical aberrations, in daylight.

Pupillary reflexes

The light reflex, evoked by light falling on the retina, produces constriction of the pupil—miosis. This miosis will affect both eyes, even if the light source falls on only one eye. The degree of miosis will depend on both the intensity of the light and on the adaptation of the eye—an eye which has already become accustomed to a certain light will respond less markedly to further light stimulus. Stimulation of both eyes at the same time produces a more rapid miosis of a greater degree. Should the stimulation from a certain light source be maintained, a degree of dilatation will take place, until the pupillary size is that shown normally for that particular intensity. Full constriction of the pupil under conditions of intense light is reached more rapidly than is full dilatation—mydriasis—under conditions of darkness.

The light reflex is initiated by the rods and cones, the impulse being sent via the optic nerve to the superior corpora quadrigemina and thence via the oculomotor nerves to the ciliary ganglion, the ciliary nerves and the sphincter pupillae. Pupillary dilatation is effected by the sympathetic nerves, via the superior cervical ganglion, the gasserian ganglion and the ciliary branches of the nasociliary nerve.

The near reaction produces miosis when looking at a near object, in man. In the dog, however, accommodation produces dilatation of the pupil.

The trigeminal reflex, evoked by stimulation of the cornea, conjunctiva or eyelids, produces constriction of the pupil.

The psychosensory reflex produces mydriasis in association with fear, pain, anger or excitement.

THE ACTION OF DRUGS ON THE PUPIL

Pupillary dilatation may be produced by cycloplegic drugs, such as atropine, homatropine, eumydrine and hyoscine, which act as parasympathetic antagonists by paralysing the nerve endings of the third cranial nerve in the sphincter pupillae and also in the ciliary muscle. These are, therefore, parasympatholytic drugs, and of these, the only mydriatic, as distinct from cycloplegic, is eucatropine hydrochloride.

Sympatheticomimetic drugs, producing pupillary dilatation, include phenylephrine hydrochloride, adrenaline and cocaine.

Pupillary constriction, due to parasympathetic stimulation, may be produced by such drugs as acetylcholine, choline, pilocarpine and muscarine. Eserine, prostigmine and di-isopropyl fluorophosphonate (DFP) produce miosis by preventing the breakdown of acetylcholine by choline-esterase. Constriction due to the stimulation of smooth muscle may be elicited by histamine, ergot and morphine.

Mydriasis and Miosis

Mydriasis will be exhibited following the use of drugs in the dog, as outlined above; when the lens or cornea have increased density and thus hinder the passage of light to the retina; where there is retinal degeneration; hypertension resulting from injury to the eyeball; luxation or subluxation of the lens; poisons such as belladonna or strychnine; and in hysterical states.

Unilateral mydriasis may result from disease, injury to or neoplastic conditions involving the oculomotor nerve. Involvement of both oculomotor nerves will produce bilateral mydriasis. Lesions of the cerebral cortex do not produce mydriasis. The condition of *anisocoria* or unequal size of the two pupils, must always be regarded as pathological. A persistent unilateral mydriasis is usually indicative of glaucoma.

Miosis will be produced by drugs, as outlined above; in cases of acute keratitis, corneal ulceration and uveitis; when the intraocular pressure is lowered; in some diseases of the brain and spinal cord; and following the use of compounds containing morphine.

A pupil of normal size that fails to either dilate or contract is usually indicative of posterior synechia, or atrophy of the iris.

INJURIES TO THE UVEA

The iris may become lacerated as the result of trauma or iridodyalysis may occur. In either case, a hyphaema or fluid level of blood in the anterior chamber is likely to be the sequel.

Either direct or indirect injury might cause haemorrhage from the iris, and, in most cases, the resulting hyphaema will be absorbed within a few days, without complications, and without treatment. In such cases, atropine should not be administered, for the subsequent dilatation of the pupil is likely to cause narrowing of the filtration angle as well as a limiting the area of iris available through which reabsorption can take place. Extensive or repeated haemorrhages may result in secondary glaucoma.

Haemorrhages of the choroid are normally reabsorbed slowly. Although uncommon, they will occasionally be seen, on fundal examination, as dark brown masses underneath an elevated retina.

Injury to the iris may occasionally be manifested as an iridodyalysis, the tearing away of the iris root from the ciliary body. The resulting distortion of the iris shows as a black segmental hole at the periphery and an alteration in the pupillary shape due to the pull of the pupillary sphincter. The periphery of the lens may sometimes be seen through the gap, together with a segment of the ciliary processes. All wounds of the iris, however caused, show little tendency to repair, probably due to the rapid removal of fibrin by the aqueous humour.

Haemorrhages within the iris have recently been reported associated with tropical canine pancytopaenia.

PROLAPSE OF THE IRIS

Deep penetrating wounds of the cornea may result in prolapse of the iris and its incarceration in the wound (Figs. 174, and 131, p. 156). Similarly, prolapse may follow intraocular procedures, where a limbal or corneal incision has been used, particularly in those cases where adequate wound suturing has not been employed.

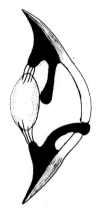

FIG. 174. *Iris prolapse.*

Only in the very earliest of cases can a prolapsed iris be persuaded to return to its normal position by the application of miotic drugs such as eserine; in a few other early and mild cases, the iris can be repositioned by means of a repositor (Fig. 173) and the cornea sutured. After a very short time, however, the prolapsed iris becomes firmly adhered to the lips of the wound and simple repositioning is no longer possible. When this occurs an abscission (cutting off) of the protruding part of the iris may be necessary, the remainder of the iris being returned to the anterior chamber and the wound repaired. Such a procedure in the dog, however, is likely to be followed by extensive haemorrhage and hyphaema; in many instances it is preferable to leave the prolapse in position, protecting the wound by means of a conjunctival flap until such time as the wound has healed and the prolapsed part sloughed away. A resulting anterior synechia is inevitable, but this is often preferable to an intractable intraocular haemorrhage and the ensuing complications.

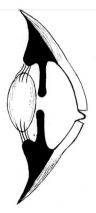

Fig. 175. *Keratocele.*

DISEASES OF THE UVEAL TRACT

Congenital abnormalities of the iris

Most congenital abnormalities of the iris, whilst encountered from time to time in the dog, are uncommon; some are extremely rare. Although the majority are of little clinical importance, they do, nevertheless, form an interesting group of defects.

Albinism is seen particularly in the Collie, Shetland Sheepdog and Great Dane, and hereditary factors may be involved (Fig. 176). There may or may not be associated retinal albinism, but the condition is rarely associated with defective vision.

Heterochromia iridium, in which the two irises show a marked difference in colour, is not uncommon, and has no pathological significance (Fig. 177). In some cases, the difference in coloration is confined to a section of one iris; a difference in the coloration of the iris is apparent, producing spots of a colour other than the basic colour of the iris.

Anaridia or complete absence of the iris, is rare. In some instances, the whole iris may be absent, exposing the margin of the lens and its zonule

(Fig. 178). In such cases, there may be associated retinal defects, or photophobia may be exhibited. In most cases a thickened iris root is present, which, since it lies in the filtration angle of the anterior chamber, may lead to glaucoma.

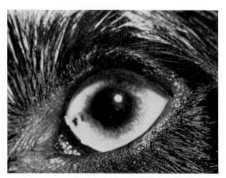

Fig. 176. *Albinism of the iris.*

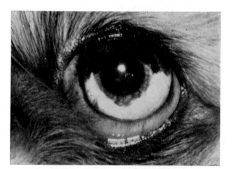

Fig. 177. *Heterochromia iridium.*

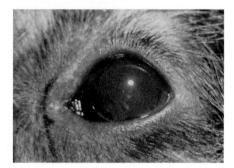

Fig. 178. *Anaridia.*

Coloboma, a condition where part of the iris is lacking, is not uncommon. It produces many variations in pupil size and shape. Colobomata, which may be hereditary in origin, are developmental defects due to imperfect closure of the foetal cleft, and therefore tend to occur along the lower nasal or lower temporal sectors of the eye. Since the foetal fissure is normally closed before the formation of the iris, those occurring in this organ are atypical and may occur in any meridian.

Colobomata of the iris may be unilateral or bilateral, and may involve whole sections of the iris. More commonly, a wedge-shaped or circular section may be missing; or several portions of the pupillary edge may be deficient, giving the pupil a trifoliate, oblong or square outline. Such defects are normally termed notches (Fig. 179A). On other occasions, the edge of the pupil may be intact, but one or more apertures may appear in the width of the iris, sometimes exposing the periphery of the lens or the zonule—the so-called 'hole in the iris' (Fig. 179B). In other cases, the coloboma is confined to the iris root—iridodiastasis.

Persistent pupillary membranes are encountered regularly in the dog's eye (Fig. 180). Embryologically, the membrane is derived from the iris mesenchyme, constituting the anterior vascular sheath for the lens, and forming a delicate membrane stretching across the pupil. The membrane persists in early postnatal life, but atrophies and normally disappears by the age of 5 weeks. Where the atrophy is not complete, parts of the membrane persist as fine strands attached to the lesser circle of the iris. These strands may be attached only to the anterior surface of the iris, or may span the

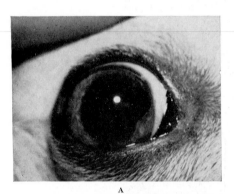 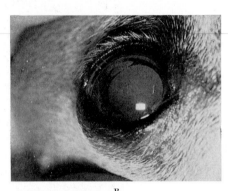

A   B

Fig. 179. *Coloboma of the iris showing* A *notches,* B *hole in the iris.*

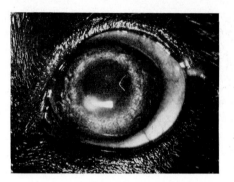

Fig. 180. *Partial persistent pupillary membrane.*

pupil. In other cases, they are inserted into the anterior lens capsule, or may form congenital anterior synechiae, running from iris to the posterior surface of the cornea. These membranes are normally of no significance and cause no inconvenience to the animal concerned.

In rare instances, remnants of the capsulo-pupillary vessels, which pass around the equator of the lens, uniting the pupillary membrane with the posterior vascular sheath of lens (derived from the hyaloid supply), may persist. When present, they occur as strands of connective tissue passing from the lens equator to the limbus, and their presence may be responsible for the development of coloboma of the iris or lens.

An inherited form of persistent pupillary membrane, probably associated with an autosomal dominant gene, has been described in the Basenji by Dr. Roberts. Both sexes are affected. In severe forms, bands arise from the minor arterial circle of the iris and cross the pupil to insert in other parts of the circle, or pass from iris to cornea, or from iris to lens. The mildest forms show star-shaped scars in the cornea, in the region of Descemet's membrane, which may be visible only by biomicroscopy. Some dogs show dense scars in the cornea; in other cases, only a prominence of all or part of the embryonic vessels is exhibited. Dogs showing minor lesions only may produce stock exhibiting larger lesions, and affected stock tends to show a high increase of embryonic defects of the median or paramedian suture lines, such as hernia.

Epicapsular stars, star-shaped, pigmented deposits on the anterior lens capsule, representing a residue from the foetal pupillary membrane, are occasionally seen in the dog.

Iridodenesis, or trembling of the lens, may, on rare occasions, be exhibited in the young Sealyham or Wire-haired Fox Terrier, indicating a weakness in the suspensory ligament of the lens, and being a certain sign of luxation of the lens at a later date.

Iris cysts of congenital origin are rare. Pigmented, they appear as black nodules attached to the iris and hanging in the anterior chamber, sometimes occluding the pupil. On other occasions they may be seen, through the thickness of the iris, attached to the posterior surface, appearing as irregularly circular areas of increased density (Plate V, Fig. 1, facing p. 224). Such cysts arise from the posterior pigmented layers of the iris and originate through a persistence of one stage in embryonic development, where the cavity in the optic cup fails to close completely. Congenital iris cysts may be single or multiple, and may vary in size from $\frac{1}{4}$ to 1 ml. Occasionally they may become detached from the iris and float free in the anterior chamber. Most appear semitransparent and show a fine pigmented reticulum on the surface; others may be opaque and darkly pigmented. Cysts, whether fixed or free, normally cause no discomfort or other change within the eye; but sometimes an iridocyclitis may develop, or multiple free cysts may lead to secondary glaucoma from blockage of the filtration angle. Such cysts may be removed through a limbal incision, allowing them to float out with the escaping aqueous. Cysts attached to the iris are normally best left alone, for their removal might lead to excessive haemorrhage from a damaged iris.

UVEITIS

Inflammation of the iris (iritis), ciliary body (iridocyclitis) and choroid (choroiditis) are conditions that are usually coexistent, although any one of the three parts of the uveal tract may be affected primarily. Nevertheless, the adjacent tissues of the tract are always involved in an inflammatory

15

reaction of one part, even though this may not be clinically obvious. It is, however, not always possible to differentiate the various conditions clinically. On the other hand, it is most important to distinguish between an acute iritis and an acute glaucoma, for the treatment of these two conditions will be very different.

Clinical signs. The signs of an anterior uveitis may be somewhat variable, and will often be unilateral. Cases of iritis exhibit an engorgement of the episcleral vessels, particularly in the region of the ciliary body, producing

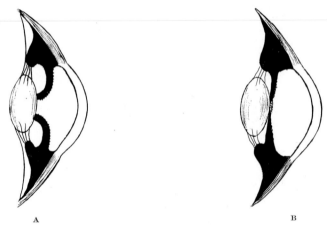

A   B

FIG. 181. A *Secluded pupil*, B *occluded pupil.*

brick-red circumcorneal injection, as distinct from the conjunctival injection of a conjunctivitis. If, however, the congestion is marked, some engorgement of conjunctival vessels may also be noted. The pupil is contracted, due to spasm of the sphincter and engorgement of the iris with blood, and the iris is immobile, dull and swollen (Plate V, Fig. 2, facing p. 224). In the early stages, the presence of cells floating in the aqueous may be detected with a slit-lamp, and later leucocytes may gravitate to the bottom of the anterior chamber, producing a hypopyon. Such a condition is most likely to be seen in cases of iritis following deep corneal ulceration. The increased protein content of the aqueous produces atypical opalescence—the 'aqueous flare'. Occasionally, the formation of keratic precipitates (K.P.s) may be seen —small masses of leucocytes, visible as greyish spots on the posterior surface of the cornea. These precipitates are produced by leucocytes circulating in the aqueous becoming adhered to the oedematous corneal endothelium, which is continuous with the endothelium of the iris. In some cases, the root of the iris may adhere to the corneal endothelium at the filtration angle, due to the existence of congestion of the tissues and adherent exudate. Such anterior peripheral synechiae may hinder aqueous drainage and lead to glaucoma. At the same time, exudates may form on the anterior surface of the lens, to which the iris may adhere, particularly at the pupillary margin, producing posterior synechiae. In the early stages of an exudative iritis, these synechiae may affect only small areas of the iris margin, but at a later stage, the whole of the pupillary circumference may become adhered to the lens, producing a *secluded pupil* (Fig. 181A). In other cases, where the pupillary aperture is small, the pupil may become blocked with exudate, producing an *occluded pupil* (Fig. 181B). In either case, the aqueous which is being secreted by the ciliary body and posterior surface of the iris is unable to find its way into the anterior chamber. In this event, the posterior chamber will become distended and the iris will become ballooned forwards, the so-called *iris bombé* (Plate V, Fig. 3, facing p. 224). Some rise of intraocular pressure is likely to follow pupillary adhesions of this type in cases of acute

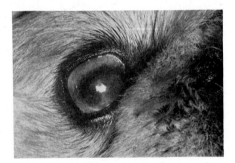

Fig. 182. *Phthisis bulbi.*

iritis, but in more chronic cases, tension is more likely to be low, either due to atrophy of the ciliary body and deficient aqueous production, or due to the posterior surface of the iris becoming completely adhered to the anterior surface of the lens. In most cases of acute iritis, in the early stages, the intraocular tension is lowered, but will rise if an iris bombé should develop, or if the filtration angle should be blocked with exudate. In cases where the ciliary body is damaged and aqueous production is diminished, the tension will be low, leading to atrophy of the eyeball and phthisis bulbi as the eyeball shrinks (Fig. 182). (Although the term 'phthisis bulbi' is more often used, this should properly be reserved for shrinkage following perforating injuries. Atrophy following damage to the ciliary body should be termed 'atrophia bulbi').

Clinical symptoms that may be exhibited in cases of acute iritis include pain, photophobia, lacrimation and blepharospasm.

Inflammation of the ciliary body (cyclitis) cannot be differentiated clinically, and most cases amount to an iridocyclitis. In cases where the ciliary body is deeply involved the engorgement is likely to be more intense, and exudate is likely to become attached to both the anterior and posterior surfaces of the lens.

Inflammation of the choroid, choroiditis or posterior uveitis, is uncommon in the dog, but may be associated with an anterior uveitis. Such cases are likely to be accompanied by exudation into the vitreous, varying from deposits on the posterior surface of the lens to dense exudation obscuring the picture of the fundus when viewed with an ophthalmoscope. Three types are said, traditionally, to occur—diffuse, disseminated and circumscribed. In the diffuse type, early changes in the colour of the fundus are, in the dog, masked, by the tapetum, but at a later stage, the optic papilla becomes white and the retina shows light-coloured spots and streaks, sometimes accompanied by areas of retinal detachment. In the disseminated type, irregular greyish spots are found, the size of the optic disc, separated by areas of normal fundus. In the circumscribed type, only a small area of the fundus is affected, producing a circular patch.

Differential diagnosis. An acute, painful, congested eye is presented in cases of acute iritis, acute conjunctivitis and acute glaucoma. Differentiation of these three conditions is important, and the following criteria may be used:

Signs	Acute glaucoma	Acute iritis	Acute conjunctivitis
Iris	Congested Dull, Discoloured	Dull Discoloured	Normal
Pupil	Dilated Immobile	Contracted Irregular	Normal
Pupillary reflex	Reduced	Reduced	Normal
Anterior chamber	Clear Shallow	Normal depth Exudate	Normal
Cornea	Oedema Insensitive	Transparent Exudates	Normal
Congestion	Circumcorneal Purple	Circumcorneal Brick-red	Conjunctival Pink
Tension	Increased	Normal (sometimes high or low)	Normal
Tenderness	Marked	Marked	Normal
Pain	Severe	Moderate	Some discomfort
Photophobia	Slight	Marked	Slight
Secretion	Lacrimation	Lacrimation	Watery, mucoid or purulent
Vision	Reduced	Reduced	Normal

Complications of iritis. Complications that may arise due to iritis include secondary glaucoma, anterior or posterior synechiae formation, secondary cataract, secondary retinal detachment, endophthalmitis, vitreous opacities and corneal opacity.

Secondary glaucoma may arise from blockage of the filtration angle with exudate, by fibrinous deposits in the angle, or by anterior or posterior synechiae. Secondary cataract may result from interference with lens nutrition. Corneal opacities due to persistent corneal oedema may be permanent.

Sympathetic ophthalmitis. Bilateral uveitis, usually following a perforating wound, involving uveal tissue in one eye only, occurs in man but has not been recorded in the dog.

Aetiology of uveitis

Uveitis may be either secondary, or exogenous in origin, or may be primary or endogenous.

Exogenous uveitis may follow perforating wounds of the cornea or eyeball, or may be a sequel to corneal ulceration or intraocular surgical manipulations. Such cases may result in an endophthalmitis which, in turn, may result in either a panophthalmitis or a phthisis bulbi. Such cases of uveitis are secondary to some exogenous infection, or may be the result of the spread of allergic inflammation.

Endogenous uveitis may be either infective (granulomatous) or allergic (nongranulomatous). Granulomatous uveitis is usually chronic, associated with tissue destruction and replacement with granulation tissue. In such cases, specific organisms invade the uvea. Little is known about specific causes of uveitis in the dog, but many organisms have been incriminated in various case reports. These include virus hepatitis, distemper virus, leptospirosis, toxoplasmosis, cryptococcosis, coccidioidomycosis, blastomycosis and tuberculosis. Many cases of choroiditis or choroidoretinitis are probably associated with toxoplasma. Nongranulomatous uveitis is usually acute, producing the typical acute iritis, and may be considered to be an allergic reaction to bacterial allergens, produced at a focus of infection elsewhere in the body. Such a focal infection may exist in teeth, tonsils, sinuses, prostate gland or uterus.

Treatment of uveitis

Prompt dilatation of the pupil should be effected by the use of atropine, or one of its substitutes; administration may be by means of a 1 % solution or ointment, or subconjunctival injections may be used if a more rapid effect is required. Mydriasis paralyses the ciliary muscles, thus relieving pain from muscle spasm, and giving rest to the uveal musculature; in addition, a dilated pupil will prevent the formation of central posterior synechiae.

In cases of nongranulomatous uveitis, where there is no actual infection of the uvea, corticosteroids will limit the inflammatory response and may be administered locally or subconjunctivally; in very severe cases, systemic corticosteroids may be employed.

Specific treatment must be employed for any underlying causal disease, and, in cases of uveal infection, subconjunctival antibiotics should be considered.

Paracentesis of the anterior chamber will reduce the severity and duration of an attack, by allowing the entry of fresh aqueous with a high antibody content. The operation may be repeated daily, but the increased

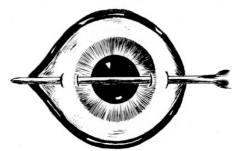

Fig. 183. *Operation for iris bombé.*

fibrin content of the aqueous produced after repeated paracentesis may be responsible for the formation of adhesions. This technique is of particular value where an early secondary glaucoma develops due to blockage of the filtration angle.

Iridectomy is sometimes advocated in cases of acute uveitis, but this is contraindicated in the dog because of the ensuing haemorrhage and the trauma inflicted on an already inflamed tissue. In cases where an iris bombé has formed, however, it may be necessary to perform an iridotomy, transfixing the ballooned iris with a narrow cataract knife, introduced at the limbus, so that the resulting puncture holes in the iris allow the escape of aqueous from the posterior into the anterior chamber (Fig. 183).

Protein shock therapy, by the use of foreign proteins, has been suggested as a useful additional measure, particularly in slowly progressive types. Sedatives may be given to relieve ocular pain, and the salicylates may be of value in the allergic type of uveitis.

DEGENERATIONS OF THE UVEA

Essential iris atrophy is a rare, usually unilateral condition of unknown aetiology. Some cases may occur as a sequel to uveitis, whereas other cases may occur as a result of the increased intraocular pressure in glaucoma.

In this condition the tissues of the iris atrophy, forming large adjoining holes, until eventually most of the iris tissue is lost. In such cases, peripheral anterior synechiae are likely to form, leading to a glaucoma. In most cases, therefore, where an iris atrophy and a glaucoma are both present, it is difficult to decide whether the atrophy is the cause, or the result of, the increased tension.

Iris erosion or iridoschisis, may appear in old animals as a senile dystrophic change. The erosion usually effects both eyes, producing similar, but more diffuse, lesions to those seen in essential iris atrophy.

Iris cysts are uncommon in the dog and although usually benign, they may lead to either an iritis or a glaucoma. Cysts of the posterior epithelium of the iris, resulting from inflammatory changes, may appear in the pupillary margin, and must be distinguished from melanomata. Implantation cysts may appear on the anterior surface of the iris, when active epithelial cells are transplanted on to this area from perforating wounds or operative incisions.

TUMOURS OF THE UVEA

Tumours of the uveal tract, although relatively uncommon in the dog, are not rare. They may involve the iris, the ciliary body, the choroid, or a combination of these structures. Most involve the ciliary body or extensive areas of the uvea, tumours confined to the iris only comprising less than 10% of all uveal neoplasia.

Benign tumours are less common than malignant tumours, and only a very few have been recorded in the veterinary literature. Those that have been noted include adenoma of the iris, haemangioma of the iris, and epithelioma of the ciliary processes arising from the nonpigmented epithelium. It is often difficult to be certain, clinically, that a uveal tumour is benign, but in some cases, surgical removal is possible, without recurrence.

By far the most common pigmented malignant tumour is the malignant melanoma, which usually affects the ciliary body, but may sometimes be situated in the choroid or iris, or may involve the whole tract. In most cases, only one eye is affected and secondary glaucoma may develop. A malignant melanoma affecting the uveal tract may be primary, or may arise as a metastasis from some other area such as the oral mucosa. Primary malignant melanoma is itself likely to metastasise to such areas as the brain, lungs, heart or kidneys, or it may invade the sclera producing extrabulbar extension of the growth (Fig. 184). In a few cases, where only the iris is affected, it may be possible to carry out treatment by means of an iridectomy. In most cases, however, enucleation is indicated, before metastasis has taken place.

Other primary malignant tumours of the iris, that have been recorded, include lymphosarcoma, adenocarcinoma, sarcoma and melanocarcinoma.

Primary malignant tumours of the ciliary body that have been noted include carcinoma (Plate V, Fig. 4), leiomyosarcoma and melanosarcoma.

Secondary malignant tumours have been noted on many occasions, and these include neurogenic sarcoma and angiosarcoma of the iris, adenocarcinoma (from tonsil and pancreas) of the ciliary body, rhabdomyosarcoma and adenocarcinoma (from the kidney) of the choroid.

Involvement of the uveal tract by lymphosarcoma may occur as a late manifestation of the disease. In most instances, the anterior uvea is involved, and this may lead to glaucoma and infiltration of the cornea. Primary lymphocytic lymphosarcoma, affecting the iris and ciliary body of both eyes, has also been recorded.

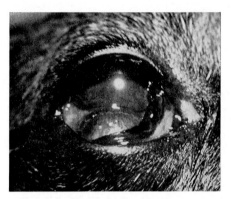

FIG. 184. *Exteriorized uveal melanoma.*

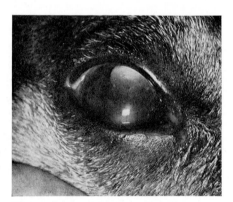

FIG. 185. *Distortion of pupil from uveal tumour.*

Secondary involvement of the uveal tract by the transmissible venereal tumour has also been noted, and it has been concluded that the eye may be a site of predilection of metastases of this particular tumour.

Recognition of uveal tumours is usually straightforward, for in most cases, the cornea remains clear, at least in the early stages. The presenting signs will, of course, vary with the type of tumour, its position, and its rate of growth. In most cases, some irregularity of the pupil will be presented together with some loss of the anterior chamber (Fig. 185); the iris will show thickening or folding, with increased pigmentation; there will usually be some episcleral congestion and a rise in intraocular pressure; and the sclera may become ectatic at the site of the tumour if this is in choriod or ciliary body.

SURGERY OF THE IRIS

Because of the highly vascular nature of the iris of the dog, surgical interference with this structure is likely to result in severe haemorrhage. Difficulty may be experienced in many cases in controlling this haemorrhage,

PLATE V

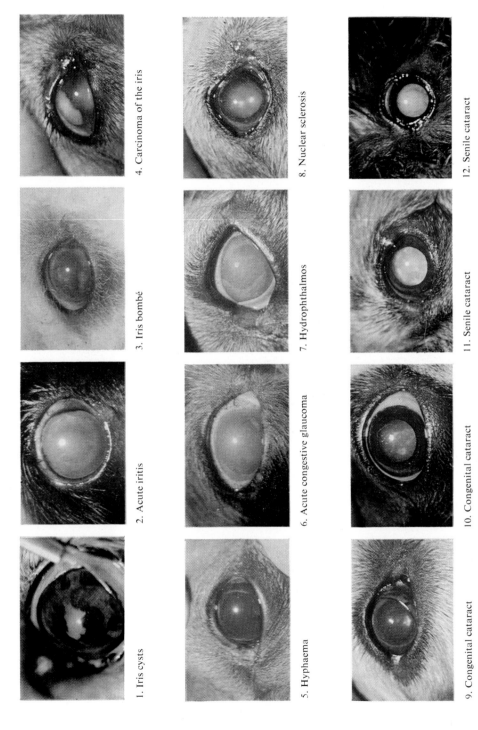

1. Iris cysts

2. Acute iritis

3. Iris bombé

4. Carcinoma of the iris

5. Hyphaema

6. Acute congestive glaucoma

7. Hydrophthalmos

8. Nuclear sclerosis

9. Congenital cataract

10. Congenital cataract

11. Senile cataract

12. Senile cataract

and operations upon the iris should be avoided unless strictly necessary for the well-being of the eye. All surgical interferences involving the use of cutting instruments upon the iris are contraindicated, and an electrocautery or diathermy should be used for this part of the operation. Some difficulty may be experienced in using such instruments whilst, at the same time, avoiding their adhesion to the iris; should adhesion occur, the release of this is likely to result in further haemorrhage.

Iridectomy

The removal of part of the iris, iridectomy, is a technique used in some instances of cataract removal, to increase the operational area; in the removal of cysts or neoplasms from the iris; in cases of prolapse of the iris; in

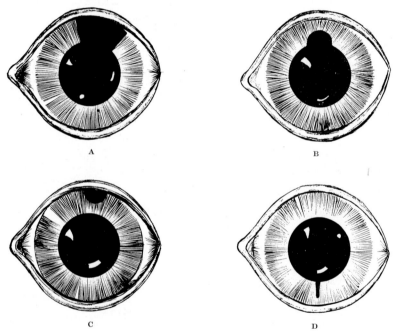

FIG. 186. *Iridectomy.* A *complete*, B, *pupillary*, C *peripheral*, D *sphincterectomy*.

some glaucoma operations; and in cases of occlusio pupillae. An iridectomy may be complete, pupillary or peripheral. Complete iridectomy signifies that a segment is removed from the pupillary border to the base of the iris (Fig. 186A). Pupillary iridectomy signifies that a portion is removed from the pupillary margin (Fig. 186B). Peripheral iridectomy signifies that part of the root of the iris is removed (Fig. 186c).

The eye is prepared, the lids retracted and the eyeball fixed as for any intraocular operation. With the eye held slightly forward, a keratome incision is made into the anterior chamber, just in front of the limbus, and the keratome is passed into the anterior chamber, parallel to the iris. On withdrawal, the blade is held slightly forward, and removed quickly, so that little aqueous is lost.

Complete iridectomy. Curved iris forceps, such as Lang's (Fig. 187), are passed into the keratome section with their blades closed, and moved towards a point about 2 mm from the pupil margin. The blades are then opened, and the iris grasped with the teeth of the forceps and withdrawn

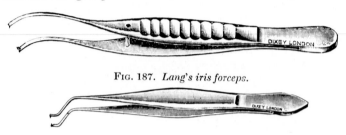

Fig. 187. *Lang's iris forceps.*

Fig. 189. *Barraquer's iris forceps.*

from the wound. To produce a narrow iridectomy of 3 mm or less, the electrocautery is applied along a line joining the centre of the cornea with the centre of the keratome incision. To produce a broad iridectomy of 4 mm or more, the electrocautery is applied parallel to the keratome incision. After the iris has been excised any blood is soaked up with sponges, and if necessary the anterior chamber is irrigated with warm saline. An iris repositor is passed into the incision to replace the iris by stroking towards the centre of the pupil, following which sterile air is injected into the anterior chamber, and atropine is applied.

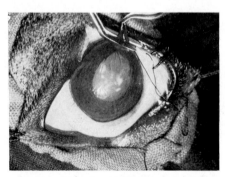

Fig. 188. *Iridectomy.*

Peripheral iridectomy (Fig. 188). Removal of a part of the iris at its base is a technique employed in certain glaucoma operations, particularly the trephine operation; in cataract surgery, to reduce the risks of iris prolapse; and in cases of iris prolapse.

Double-curved iris forceps, such as Barraquer's (Fig. 189), are passed into the incision, and engaged at the root of the iris. A small fold of the iris is lifted from the wound, and a small portion of the iris excised at its root.

Iridotomy

The division of part of the iris may be used in cases of synechiae formation; in an iris bombé; to produce an artificial pupil in cases of occlusio pupillae; or, as a sphincterectomy, to facilitate intracapsular cataract removal and prevent a drawn-up pupil (Fig. 227, p. 279).

Synechiotomy

The division of anterior synechiae may be employed where synechiae are responsible for gross distortion of the pupil and subsequent loss of vision. In this operation, a knife-needle with a 4 mm cutting edge is employed. This is passed into the anterior chamber at the limbus, and the blade carried across so that its sharp edge is in contact with the synechia. The adhesions are severed by sweeping and sawing movements, and the knife withdrawn quickly to avoid loss of aqueous.

CONGENITAL ABNORMALITIES OF THE CHOROID

Absence of the tapetum lucidum. Complete or partial absence of the tapetum lucidum has been recorded in dogs with a dapple coat colour, often associated with other minor ocular abnormalities. The breeds in which this has been noted include the Collie, the Dachshund and the harlequin Great Dane. Some cases have been associated with microphthalmos, general hypoplasia of the uvea or hypoplasia of the choroid.

Coloboma of the choroid. Typical coloboma of the choroid occur in the area of the embryonic foetal fissure, due to arrested development and imperfect closure. Variable in size, they may extend from optic nerve to iris, with a sector-shaped gap running through choroid, ciliary body and iris, and causing an indentation in the lens; or they may involve only a section of the choroid or produce a localized patch in the fundus.

The edges of a choroidal coloboma are normally well-defined, with a floor composed of sclera, which may be ectatic.

Atypical colobomata—clefts appearing in areas other than that of the foetal fistula—may be seen on rare occasions. It has been suggested that such developmental aberrations may result from intrauterine choroiditis during the latter half of pregnancy, possibly due to infection with toxoplasmosis.

14

THE ANTERIOR CHAMBER

THE AQUEOUS HUMOUR

The aqueous humour fills the prelental space of the eyeball, that is, the anterior and posterior chambers. The anterior chamber, which comprises approximately one-fifth of the whole cavity of the eyeball, is bounded in front by the posterior surface of the cornea, and behind by the anterior surface of the iris and the lens in the pupillary opening. The posterior chamber, situated between the posterior surface of the iris and the suspensory ligament of the lens, is very small in the dog, due to the close proximity of the iris to the lens, maintained in close contact with one another.

The aqueous humour, acting as the essential tissue fluid of the eye, furnishes nutrients for the cornea and lens, and is responsible for the entire metabolic changes in these tissues. In addition, it affords support for the cornea; is partly responsible for the correct shape of the eyeball; and by the maintenance of an exact flow, ensures correct and constant level of pressure within the eyeball. The aqueous is not static, but in order to maintain the supply of nutrients has to be constantly formed, removed and replaced.

In composition, the aqueous, which is clear and colourless, roughly corresponds to plasma, except that the protein content is considerably lower. The aqueous is therefore more dilute than plasma. In addition to protein, other contents include fats, sugar, urea and the salts of such ions as sodium, potassium, calcium, magnesium, chloride and phosphate. In addition, hyaluronic acid is present, and also ascorbic and lactic acids, these last two in quantities greater than in plasma. The osmotic pressure is slightly higher than that of plasma.

Secondary aqueous, or plasmoid aqueous, the new fluid that is formed if the aqueous is lost, either through trauma or by surgery, shows a marked increase in protein content, and its composition more nearly corresponds to that of plasma. In appearance it is slightly opalescent and it contains fibrinogen and immune bodies.

The formation of aqueous has been the subject of many theories in the past. A steady flow of aqueous is maintained, from the arterial capillaries, through the anterior chamber and on to the veins by hydrostatic pressure. The fact that there is such a steady flow is shown by the rise of pressure that will follow any obstruction at the filtration angle, and by the way that fluid will collect behind the iris, forming an iris bombé, if the passage of the aqueous through the pupillary opening is closed. In addition to the steady flow, thermal circulation also takes place within the anterior chamber.

The generally accepted theory is that aqueous is formed by the processes of the ciliary body by both secretion and diffusion. It is therefore formed

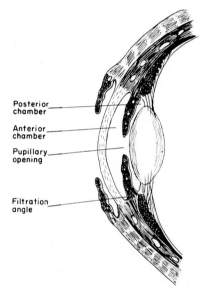

Posterior chamber

Anterior chamber

Pupillary opening

Filtration angle

FIG. 190. *The anterior and posterior chambers.*

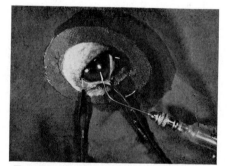

FIG. 191. *Irrigation of the anterior chamber.*

in the posterior chamber, where it flows between the posterior surface of the iris and the anterior surface of the lens into the anterior chamber. Driven out by hydrostatic pressure, it drains directly into the trabeculae at the filtration angle—the recess formed by the junction of the cornea, sclera, ciliary body and ciliary border of the iris, in the anterior chamber. In this area, loose fibrous tissue occurs—the pectinate ligaments—connecting the iris to the cornea. The pectinate ligaments form the framework of the trabeculae, the spaces formed by the trabecular network being known as the Spaces of Fontana. These spaces are comparatively large in the dog, allowing the passage of large particles. A definite drainage canal such as occurs in man (the canal of Schlemm) is not present in the dog. In the latter, the trabecular network is in contact with a venous plexus—the scleral venous plexus or Circle of Hovius—composed of a network of interlacing veins running between the trabecular fibres. The aqueous passes through the trabeculae into the trabecular veins, and hence through the sclera into the episcleral veins and on to the general circulation.

The blood-aqueous barrier. The difference in composition of the aqueous and the plasma indicates the existence of a selective barrier. This is formed by the anterior iris surface, the ciliary epithelium and the retina. Its clinical importance lies in the fact that drugs such as antibiotics, introduced into the body, do not readily pass this barrier and blood levels of any particular substance are no indication of the intraocular level obtained.

Intraocular pressure. The normal intraocular pressure in the dog lies between 16 and 30 mm Hg, considerable variation in the normal occurring in this animal. The maintenance of normal pressure within the eyeball is essential for the health and function of the eye. If the pressure is unduly raised the cornea will become waterlogged; if unduly lowered, folds will develop in Descemet's membrane. In addition, in the dog, the walls of the eyeball readily yield to increases in intraocular pressure, producing a hydrophthalmos.

The intraocular pressure may be measured experimentally with a manometer, by means of a needle inserted into the anterior chamber. This is not possible in clinical practice, and a more usual method is to measure the pressure indirectly by assessing the impressibility of the cornea and sclera. For routine work, digital palpation, with practice, gives a reasonably reliable estimate of the resistance encountered. A more accurate estimation may be obtained by the use of a Schiøtz tonometer, which calibrates the extent to which a plunger, under a known weight, will sink into the cornea.

The measurement of intraocular pressure by digital palpation or by a tonometer is influenced by the rigidity of the cornea and sclera, and some authors have distinguished between intraocular pressure and tension; intraocular pressure referring to manometric measurement of the pressure of the intraocular fluid, and tension referring to the digital or tonometric measurement of the tension of the tunics of the eye.

Hyphaema

The presence of blood in the anterior chamber, either filling the chamber, or producing a fluid level, is known as hyphaema (Plate V, Fig. 5, facing p. 224).

Most cases result from direct or indirect injury to the iris, often of a minor nature, and such haemorrhages are normally absorbed within a few days. No treatment is required in simple cases, and no untoward sequel is likely to result. Only when the haemorrhage is copious or continuous is a secondary glaucoma likely to develop. In such cases, treatment with miotics and carbonic anhydrase inhibitors is indicated and, in cases where the glaucoma persists, or the hyphaema does not resolve, washing out of the anterior chamber will be required.

Other cases of hyphaema may result from surgical interferences, particularly those involving deliberate or accidental damage to the iris or ciliary body. Hyphaema may also be exhibited in some cases of lymphosarcoma or, rarely, in cases of lymphatic leucosis. Intraocular haemorrhage has also been reported in cases of optic disc ectasia and leishmaniasis.

Irrigation of the anterior chamber may be performed through a paracentesis incision, flushing the chamber with saline (Fig. 191). In cases where the hyphaema quickly reforms after such a procedure, indicating capillary leakage, systemic coagulants and vitamin K are indicated.

In the absence of further haemorrhage, blood in the anterior chamber tends to clot quickly in the dog. Such a clot may become organized and form adhesions, leading to iridocyclitis or even phthisis bulbi. In such cases, surgical removal of the clot is indicated, performing a small limbal incision, and removing the clot with forceps, followed by irrigation to remove small residues. If the incision required is large, the cornea must be sutured; small incisions may be covered with a conjunctival flap. Care must be taken, when manipulating instruments in the anterior chamber for the removal of blood clots, so as not to damage the corneal endothelium, or permanent opacities are likely to result.

Recently, a human plasminogen activator (Urokinase, Leo Laboratories) has become available for the treatment of hyphaema. Urokinase is an enzyme with the specific action of converting plasminogen to plasmin. Clots exposed to the action of plasmin dissolve and can be removed by irrigation. In the dry state, the enzyme is stable, and solutions are prepared immediately prior to use and injected into the anterior chamber via a small limbal incision. Dissolution of the clot takes 5 to 15 minutes. Unfortunately, the high cost of this preparation is likely to limit its use in veterinary ophthalmology.

Parasites in the anterior chamber

A case has been recorded (Schnelle and Jones) where the helminth parasite, *Dirofilaria immitis*, occurred within the eye. The presenting signs were photophobia, cloudiness of the cornea, with vascularization and a small pupil. The worm was visible in the anterior chamber.

Similarly, Henry and Lesbouyries recorded the occurrence of a strongyle (*Angiostrongylus vasorum*) in the anterior chamber.

GLAUCOMA

By glaucoma is meant an increase in intraocular pressure. Glaucoma, or ocular hypertension, may, therefore, be indicative of a condition that leads to excessive aqueous production, or of one in which there is an inadequate aqueous drainage. Those cases that cannot be attributed to any definite lesion within the eye are termed primary glaucoma; those that follow a specific eye disease (such as lens luxation) are termed secondary glaucoma. Congenital cases, in which the rise in intraocular pressure is dependent on some malformation of the eye, are generally referred to by the term buphthalmos.

Primary glaucoma

Primary glaucoma would appear to occur only in the Cocker Spaniel in the U.S.A. There is no evidence that such a condition occurs in this breed in Great Britain, nor is there any definite evidence that other breeds of dog can be so affected. Many cases of primary glaucoma that have been noted in the past are undoubtedly of secondary origin, although it is possible that primary glaucoma occurs in Great Britain in the Bassett Hound.

However, in the American Cocker Spaniel undoubtedly an hereditary predisposition to glaucoma exists in some strains, although the mode of inheritance is still obscure. The disease would appear to be more prevalent in females than in males, and the initial involvement appears more often in the left eye. In most cases, the second eye will become involved within one year, although this period may be as short as a few days in some cases. Most cases occur during the period from October to May.

There is some evidence that the predisposition to attacks of acute congestive glaucoma results from a narrow angle between the iris and the cornea, the narrow angle causing obstruction to the escape of aqueous from the anterior chamber. Studies in the U.S.A., by gonioscopy, have shown a narrow or closed angle to be present in affected eyes and in unaffected eyes in the same animals.

In the absence of subjective symptoms, the early diagnosis of primary glaucoma may be made only when there is no other discernible secondary condition within the eye that could lead to an increase in tension.

Secondary glaucoma

Secondary glaucoma, occurring as a complication of some other ocular disease or of damage to the eye, may have either a neurovascular or a mechanical origin. It can result from the obstruction of flow of the aqueous humour; from an increased production of aqueous; or from a combination of both factors.

Secondary glaucoma is fairly common in dogs and, as luxation or subluxation of the crystalline lens is the most common cause, it will be seen most frequently in those breeds in which dislocation of the lens is commonly encountered. Other known causes include uveitis, anterior and posterior synechiae formation, iris atrophy, intraocular neoplasia, intraocular infection, lenticular intumescence and hypermature cataract formation; it may also follow cataract extractions.

Diagnosis of the exact cause of glaucoma is often problematical and a definitive diagnosis is not always possible. In some, advanced, cases, structural alterations within the eye may prove to be the result of, and not the cause of, the glaucoma.

Subluxation and luxation of the lens. The movement of the lens brings it into contact with the ciliary processes, and the subsequent irritation and oedema leads to increased aqueous formation. With anterior luxation, the root of the iris may press against the cornea, partially blocking the filtration angle. If the lens is wholly within the anterior chamber it may itself interfere with the flow of aqueous. A posterior luxation may cause vitreous to be pushed forward into the pupillary space. In other cases, glaucoma may be produced by an induced uveitis. It is thought that some primary cases in Cocker Spaniels may develop luxation later, through prolonged tension increase and stretching of the ocular structures.

Uveitis. This may be a secondary cause of glaucoma or may result in synechiae which produce glaucoma.

Anterior and posterior synechiae. Anterior synechiae, that is adhesions of the iris to the posterior surface of the cornea, result from anterior uveitis or from a perforating corneal wound. Posterior synechiae, that is adhesions of the pupil margin to the anterior lens surface, arise from inflammation of the iris or ciliary body.

Anterior synechiae may obliterate the angle of the anterior chamber. Posterior synechiae prevent the forward passage of aqueous. This is particularly so where the whole of the pupil margin adheres to the lens. In such cases, the resultant iris bombé causes the root of the iris to be pressed against the cornea with subsequent blockage of the angle.

Essential iris atrophy. Although somewhat rare, cases of iris atrophy may result in blockage of the angle with iris debris. Other cases of iris atrophy may be the result of prolonged increased tension within the eye.

Intraocular neoplasia. Both benign and malignant tumours of the uvea may result in blockage of the filtration angle.

Intraocular infection. Any endophthalmitis may cause blockage of the drainage mechanism with debris and cellular exudate; or may result in intraocular adhesions and subsequent secondary glaucoma.

Lenticular intumescence. The swelling or intumescence of the lens, which occurs during the development of a cataract, may result in the anterior chamber becoming shallow and the swollen lens pressing the iris against the trabecular wall. This is likely to lead to a secondary glaucoma only in those eyes exhibiting a narrow drainage angle.

Hypermature cataract. Secondary glaucoma, in such cases, is dependent on liquified lens material leaking out into the anterior chamber, through the

16

capsule of a hypermature, or Morgagnian, cataract. This lens material will provoke a phagocytic response and the engorged cells, having ingested the material, may be carried to the filtration angle where they may cause mechanical blocking. In cases in which rupture of the lens capsule takes place, there may also be irritation from lens particles, or an increase in the protein content of the aqueous may alter the osmotic pressure difference between aqueous and plasma.

Postoperative causes. Glaucoma may follow cataract extraction, due either to iris prolapse, hyphaema, the presence of cortical lens remnants, incarceration of the lens capsule, vitreous prolapse, postoperative uveitis or postoperative oedema.

Wounds, whether traumatic or operative, may produce adhesions and subsequent drainage block; or a downgrowth of epithelium into the wound, so that eventually these cells line the whole anterior chamber, preventing filtration.

Clinical signs

Acute congestive glaucoma is sudden in onset and all the congestive signs are pronounced (Plate V, Fig. 6, facing p. 224). This is the type normally found in the dog, and corresponds to the 'narrow-angle glaucoma' in man. The prodromal stage, the symptoms of which are entirely subjective, is of course absent in the dog, and the stage of evolution is usually sudden in onset. Transient attacks may go unnoticed by the owner, and cases may be presented only when the signs are so exaggerated that the success of treatment is in jeopardy. No one case will exhibit all the characteristics of intraocular tension rise, and cases of primary glaucoma will tend to differ in detail from cases of secondary glaucoma. Certain characteristics are, however, common to all types.

The affected eye is extremely painful, the lids are half closed and the third eyelid is prominent. Examination may be difficult due to blepharospasm, and narcosis or anaesthesia may be required in order to complete the examination. Pain, due to pressure on the ciliary nerves, is not a constant feature, and is, to a certain extent, dependent upon the duration of the pressure rise. Where tension has been exhibited for any length of time, pain is less likely to be shown, but in most cases some pain is apparent on digital palpation.

The cornea, which is frequently insensitive, is cloudy due to oedema and small punctate opacities are often present. Again, this cloudiness of the cornea is more likely to be exhibited in the acute congestive case. In early conditions, the cloudiness of the cornea is reversible if the pressure is decreased; where opacities develop, however, due to folds in Descemet's membrane (a *striate keratitis*), some permanent opaque remnants are likely. Oedema, or opacities, of the cornea may make observation of the fundus difficult or impossible.

The conjunctiva is congested, particularly in chronic cases and those accompanied by hydrophthalmos, and some chemosis may be present. A constant feature in any case of tension rise is congestion of the episcleral vessels, due to distension of the anterior ciliary veins.

A further constant feature is dilatation of the pupil which is insensitive to light. This dilatation is due to pressure on the ciliary nerves, pressure on the sphincter and sympathetic irritation. Where tension is exhibited for any length of time, posterior synechiae may form between the pupillary margin and the anterior lens capsule; when this occurs the pupil will remain dilated even though the pressure be normalized. Full dilatation may cause an alteration in the reflectivity of the eye, and this may especially be noted in cases of acute congestive glaucoma, due to a turbidity of the intraocular media.

Digital tonometry reveals a marked increase in intraocular pressure, and, in unilateral cases, a comparison may be made with the other eye. Alternatively, a tonometer may be used to produce a more accurate estimation of intraocular pressure. In the early stages of glaucoma, little or no loss of vision may be noted, but in more advanced stages or where there are corneal changes, some alteration in visual acuity may be noticed. Transient blindness, in early cases, is reversible if the pressure is reduced. Such blindness may be due partly to cloudiness of the cornea and refractive media, and partly to retinal ischaemia produced by the rise in tension. Tension rises of any great degree, or of any great duration, are likely to lead to permanent damage to vision.

In all cases in the dog, in which a pressure increase is maintained for any length of time, a *hydrophthalmos* is likely to occur whether the glaucoma be primary or secondary in origin (Plate V, Fig. 7, facing p. 224). This enlargement of the eye, due to a gradual stretching of the globe, is sometimes slow and at other times rapid. The progressive enlargement leads to distortion of the cornea and eventually to an exophthalmos. Subsequently, other changes such as interstitial vascularization, pannus formation, pigment deposition or dystrophy may take place in the cornea.

In those patients in which examination of the fundus is possible, atrophy of the optic disc is likely to be noted, the disc becoming greyish, with constriction of the emerging vessels, so that the retina becomes atrophic and devoid of vessels. Some cases, but not all, will show cupping of the optic disc —a depression of the optic nerve head—visible with an ophthalmoscope and produced by a backward yielding of the lamina cribosa, the weakest part of the sclera, where it is perforated by the optic nerve. This does not appear to be a constant feature of glaucoma in the dog, and is most likely to be seen in early acute cases. The cupping appears as a depression of the optic disc, with the blood vessels passing over the edge of the disc, to be only faintly visible at the base of the depression.

Atrophic changes may take place in the iris in chronic cases, so that the iris appears fragmented and thin, and iris pigment may become deposited on the lens capsule or may appear in the anterior chamber.

If not treated, the acute phase may subside, leaving some loss of vision, but further attacks will inevitably take place at a later date. Chronic congestive glaucoma may result from previous acute attacks. The changes in the eye are similar to the acute form, but less intense, and some vision may remain. Noncongestive glaucoma, the so-called 'wide-angle glaucoma' of man, does not appear to have been recorded in the dog.

Absolute glaucoma

Absolute glaucoma will result in complete loss of vision as it develops. The congestive signs are no longer present, although the episcleral veins are

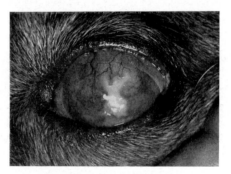

FIG. 192. *Absolute glaucoma.*

more prominent. The pupil remains fully dilated and the cornea is usually clear. Atrophy of the iris and the disc is evident and increased intraocular tension is noticeable. Pain is either absent or periodic and the eye will appear proptosed due to the development of hydrophthalmos (Fig. 192).

Absolute glaucoma is followed by degeneration. The cornea may ulcerate and panophthalmitis may result from corneal perforation. Alternatively, corneal opacities and secondary cataract may develop and the eye becomes soft and shrinks due to atrophy of the ciliary epithelium and the non-formation of aqueous humour.

MEDICAL TREATMENT

The treatment of glaucoma, which may be either medical or surgical, is often unsatisfactory and the development of a hydrophthalmos will often necessitate the enucleation of the eye. Medical treatment is of value in acute congestive attacks, to normalize tension, and is of value preoperatively to make the eye softer and less congested. Medical treatment is often unsuitable as a permanent measure, firstly because it must often be maintained indefinitely, and secondly because the condition tends to recur as soon as treatment is stopped. In acute cases, following the return to normal tension after medical treatment, resort to surgery should not be delayed.

Medical treatment is based on two factors—miotics, to open the angle of filtration and the posterior venous chambers, and to constrict the blood supply of the ciliary body; and drugs given internally—the carbonic anhydrase inhibitors—to inhibit the formation of aqueous. Miotics, of course, can only be successful if the iris is mobile, and not adherent to the lens capsule. Carbonic anhydrase inhibitors do not affect the outflow of aqueous, only its formation, and should be used in combination with miotics. The inhibition of aqueous formation will result in some lowering of the intraocular pressure; in these circumstances, miosis will be more readily achieved.

Miotics that have been used in the past include eserine and pilocarpine, but the degree of miosis that they will produce in glaucomatous eyes is very limited. Newer miotics, such as di-isopropyl fluorophosphonate and demacarium bromide, are more effective, and will often lower, if not normalize, tension, particularly if combined with an inhibitor drug.

The recommended scheme, using DFP, is one drop (0·05 ml) every hour for 4 to 6 installations, followed by twice daily applications which may be maintained for long periods. DFP inhibits cholinesterase, thus enhancing the effect of the natural acetylcholine on the muscles of the uveal tract. It is normally used as a 0·05 to 0·1% solution in oil, aqueous solutions being unstable.

Other powerful miotics, such as demacarium bromide (Tosmilen) and echothiopate iodide (Phospholine iodide) are water-soluble, and exert even a greater effect. Infrequent installation is required, and miosis may often be maintained by one application daily or even every other day.

Topical treatment must in all cases be supplemented by the use of carbonic anhydrase inhibitors. These anti-enzymes reduce the production of aqueous and thus lead to a lowering of the intraocular tension.

Acetazolamide (Diamox) is given in a dose, for a 9 to 14 kg dog, of 125 mg every 8 hours for 3 doses, followed by 125 mg every 12 hours. Side-effects may be exhibited and include nausea, vomiting, anorexia and polyuria. In some cases, these may be controlled by the oral administration of potassium bicarbonate, but, in other cases, it may not be possible to use this drug for prolonged periods.

Dichlorphenamide (Daranide) is given at the rate of 25 mg every 8 hours, for a 9 to 14 kg dog.

Ethoxolamide (Cardrase) may be given to a 9 to 14 kg dog in a dose of 62·5 mg every 8 hours for three doses, followed by this amount every

12 hours. Undesirable side-effects are less likely to follow the administration of these latter two preparations.

These inhibitors, which may be maintained for long periods if necessary, seem to have a variable effect in the dog, being sometimes effective for months, and sometimes only for weeks. Their use is suggested in the initial stages of glaucoma and as a preliminary to surgery.

Urea administered intravenously (Urevert) will produce a dramatic lowering of intraocular pressure and is of value in the acute case. A 30% solution is used, given at the rate of 1·0 g/kg. Glycerine given orally, at the rate of 1·5 ml/kg, has a similar effect in many cases.

SURGICAL TREATMENT

Whilst medical treatment is useful in the early stages, its effect is sometimes only transient, and surgical interference is indicated in order to lower the intraocular tension and preserve vision. Specific surgical procedures are obviously necessary in certain types of secondary glaucoma, as for example in luxation of the lens. In cases of absolute glaucoma, preservation of the globe is sometimes preferred by dog owners to enucleation. Many cases have reached the stage of being absolute before they are presented for treatment, nevertheless many owners will prefer the globe to be preserved if at all possible. The type of surgical interference indicated will vary according to the cause of the glaucoma, to the individual preference of the surgeon, and to the success or otherwise of previous operations.

The principle of all surgical treatment is either to establish an exit for the aqueous through the sclera, or to establish a fistula, through which the aqueous can filter into the subconjunctival lymph spaces or suprachoroidal lacunae. In all instances, and certain procedures in particular, haemorrhage will be experienced if the eye is very congested and occasionally blood clots may block the artificial passage produced. In such conditions therefore, whenever possible, medical treatment should precede surgical interference and the eye should be allowed to become quiet before surgery.

Iridectomy

The classical operation for congestive glaucoma is the 'glaucoma iridectomy' in which a wide area of the iris is excised. Such an iris coloboma will not heal, and the congested iris root is thus prevented from causing obstruction to the drainage angle over the area of excision.

Results from iridectomy, in the dog, are disappointing, but this operation may be indicated in the very early stages of an acute attack of primary glaucoma. In such conditions, where there is a narrow filtration angle, this procedure will help by deepening or opening the filtration angle and allow aqueous escape to the trabeculum. Unless performed in the early stages anterior peripheral synechiae will develop and, whenever this technique is employed, the establishment of permanent drainage by means of a filtering operation will need to be performed at a later date.

An iridectomy is also of value if the cause of the glaucoma is an iris bombé, where it will provide a passage for circulation between anterior and posterior chambers. In such cases, a simple iridectomy through the pupillary border is usually sufficient.

In instances of primary glaucoma, where it is felt that the second eye will be similarly involved at some time in the future, it may be thought advisable to perform a prophylactic iridectomy in the normal eye. However, the fact that the operation is not always successful in preventing an attack in the second eye, and the ever-present risk of haemorrhage in this particular operation, may mean that such a procedure is rarely indicated.

The operation is best performed *ab externo*—a transfixion operation at the limbus is likely to prove hazardous, due to the shallow anterior chamber that is so often present, and due to the placement of the iris root in the filtration angle. A conjunctival flap is turned down over the upper quadrant and an incision is made into the anterior chamber for about 5 mm concentric with and just posterior to the limbus. As the blade of the keratome is withdrawn, the iris will normally present in the wound. It is grasped near its root and drawn well out of the incision. It is pulled first to one side and this limb divided as close as possible to the section, and then to the other side where the other limb is divided. Iridectomy in the dog is invariably followed by marked haemorrhage from the cut surface, the division being best accomplished by means of cautery. Following division of the iris, the remainder is reinserted into the anterior chamber and stroked back into place with an iris repositor, ensuring that no part of the iris remains caught in the section. Care must be taken that no damage is inflicted to the lens by the repositor. The conjunctiva is then replaced and sutured. An injection of air into the anterior chamber will assist the reformation of the anterior chamber, atropine and antibiotic drops being instilled daily until the eye is quiet; thereafter, corticosteroid drops should be used for a few weeks.

The complications that may follow glaucoma iridectomy include cataract formation, due to injury to the lens capsule by either the keratome or the repositor; or to the sudden release of aqueous; or to hyphaema formation. The latter is common and absorption may be very slow, with resultant fibrinous adhesions in the anterior chamber.

Posterior sclerotomy

This operation, in which a Graefe knife is inserted through the sclera, so that its point reaches the central part of the eyeball, after which it is rotated through 90° and withdrawn so that a little vitreous escapes, is contraindicated in the dog. The lowering of tension that will follow such an operation will be only very temporary, and there is a very great risk of either vitreous haemorrhage or retinal detachment.

Trephine operation

In this procedure, a disc of corneosclera, of approximately $1\frac{1}{2}$ mm diameter, is removed, allowing the aqueous to exit from the anterior chamber into the subconjunctival lymphatics. Such a trephine hole will become blocked with iris tissue unless a peripheral iridectomy is performed in the underlying iris, but otherwise tends to remain patent. Such an operation may be particularly useful in cases where the iris is atrophic.

The operation is performed under a conjunctival flap. This flap is raised by an incision in the conjunctiva, approximately 8 mm above the limbus, and the conjunctiva undermined downwards as far as the limbus (Fig. 193A). The flap may be usefully controlled by means of a Stallard's double-pronged hook (Fig. 194). The flap is best fashioned with scissors, and cut so that the edges slope downward towards the limbus. The undermining is best carried out by inserting closed spring scissors, and opening them under the conjunctiva. In the central area the undermining is continued to the limbus, it being ensured that the scissors are kept close to the sclera so that as thick a covering as possible is left for the trephine hole. Bleeding points may be controlled by a hand cautery.

With the flap well retracted by the hook, but without undue tension, the limbus is defined by swabbing, and a Tooke's corneal splitter (Fig. 195) is placed, at the 12 o'clock position, at the junction of conjunctiva and corneal epithelium. The edge of the splitter is used in a sweeping movement to dissect the epithelium from the limbus for a distance of about 1 mm into the cornea (Fig. 193B). When all bleeding has been controlled, the $1\frac{1}{2}$ mm diameter trephine (Fig. 196), is placed at right angles to the limbus, half over the cornea and half over the sclera, and rotated gently to cut the disc (Fig. 193C). Before perforation is completed, the trephine is tilted slightly so that a small hinge is left on the disc to prevent it entering the anterior chamber.

The trephine is removed slowly, to prevent any sudden rush of aqueous, and, on removal, a knuckle of iris will enter the hole, pushing the hinged disc to one side. The disc is then grasped with Elliot's disc forceps (Fig. 197) and removed by cutting the hinge with scissors, making sure that no damage is inflicted upon the iris (Fig. 193D). The iris is then grasped with toothed iris forceps, and a peripheral iridectomy is carried out by holding the iris as near as possible to the scleral margin of the trephine hole, making sure that the incision does not include the pupil margin (Fig. 193E). The iris is then allowed to return to the anterior chamber. It is important that no portion of the iris be allowed to remain in contact with the trephine opening, or adhesions and synechia formation will result. Haemorrhage must be controlled as far as possible, and, if necessary, the anterior chamber may be irrigated through the trephine hole.

Lastly, the conjunctiva is replaced and sutured by a continuous suture of 3/0 black silk (Fig. 193F) and atropine instilled. Satisfactory replacement of the iris may be helped by stroking the cornea downwards with a repositor.

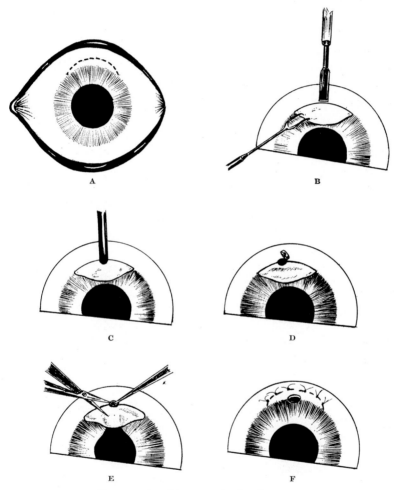

FIG. 193. *Trephine operation for glaucoma.*

Complications that might arise during or after a trephine operation include: loss of the disc into the anterior chamber, inward hinging of the disc, failure of the iris to prolapse due to faulty incising, haemorrhage, delayed formation of the anterior chamber, iritis, detachment of the choroid, blockage of the trephine hole and infection.

Button-holing of the conjunctiva may occur if the conjunctiva is per-forated during the formation of the flap, allowing the aqueous to flow through the trephine hole and into the conjunctival sac. In many instances, it is possible to alter the position of the trephine opening so that it does not lie directly above the conjunctival tear; in others if the tear is large, it may be necessary to extend it further and fashion a hooded flap.

In many instances, where the trephine disc has entered the anterior chamber, it may be extracted with a fine scleral hook. In other cases, where it cannot be removed with safety, it may be left in the anterior chamber, where it will be eventually absorbed.

Failure of the iris to prolapse is usually due to incomplete sectioning with the trephine, and a suitable knife may be employed to complete the incisions. Other cases may be due to posterior synechiae.

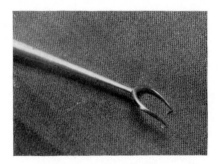

Fig. 194. *Stallard's double hook.*

Injury to the lens and subsequent cataract formation is due either to faulty instrumentation or to a sudden rush of aqueous and consequent damage to the lens capsule.

Delayed reformation of the anterior chamber, which is normally com-pleted within one week, usually indicates a choroidal detachment, possibly due to aqueous finding its way into the suprachoroidal space, but more likely due to exudation from the choroidal vessels when the intraocular tension is suddenly reduced by the incision. Such detachments normally subside in a few weeks and no treatment is indicated. Occasionally, delay in the reformation of the chamber is due to a leakage of aqueous from a fistula in the conjunctiva; such a defect can be repaired by covering it with a conjunctival flap.

Infection is a rare complication, but, when present, should be treated promptly by means of atropine and subconjunctival antibiotics.

Iridencleisis

The object of the filtering cicatrix operations is to form a permanent filtering point at the corneoscleral junction, through which aqueous may filter out under the conjunctiva. The 'wick' is formed from tissue which has been partly severed from the iris, to avoid distortion of the pupil. The iris tissue inserted into the corneoscleral section eventually becomes atrophic. The wound becomes lined with endothelial cells preventing closure of the wound and results in the formation of a filtering scar. Quite often a permanent filtering bleb is produced, which may be seen under the conjunctiva. In other instances, no such bleb is apparent, even though ten-

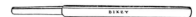

FIG. 195. *Tooke's corneal splitter.*   FIG. 196. *Lang's trephine.*

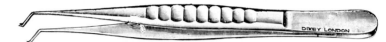

FIG. 197. *Elliot's disc forceps.*

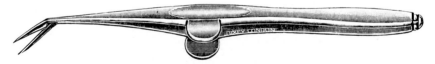

FIG. 199. *de Wecker's scissors.*

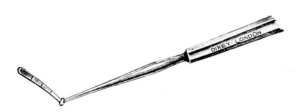

FIG. 201. *Cyclodialysis spatula.*

sion remains normal after the operation, thus suggesting that factors other than straightforward filtering are involved. In the majority of dogs, favourable results are obtained initially, but these, unfortunately, are not always maintained.

In most cases of glaucoma in the dog, this is probably the operation of choice and the indications include primary, narrow-angle glaucoma, and secondary glaucoma due either to iris bombé where there are anterior peripheral synechiae, or traumatic adhesions of the filtration angle. It is not indicated where iris atrophy is present and a trephine operation is more likely to prove successful.

The operation is performed under a conjunctival flap, as with the trephine operation, and the flap is turned down as far as the limbus (Fig. 193B). Bleeding points are controlled by cautery and the flap is retracted forward and downward. A Tooke's knife is used to clear the episcleral tissue from the sclera and, using an angled keratome, an incision is made into the anterior chamber 1 mm posterior to the limbus. If the conjunctival flap is reflected back when the point of the keratome enters the anterior chamber, the sur-

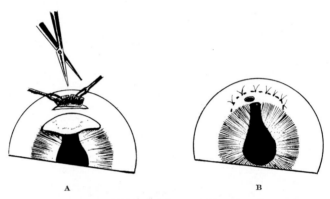

A   B

FIG. 198. *Iridencleisis*. A *stage 1*, B *stage 2*.

geon may observe the blade when making the incision, so that damage to the iris or lens capsule is avoided. With the blade parallel to the iris, the incision may be enlarged to about 5 mm allowing the aqueous to escape slowly and thus avoid damage to the lens. The keratome is withdrawn, and any haemorrhage controlled by cellulose swabs.

By depressing the keratome incision posteriorly, the iris is made to present itself in the lips of the wound and may be withdrawn by forceps or an iris hook. The iris is grasped with iris forceps at the pupillary margin, and a second grasp is taken with a further pair of forceps close to the first pair (Fig. 198A). Between these two forceps, the iris is divided with de Wecker's scissors (Fig. 199), from pupillary margin to root. The two pillars thus formed are pulled apart gently, one pillar being drawn upwards into the wound and out on to the sclera and the other pillar stroked back into its original position.

Alternatively, the two pillars may be placed at opposite ends of the scleral incision, and if necessary sutured in position, leaving enough iris tissue outside the wound to prevent closure. A third possible technique is to grasp the iris midway between pupillary margin and root and excise a triangular flap towards the root, the root itself being left intact. The flap is drawn out of the wound and placed on the sclera. The latter technique leaves a pupil of normal shape and position.

After the iridencleisis is completed the conjunctival flap is repositioned and the incision closed by a continuous suture (Fig. 198B). Atropine and antibiotic drops are instilled and maintained until the eye is quiet, following which corticosteroid applications may be used.

To prevent occlusion of a trephine hole with episcleral tissue and conjunctiva, and, to maintain filtration in an iridencleisis operation, a strip of sterile absorbable film (Gelfilm) may be used. This film, used as a strip about 6 × 4 mm, may be inserted between the scleral wound and the episcleral tissues to prevent adhesions and to ensure the formation of a bleb. The film, which will become pliable when moistened with saline, may be sterilized by dry heat at 140°C (284°F) for 4 hours. It is non-antigenic, and is absorbed within one to six months.

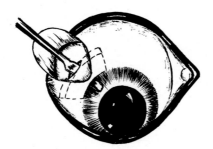

FIG. 200. *Cyclodialysis.*

Cyclodialysis

In the operation of cyclodialysis, the ciliary body is separated from the sclera, allowing the anterior chamber to become continuous with the supra choroidal space (Fig. 200).

An incision is made through the conjunctiva, and into the sclera for about 3 mm, parallel to the limbus and about 8 mm from it, the incision being deepened until the black uvea is seen. A cyclodialysis spatula (Fig. 201) is then inserted into the incision, so that it lies between the sclera and the choroid, with the tip pressed well against the overlying sclera. When the tip of the instrument appears in the anterior chamber, it is swept round 90° on either side, thus separating the root of the iris from the sclera for as great a distance as possible. It may then be withdrawn and reinserted in a different direction and the procedure repeated, so that two-fifths of the ciliary body is dialysed.

Although the operation of cyclodialysis has been advocated for use in the dog, and it may be of value in some cases where there are peripheral anterior synechiae, it is likely to be accompanied by considerable haemorrhage.

Cyclodiathermy

In this technique, a diathermy current is applied to the ciliary body, through the sclera, using either penetrating or nonpenetrating electrodes. The ciliary body is thus partly coagulated over half its circumference, with a resultant loss of secretory function.

The main indications for the use of cyclodiathermy would appear to exist in those cases in which excessive haemorrhage is to be expected, following the application of any of the techniques already described; or where a filtering operation has not resulted in a sufficient lowering of tension; or if other techniques have failed to produce any improvement.

Nonpenetrating cyclodiathermy may be performed either through the

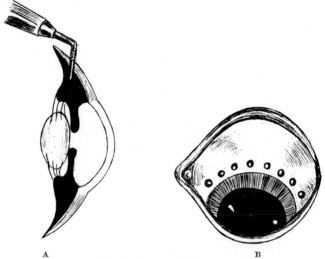

A   B
Fig. 202. *Cyclodiathermy.*

conjunctiva, or after the formation of conjunctival flaps; the former produces some charring of the conjunctiva which is of little consequence. In this technique, an electrode of 2 mm diameter is used, and a series of applications made in a row extending along a line about 4 mm from the limbus (Fig. 202). Alternatively, retrociliary applications may be made, placing a single row of applications about 7 mm behind the limbus, and extending over as great a circumference as is possible. In each case a current of 70 mA is applied for 7 seconds.

Perforating cyclodiathermy may be performed with a fine 1 mm electrode, using about 10 to 15 applications, evenly spaced in two rows, about 6 and 8 mm behind the limbus. In this case, a current of 70 mA for 4 seconds is used for each application.

Following cyclodiathermy, atropine is applied. There may be some loss of fluid from the areas of application, some chemosis and some postoperative rise in tension. The tension will soon subside, and chemosis may be controlled by the use of corticosteroid applications.

The operation of cyclodiathermy may be repeated as necessary, and may prove to be a useful technique for the maintenance of normal pressure in hydrophthalmic eyes. Sometimes, however, particularly if the procedure is repeated, hypotony and phthisis bulbi may result.

Lendectomy

Lendectomy is indicated where there is glaucoma due to subluxation or luxation of the lens, lens intumescence, or when it is secondary to a lens-induced uveitis.

OTHER TREATMENTS

Absolute glaucoma

The pain often associated with absolute glaucoma may be relieved by the injection of 1 ml pure alcohol by the retrobulbar route, or alternatively, a reduction in intraocular pressure may be obtained by the use of cyclodiathermy.

Congenital glaucoma

Congenital glaucoma, or buphthalmos, is very occasionally seen in puppies, due either to malformation of the filtration angle or to obstruction of the filtration angle from persistent foetal tissue. One or both eyes may be affected, and marked distension of the eyeball will be apparent, together with scleral ectasia. The intraocular pressure is normally only slightly increased (due to the stretching of the eyeball), the cornea appears hazy due to oedema, and cupping of the optic disc may be observed. In due course, some drainage may become established, but the eye will remain distended and cloudy.

In cases of buphthalmos, paracentesis of the anterior chamber will afford only temporary relief, and the normal drainage operations will rarely prove adequate. Where there is gross distension of the eyeball, or marked damage to the cornea, surgery is seldom worthwhile. In less advanced cases, however, the operation of goniotomy may be performed.

Prior to surgery, the intraocular pressure should be reduced by the use of carbonic anhydrase inhibitors, and full constriction of the pupil will be required. A Saunder's needle is used and this is passed through the temporal limbus and through to the nasal angle of the anterior chamber. The needle is then swept along the angle from 45° above to 45° below the horizontal. The needle must be manipulated so as to avoid aqueous loss as far as possible, and, since marked haemorrhage is likely, the manipulation must be carried out with all possible speed, before vision is obscured. The resultant hyphaema will, in many cases, be absorbed within a few days.

15

THE LENS

ANATOMY AND PHYSIOLOGY

The lens is a biconvex, transparent body, situated between the iris and the vitreous body, and suspended within the eyeball by the zonular ligaments, connecting the equator of the lens with the ciliary body. Anteriorly, the iris rests on the lens surface; posteriorly, the lens fits into a depression in the anterior vitreous surface, the fossa patellaris.

The diameter of the lens in the dog varies between 9 and 11·5 mm, and the antero-posterior thickness averages 7 mm. The volume of the lens is about 0·5 cm³ and the proportion of lens to the entire globe varies from 1:8 to 1:10.

Although the posterior surface shows a slighly greater convexity than the anterior surface, the difference in curvature is less marked than in man. The curvature of the lens surface, and consequently the shape of the lens, is altered during the process of accommodation—the act of bringing near objects to correct focus on the retina. In the dog, the degree of accommodation possible with the normal intact lens is limited, light rays being diverged on to the retina mainly by the cornea.

Accommodation is accomplished by the contraction of the ciliary muscle. In the state of rest, the ciliary muscle is relaxed, and the suspensory ligament and the lens are under tension. Contraction of the muscle causes the ciliary body and the choroid to be pulled forward, thus displacing the ciliary processes towards the lens. The tension normally present in the zonule is thus relaxed, and this relaxation is transferred to the elastic lens capsule, allowing the lens cortex to assume a more spherical form.

The crystalline lens is composed of three structures—the capsule, the anterior epithelium and the lens substance.

The capsule, which completely encloses the lens, is a structureless, highly elastic membrane, and, as the lens is convex, may be divided into two sections, anterior and posterior, with the junction of the two parts forming the equator of the lens. The thickness of the capsule varies somewhat in different parts of the lens, being thinnest at the posterior pole, and thickest at the equator. In the dog, there is great variation in thickness between anterior and posterior capsules. The thickness of the anterior capsule is approximately 50μ and that of the posterior capsule $3 \cdot 5\mu$. Thus, in the dog, the changes in curvature of the two surfaces during accommodation are probably very unequal.

The areas of greatest thickness in both capsules are found just in front of and just behind the equator, and this area serves for the insertion of the zonular fibres of the suspensory ligament.

The anterior capsule forms the posterior boundary of the anterior chamber; the posterior capsule fits into the hyaloid fossa, or fossa patellaris, of the vitreous body. The anterior lens capsule, although comparatively thick in the dog, is, nevertheless, friable, highly elastic, and easily torn.

The anterior epithelium, situated just under the anterior lens capsule, is composed of a single layer of cuboidal cells, situated on the anterior lens surface. There is no posterior epithelium. At the equator, where the new lens fibres are being formed constantly, the cells are more elongated and tend to be arranged in rows. In this area, the thickness of the anterior epithelium is about 20μ, whereas, on the anterior surface of the lens, the thickness does not exceed 9μ.

The lens substance consists of lens fibres, $2 \cdot 5$ to 4μ thick, which are long flat elements, hexagonal in cross-section, united by an amorphous cementing substance. The fibre substance is somewhat denser on the surface of each fibre, giving the appearance of a membrane.

During embryonic development, the posterior epithelium forms the primitive fibres, and these fibres are directed in the lens from front to back. Subsequently, the epithelial cells at the equator grow and metamorphose, and the succeeding fibres come to be arranged meridionally in layers. This process continues throughout life and the lens substance comes to consist of concentric lamellae of fibres. The nuclei are lost in the older and deeper fibres, and with the continuous addition of new fibres around the old shrinking ones, the lens increases in density with age. In the young animal, the lens exhibits only a small central nucleus and the majority of the lens substance is quite soft. With age, this nucleus becomes larger and harder, and in later life, the lens is hard throughout. It is, therefore, possible to differentiate between a softer, superficial cortex, and a harder central nucleus.

The cement binding the fibres together is slightly more apparent where the ends of the fibres meet one another, forming a central strand between anterior and posterior poles of the lens. A series of branching partitions, arising from this strand, divides the lens substance into sections. The lines of separation—the *lens sutures*—appear as an upright **Y** on one side of the lens, and as an inverted **Y** on the other. The lens sutures are symmetrically placed, at an angle of $120°$ with each other, forming a star-shaped figure, the *lens star.*

17

Changes in the lens associated with age. Slit-lamp studies have shown that, at the age of 1 year, the lens is light grey in colour, with a large embryonic nucleus and poorly marked zones. At 2 years, the lens sutures are more noticeable but not dense, but, by 3 years, slight density in the sutures is apparent. By 6 years of age, some sclerosis of the lens is often noticeable.

The suspensory ligament, zonular ciliaris or zonule of Zinn, supports the lens in its position within the eye, and is composed of very numerous and dense delicate fibres which radiate from the equator of the lens capsule to the inner surface of the ciliary body. These fibres arise both from the orbicularis ciliaris and from the valleys between the ciliary processes, and are inserted into a narrow area of the lens capsule at the equator. In the dog, the fibres are attached largely to the periphery and anterior surface of the lens capsule, and little, if at all, to the posterior surface of the lens. Again, in the dog, the zonular ligaments are tough and resistant to rupture.

The lens has no direct supply from the vascular system and is, therefore, dependent upon the aqueous humour for its nourishment. Its transparency is maintained by the swelling of the gelatinous proteins contained within the lens substance. The amount of fluid absorbed by the lens substance, and therefore its transparency, depends upon the permeability of the lens capsule, the chemical nature of the lens proteins, and upon factors such as the concentration of mineral salts contained within the lens, which in turn will influence osmosis. Particularly in the young animal, the lens is dependent on the protection offered by an intact lens capsule; breaks in the capsule, allowing the entrance of aqueous humour, may result in loss of lens proteins into solution and eventually the lens may be dissolved.

The lens, being avascular, is incapable of exhibiting an inflammatory reaction; its reaction to damaging stimuli is to become opaque.

CONGENITAL ABNORMALITIES

Anterior and posterior lenticonus, characterized by conical elevations at the anterior or posterior poles, are very rare defects in the dog. Vision is defective by virtue of the myopic centre of the lens, and cataract formation is likely to be exhibited at a later stage. Diagnosis is readily made with the use of a slit-lamp.

Coloboma of the lens, an indentation forming a notch in the lens equator, is due to a defect in the zonule and is usually unilateral affecting the lower quadrant.

Lens colobomata are rare, but may result from a persistence of the embryological anastomosis between the anterior and posterior vascular sheaths of the lens.

Ectopia lentis, congenital dislocation of the lens is, like all congenital lens defects in the dog, rare. Basically, it is due to a defect in the zonule over an extensive area, allowing the lens to be pulled over to one side, presenting an aphakic crescent. In other cases, the zonule may be entirely absent, allowing complete dislocation of the lens so that this structure lies free in the anterior chamber, anterior to the iris.

Posterior polar opacities may result from the persistence of remnants of the hyaloid vascular system. Embryologically, the hyaloid supply gives rise to the posterior vascular sheath of the lens, the hyaloid artery extending from lens to optic disc. Persistence of part of the sheath may give rise to opacities which may be only pin-point in size.

CATARACT

Cataract signifies any opacity of the crystalline lens or its capsule. There are many ways of classifying cataracts, such as congenital or acquired; anterior or posterior; hard or soft; and so on. From the clinical point of view, the best classification is probably as developmental, senile, secondary, complicated and traumatic.

Cataracts may also be classified according to the site of the opacities within the lens substance. Thus, an opacity may be termed nuclear, cortical (peripheral or axial), capsular (anterior or posterior), subcapsular or, if localized to the axis, polar (Fig. 203). A mature cataract is one in which the whole of the lens substance is opaque; an immature cataract is one in which there is still a considerable amount of clear lens material.

Aetiology

Occasionally, a cataract may have a definite and known cause; others may be regularly produced by certain experimental agents. In the vast majority of cases, however, the aetiology remains obscure.

As has already been stated, the transparency of the lens depends upon its water content and the state of the lens proteins. During the development of opacity, certain chemical changes take place within the lens substance, and these include an increase in the water content and the calcium content, and a decrease in the potassium, protein, ascorbic acid and glutathione levels. With the loss of glutathione the oxygen consumption falls and the percentage of ash in the nucleus becomes greater than that in the cortex. Although, in the early stages, the water content increases, this falls as the cataract becomes mature.

Many theories have been advanced to explain the development of cataract. Most cataracts encountered in the dog are due to senility and being a sign of old age may be physiological in origin. They may be due to decreased permeability of the lens capsule, leading to nutritional deficiencies; lowered metabolism; accumulation of waste products; and general dehydration. Hereditary factors may be involved, and other changes may be produced by the effect on the lens protein of absorbed radiation, generalized arteriosclerosis, endocrine dysfunction and chemical toxins.

With the exception of certain breeds, it is doubtful if cataract is often of hereditary origin in the dog, except in association with other ocular changes, such as occur in hereditary progressive retinal atrophy. There is little support today for theories based on immunological factors, associated with the antigenic activity of a-crystallin; and functional theories, based on refraction and the strains of accommodation, are hardly likely to be applicable to the dog.

Metabolic disorders may be operative in the production of cataract; and disturbances in the ciliary body, and, therefore, changes in the aqueous humour, might be involved. Any factor altering the permeability of the lens

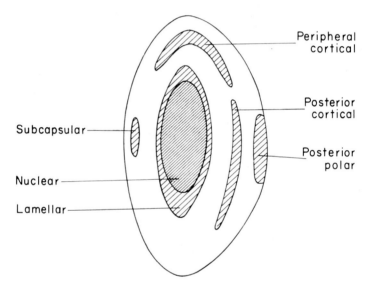

FIG. 203. *Types of cataract.*

capsule would also be of significance, either by increasing the permeability, and thus allowing the entrance of any toxic substances from the aqueous, or decreasing the permeability, and thus allowing the accumulation of waste products and interfering with nutrition. Cases of punctate cataract have been described—*tetanic cataract*—associated with hypocalcaemia, hypoparathyroidism and renal insufficiency.

Vitamin deficiencies might possibly be involved, and experimental cataracts may be produced in this way. Those vitamins most likely to be involved are B_1, B_2, and C. Endocrine disorders, particularly diabetes mellitus, may also be associated with cataract formation. Experimentally, poisons such as thallium and naphthalene can produce cataracts.

Trauma, causing injury to the lens capsule, and subsequent absorption of áqueous and swelling of the lens fibres, will also cause cataract; heat and cold, and excessive exposure to ultraviolet light, can also produce lens opacities.

Congenital cataract may be due to a failure of the hyaloid artery to regress; to an abnormal arrangement of the lens fibres; to a layer of droplets deposited between the cortex and the nucleus; to maternal illness; or to hereditary factors.

Stages of development

(1) *Incipient.* In this stage there is some evidence of a commencing opacity, but vision remains normal.

(2) *Immature.* The lens is largely, but not entirely, opaque, with clear fibres surrounding the opacity. The light reflex from the fundus remains normal. The lens may become intumescent, or swollen with absorbed water; on rare occasions this may interfere with aqueous drainage.

(3) *Mature.* In this stage, the lens becomes smaller and totally opaque; the light reflex may be impaired or absent.

(4) *Hypermature.* Further water is lost and the lens becomes smaller, with desiccation of the nucleus. In some cases, a thickened lens capsule will prevent loss of water, but, as the cortex is liquefied, the nucleus falls to the bottom of the capsule, leaving the upper part of the capsule full of clear fluid—a Morgagnian cataract.

Developmental cataract

Developmental cataracts are those in which the lens is affected during development, with consequent loss of transparency. The origin of such opacities is usually obscure; hereditary factors may be involved, or the condition may be due to some nutritional or inflammatory change that has occurred during development. Cataract of inherited origin has been demonstrated in the Beagle, Alsatian, Golden Retriever, Staffordshire Bull Terrier, Pointer and Boston Terrier, and probably occurs in other breeds as well (Fig. 204).

Most congenital cataracts are bilateral, and, as they develop before the development of the cortex, they tend to occur in the nucleus or capsule. They are sometimes complete but are more often partial, and may be so slight as to cause no apparent interference with vision. Congenital cataracts have well-defined edges, and it is not usual for there to be any further increase during life. Many are of pin-point size, and commonly affect the area on the lens around the anterior or, more commonly, the posterior Y suture —the sutural or stellate cataract. Anterior polar cataracts may be associated with persistent pupillary membranes; posterior polar cataracts are usually associated with a persistence of the remnants of the hyaloid artery.

Degenerative cataracts, affecting dogs from birth up to the age of 6 years, are the result of degenerative changes taking place within the substance of the normal lens. Such juvenile, or pre-senile cataracts are often bilateral ultimately, but will usually affect one lens before the other. The onset is often slow, and the loss of transparency gradual. (Plate V, Figs. 9 and 10, facing p. 224.)

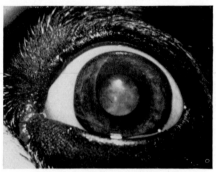

FIG. 204. *Developmental cataract.*

Senile cataract

Cataracts of this type are common in the dog, many over the age of 9 or 10 being affected to some degree. The senile lens tends to become opaque with increasing age, but many cases show little visual impairment, and the progress of the cataract may, in many cases, be slow. Senile cataracts may appear in both nuclear and cortical forms, and any part of the lens substance or its capsule may be affected (Plate V, Figs. 11 and 12, facing p. 224).

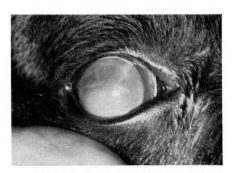

FIG. 205. *Senile nuclear cataract.*

Nuclear cataract or hard cataract is the result of normal sclerosis of the lens nucleus, associated with increasing years (Fig. 205). With age, the nuclear fibres become more and more compressed, and, eventually, the central fibres may become opaque; this may spread slowly towards the periphery until the whole of the nuclear substance is affected. Discoloration of the nucleus may take place in some cases, so that it appears at first cloudy, and later yellowish or even brown.

Cortical cataract or soft cataract is more commonly seen in the aged dog, the opacities being due to the accumulation of fluid within the lens cortex (Fig. 206). The fluid tends to form in droplets and vacuoles and tends to collect between the lens fibres, producing radial clefts between the lamellae. These changes occur most frequently around the lens sutures, particularly in the anterior cortex causing, at first, an irregular cloudiness, and later, definite opacities. Many patterns may be formed by such opacities, either showing as radial spokes, or granular deposits, or as more well defined opacities.

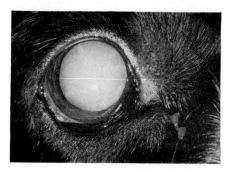

Fig. 206. *Senile cortical cataract.*

Secondary cataract

Diabetic cataract may appear as a pre-senile form, at the age of four or five years; or may appear as a diffuse subcapsular opacity, anterior or posterior, at the age of two years or so. Such cataracts are usually bilateral, and tend to progress rapidly, being floccular in appearance. In time, the whole lens may become opaque, but, as the subcapsular type is due to oedema, early cases may be reversible with treatment. Other cases may arise even during insulin treatment.

Complicated cataract

These are the result of a disturbance in the nutrition of the lens, associated with various intraocular diseases and may appear with anterior uveitis, glaucoma, luxation or subluxation of the lens, posterior uveitis, intraocular tumours or retinal detachments. They tend to affect the posterior capsule in the early stages, and gradually affect the whole of the lens substance.

Traumatic cataract

Any break in the continuity of the lens capsule will allow aqueous to permeate within the lens substance, forming an opacity whose size is dependent upon the extent of the capsular damage. If the tear in the capsule is large, the majority of the lens substance will be dissolved, leaving an empty, thickened, wrinkled capsule. If the break is small, the opening may become plugged with swollen lens fibres, thus producing only a localized opacity.

An iritis, and subsequent adhesions between iris and lens capsule, may be produced by any lens material that is liberated into the aqueous; or a glaucoma may result from interference to aqueous drainage by the lens material.

Cataract may also be caused by perforating injuries, intraocular foreign bodies, or by concussion. Similarly, severe electric shocks or excessive exposure to γ-rays or X-rays may be responsible for opacity.

Contusions of the eye may be responsible for the deposition of pigment from the iris on to the anterior lens capsule; this is normally of no consequence, although, on occasion, may be so marked as to interfere with vision.

After-cataract

This is the name given to opaque lens fragments remaining in the pupillary opening after the lens has been removed by extracapsular extraction (Fig. 207). This type of extraction invariably leaves some soft lens material in the anterior chamber, and, on occasion, this may remain *in situ* between the

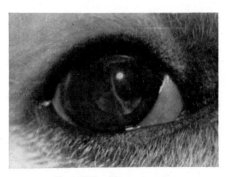

Fig. 207. *After-cataract.*

intact posterior capsule and the remains of the anterior capsule at the periphery of the lens. Sometimes it will form a complete ring—Soemmering's ring; in other cases, fibrin deposition, either from an iritis or from intraocular haemorrhage, covers the lens remnants and prevents further absorption by the aqueous. On other occasions, the posterior capsule becomes thickened by proliferating epithelial cells; this, in turn, may lead to hyaline bands on the posterior capsule, or the new cells may become vacuolated producing soap-like bubbles—Elschnig's pearls.

CLINICAL SIGNS

In a congenital cataract, the lens is soft and the contents fluid. The lens will appear bluish-white or milky.

In early senile cataract, the subjective symptoms are of course absent, but there may be early impaired vision. Often there will be polyopia, resulting in blurred vision, so that the dog will shy or bark at imaginary objects. Later, the vision becomes more impaired, and this is associated with an observable opacity of the lens. Nevertheless, many dogs are able to see quite well, despite marked changes in the lens substance.

An early senile cataract will often appear as a grey, diffuse radiation in the lens substance, and this must be distinguished from the grey opalescence of the normal senile lens. Using an ophthalmoscope, a normal senile lens will appear transparent, whereas a cataract will appear opaque.

In an incipient cataract, minute globules will sometimes appear beneath the lens capsule.

The lens is swollen in an immature cataract, causing the anterior chamber to be shallow. On reaching maturity, the lens is normal in size and uniformly opaque, being either white or grey in appearance. Later, it becomes smaller and pearly-white. The rate of development is very variable.

When examined with a slit-lamp, complicated cataracts exhibit a polychromatic lustre, and there is a poor light reflex.

The depth of the lesion may be assessed using an ophthalmoscope. If the observer's eye is moved laterally, central opacities will remain stationary, anterior opacities will move against the examiner, and posterior opacities will move with the examiner. A slit-lamp is also of value in determining the extent and depth of the lesion.

MEDICAL TREATMENT

Coagulation of the lens protein is irreversible; the only reversible changes are those few cases associated with changes in the blood chemistry and hydration of the lens, where the blood chemistry can be adjusted rapidly.

Various medical 'cures' have been claimed from time to time, but it is very doubtful if any of these have the slightest effect in influencing the course of the disease. Similarly, there is no known method of preventing the development of a cataract, and the only known satisfactory treatment is surgical removal of the lens. Recently, however, a report on the use of selenium-tocopherol in the treatment of senile lenticular sclerosis indicated that this line of treatment might prove helpful.

SURGICAL TREATMENT

History. The surgical treatment of various eye diseases in animals has been practised for many years, and there are reports from very early periods of eye operations performed on the dog.

Those operations involving the ocular adnexa or the superficial parts of the eye have evolved into highly successful techniques, and have become standard procedures in veterinary surgery. Intraocular surgery, however, has progressed far more slowly and, even today, there is a wide divergence of opinion regarding the value and practicability of operations involving the interior of the eye of the dog.

The extraction of the cataractous lens from the dog has been performed by many veterinary surgeons over the past seventy-five years, with varying degrees of success. Many failures have been experienced, which, in part at least, have been due to the limited facilities available at the time, the lack of suitable anaesthesia, inadequate instrumentation, and a lack of knowledge of the anatomy and physiology of the canine eye. The number of unsuccessful terminations has undoubtedly discouraged many surgeons in the past, and little advance was made in canine cataract surgery until the second half of the present century.

Methods of cataract removal. Many surgical techniques have been devised in the past for the relief of cataract, the object of all of them being to remove the opaque lens from the pupillary opening. Cataract surgery, as practised in ancient times, consisted of the reclination, depression or 'couching' of the lens. Today, however, this operation has very little indication, except, possibly, in some cases of posterior luxation of the lens, where the dislocated lens is occupying part of the pupil; in such a case, extraction of the lens may result in considerable vitreous loss.

Linear or curette extraction is a technique for extracting a cataract by means of a keratome incision through which the opaque lens material is expressed into a curette, the residue in the anterior chamber being washed out with an irrigator. The extraction of all lens matter by this technique is sometimes difficult; material left adherent to the underside of the iris is liable to form dense after-cataract.

Discission, the breaking up of the lens cortex and nucleus by a needle, is a useful technique in the treatment of congenital cataract. For the majority of cataracts, however, either developmental or senile, an extraction technique will be required.

Extracapsular and intracapsular extraction

In the surgery of cataracts, the lens may be removed by either extracapsular or intracapsular methods of extraction. In extracapsular extraction, the anterior lens capsule is opened and the lens is expressed through this opening, removing the nucleus and as much of the cortex as possible, but leaving the thin posterior capsule intact. In intracapsular extraction, the lens is removed intact in its capsule, after rupturing the suspensory ligament that holds the lens in position. The lens may be extracted either by forceps applied to the anterior lens capsule; by an erisiphake, an instrument applied to the anterior lens capsule through which suction is made mechanically; or by pressure applied to the globe externally.

The advantages of the extracapsular method are threefold. First, less skill in the manipulation of the lens is required than in the intracapsular method. Secondly, as the posterior lens capsule is left intact, there is less risk of vitreous loss; the posterior capsule remains as a support for the hyaloid membrane. Thirdly, as the zonule is left intact, the operation is less traumatic, and there is less risk of damage to the iris or ciliary body.

Extracapsular extraction has several distinct disadvantages. First, there is a tendency for further clouding of the pupil post-operatively by fibrinous deposits, and for the formation of iridocapsular synechiae. Secondly, the posterior capsule itself may lose transparency. Thirdly, as it is difficult to remove all lens material, and leave a clear, transparent pupil, an iridocyclitis may develop, due to irritation from lens fragments left in the anterior chamber; such remnants are far more likely to cause an exaggerated reaction in the older dog. Fourthly, a poorer visual result is more likely after an extracapsular operation than after an intracapsular extraction.

The intracapsular operation will avoid these complications, the ideal being to extract the lens with its capsule intact, and, if possible, to leave the hyaloid membrane intact, thereby avoiding vitreous loss. There are, however, several disadvantages with this method. An intracapsular extraction involves the detachment of the lens from its zonule, and, consequently, considerable intraocular instrumentation. The zonular fibres are often very resistant, particularly in the younger animals, and rocking methods, as commonly practised in human techniques, are not likely to be successful; rather are they likely to rupture the anterior lens capsule and the hyaloid membrane, resulting in some lens material and part of the capsule remaining in the vitreous humour or in the anterior chamber. The use of instruments and the push-and-pull manoeuvres that have to be employed may also result in iridocyclitic injuries and subsequent haemorrhage from the iris or ciliary body. There is some evidence that the suspensory ligament of the lens and the hyaloid membrane in the dog are continuous; rupture of the zonule, therefore, may result in vitreous loss, and a serious loss might result in failure of the operation. A final consideration is that excessive traction may result in retinal detachment.

To date, the extracapsular method has been mainly preferred, as it has been considered less dangerous from the point of view of haemorrhage and vitreous loss. It is, however, usually agreed that results have not been so favourable, in other respects, as with the intracapsular method.

Similarly, it is felt that the intracapsular method is ideal, but unfortunately, for the reasons outlined above, more difficult to perform and entailing a greater risk.

The present position of cataract extraction in the dog is summarized by W. G. Magrane when he states: 'The percentage of success could certainly be increased were an uncomplicated intracapsular extraction possible in every instance. There is no doubt that, whether it be man or dog, the intracapsular extraction is to be preferred if postoperative complications are to be kept to the minimum'.

Various techniques have been developed to assist in the performance of successful intracapsular extractions. Consideration must be given, not only to the factors involving general management and general surgical technique, but also to the factors responsible for failure in cataract extractions—be they extracapsular or intracapsular—and to those special factors which are involved especially in the intracapsular operation.

Aphakic vision in the dog

The absence of the crystalline lens, following its surgical removal, is known as aphakia. The value of cataract extraction and the subsequent aphakic vision in the dog has often been doubted in the past. Attempts have been made to fit spectacles to this animal, but apart from the obvious difficulties that will be met in both designing a suitable appliance and persuading the patient to tolerate its application, it seems to be generally agreed that most dogs would tend to concentrate their gaze upon the spectacles rather than endeavour to look through the lenses.

Provided that all other parts of the eye are functioning normally, then it should, theoretically, be possible for an animal deprived of the lens to distinguish light from darkness and to visualize large objects. Clinical evidence suggests that the aphakic dog recovers some power of receiving light, and that there is a reasonable return of vision without the need for artificial lenses. The dog has great capabilities of adaptation to errors of vision and, although an intralenticular implant might be of value, reasonable results can be expected without the use of either spectacles or implants.

It is possible that lack of success in the past has been associated with poor surgical results rather than with the failure of aphakic vision to be of value to the dog; such poor results in the past are no justification for rejecting cataract extraction in the dog.

The removal of the lens from the eye will result in a loss of refractive power and a loss of accommodation, thus changing the focusing point of the optical system. In the dog, the degree of accommodation possible, with the normal intact lens, is limited, therefore the loss of the lens is of less significance than in man. Light rays are diverged on to the retina mainly by the cornea, and the loss of the finer adjustments, accomplished by the lens, is not of importance to the dog.

Although a degree of myopia is considered normal in the dog, investigation has shown that, whereas this is often so in the brachycephalic breeds, a degree of hypermetropia is more commonly found in the dog, particularly those which hunt by sight. Myopia, when present in the dog, is usually of the degree of — 1 to — 3 D., and in such cases, the loss of the lens is likely to have less effect than in the hypermetropic or emmetropic animal.

Following surgery, a variable period for the adjustment of the vision is required. Such adaptation is possible in the dog, and the return of ambulatory vision justifies the performance of cataract operations. The dog has no need for fine optical discrimination, and as the operation in the human produces a dramatic improvement in vision, even before spectacles are provided, there would appear to be no viable optical objection to the performance of cataract surgery in the dog.

Factors responsible for surgical failure

Many factors are operative in the production of unsuccessful cataract extractions; in some cases, more than one factor is involved. First, the general factors that must be considered before intraocular surgery is contemplated, may be summarized as follows:

(1) The careful selection of cases.

(2) Surgical dexterity and suitable temperament on the part of the operator.

(3) Adequate and suitable preoperative preparation of the patient.

(4) Anaesthesia which is both adequate and suitable for intraocular surgery.

(5) Correct postoperative management.

Secondly, those factors concerned with the anatomy and physiology of the canine eye which render cataract surgery particularly difficult in the dog. These may also be summarized:

(1) Surgical approach to the canine eye is rendered difficult by the conformation of the head, and the position of the eyeball and orbit.

(2) The palpebral fissure is small, and the eyelids tend to encompass the cornea, making intraocular instrumentation difficult.

(3) The prominence of the inferior and lateral segments of the orbital ring hinders the approach to the eye.

(4) Anaesthesia tends to produce rotation and retraction of the globe within the orbit. Any retraction of the eyeball causes the nictitating membrane to protrude over the cornea, and this produces a mechanical hindrance to the approach (Fig. 208).

(5) The union between the bulbar conjunctiva and the sclera is loose, thus making fixation of the eyeball difficult, and causing the conjunctiva to spread over the limbus, thus obstructing the incisional site.

(6) Incisions encroaching upon the sclera will invariably result in haemorrhage.

(7) The lens of the dog is both large and thick, necessitating an extensive corneal incision; this may lead to excessive tissue reaction, infiltration of the cornea and difficulties in healing.

(8) Contraction of the iris, and a lessening of the pupillary opening, whether or not mydriasis has been established preoperatively, will invariably follow the opening of the anterior chamber and the escape of aqueous humour. This may greatly hinder the approach to the lens and zonule.

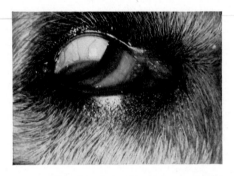

Fig. 208. *Rotation of the globe under anaesthesia.*

(9) The highly vascular nature of the canine iris will result in considerable haemorrhage if this structure, or the ciliary body, should be intentionally or accidently damaged during the operation.

(10) The resistant nature of the canine zonule makes this structure difficult to detach from the lens, and the necessary manoeuvres to accomplish this stage in the operation may result in damage to the ciliary body or rupture of the lens capsule.

(11) The nature of the hyaloid membrane and its relationship to the posterior capsule of the lens renders vitreous loss likely.

Complications that might arise during the operation, dependent upon the anatomical considerations that have been mentioned, are therefore, haemorrhage from the incision; haemorrhage from the iris or ciliary body; rupture of the lens capsule; posterior dislocation of the lens due to manipulation; and vitreous loss.

The selection of cases

It is fairly certain, from early reports in the literature of cataract extraction in the dog, that many failures were due, not only to improper technique but also to the faulty selection of cases.

The extraction of the cataractous lens is indicated in those dogs which are blind or almost blind, as a result of cataract formation, where a dense, diffuse cataract of both lenses is present. It is also indicated in cases where the cataract affects only one eye, but where the other eye is rendered blind from some other pathological condition.

There would seem to be no indication, in the dog, in undertaking cataract surgery unless the vision is lost or is seriously impaired; or when only one lens is affected, the other appearing to be perfectly normal. It has been observed that some degree of vision is retained in the dog even though it may exhibit a cataract of both lenses, and apparently of a dense nature. Surgery should be performed when this is indicated by the patient's behaviour as well as by the appearance of the lenses. It is important, however, that surgical interference is not too long delayed. Once blindness is present, or almost so, it is possible that degenerative changes may take place in the retina, due to inactivity, producing the condition of *amblyopia ex anopsia* —dimness of vision due to disuse of the eye.

For cataract surgery to be successful it is, of course, essential that the eye should be otherwise normal; any degenerative changes may nullify the beneficial effect to be expected from removal of the lens. Degenerative changes are most likely to be encountered in the retina, and the functional behaviour of this part of the eye may be estimated by observation of the pupillary reflex. It is essential that the pupillary response to light should be prompt and normal; the absence of this reflex, or a weak reflex, may indicate degenerative changes. It must be remembered that in some cases in which the pupillary reflex appears normal, there may be early retinal degenerative changes; in time, these changes may progress, and render the cataract operation useless in restoring vision permanently to the animal.

In the majority of cases in which surgery is contemplated it is found impossible to examine the retina by ophthalmoscopy, due to the opaqueness of the lens. Sometimes when surgery is requested for one eye, the other showing no cataractous changes, an examination of the retina in the normal eye will enable retinal changes to be detected. In all such cases, which are mainly encountered in breeds such as the Miniature and Toy Poodle, Golden Retriever and Labrador Retriever, which are known to be liable to be affected by progressive retinal atrophy, it should be considered that such changes are likely to affect the cataractous eye also. Here cataract surgery is contraindicated.

In selecting cases for surgery, the general physical condition of the patient should be determined, to ascertain its suitability for lengthy surgery, and the eye and adnexa should be examined for other disease conditions or infection. Advanced keratitis pigmentosa or interstitial keratitis should be considered to be a contraindication to the operation.

Intraocular pressure should be checked, either by digital or instrumental tonometry. In cases of hypertension, steps should be taken to reduce the pressure to within normal limits where possible, before surgery is undertaken. Some cases of cataract formation in the dog will be associated with diabetes mellitus, and an analysis of the urine should be undertaken in all cases in which surgery is contemplated.

Lastly, it is important that the temperament of the dog be taken into consideration. In view of the nature of the operation and the lengthy post-operative course, dogs with a highly nervous temperament that renders them unwilling and uncooperative patients are unsuitable for surgery of this type.

General management

Dogs requiring cataract surgery should be introduced into the hospital a few days before the operation is to take place. Such a period enables them to become acquainted with their surroundings and the staff who will be responsible for their welfare. Dogs exhibiting bilateral cataract, and on which a conjunctival flap covering the eye is to be used at the time of operation, will be without vision postoperatively; in these circumstances, familiarity with surroundings and nursing personnel will help in the maintenance of a smooth postoperative course.

Preoperative hospitalization will also allow the administration of tran-quillizing drugs to those animals that show nervousness or apprehension.

It is important that the kennelling facilities are good, and that accom-modation is provided that is clean, dust-free as far as possible, and of such a type that self-inflicted, postoperative trauma is avoided.

Preoperative preparation

During the period of preoperative hospitalization, it is advisable to check the patency of the lacrimal ducts, with fluorescein, and to correct any obstruction that might be demonstrated. The conjunctival sac should be irrigated with normal saline, and an antibiotic, in the form of drops, should be instilled two or three times daily for three or four days prior to the operation. The value of preoperative cultural examination of conjunctival swabs or scrapings is doubtful, as little is known of the normal bacterial flora of the canine conjunctiva, and results are likely to be misleading. Although no studies have been made in the dog, there is some evidence that chloramphenicol possesses the greatest power of penetration of the intact cornea, and this agent is used for the sterilization of the conjunctival sac.

Again, although no studies have been related specifically to the dog, there is evidence that antibiotics administered by oral or parenteral routes do not penetrate the physiological blood-aqueous barrier that protects the aqueous from many substances circulating in the blood; the blood level of a therapeutic agent is no guide to the levels reached in any part of the eye. On the other hand, chloramphenicol passes readily into the intraocular fluids from the blood stream. It is, therefore, prudent to administer this antibiotic prophylactically two or three days prior to the operation.

Mydriasis is essential to cataract surgery and, as a step in acquiring this desired dilatation of the pupil, a cycloplegic agent such as atropine is instilled into the conjunctival sac twice daily for four or five days before the operation. The effect of the mydriatic is often counteracted by anaesthesia, but adequate atropinization, over a period, is desirable.

The lowering of intraocular pressure, prior to intraocular surgery, is beneficial in that the eye is softer, and more easy to manipulate; the rush of aqueous on penetration of the anterior chamber is not so great, and there is less protrusion of the vitreous humour on delivery of the lens. The eye can be rendered hypotonic by the administration of a carbonic anhydrase inhibitor such as dichlorphenamide or acetazolamide, by mouth, for two or three days preoperatively. These drugs inhibit the formation of aqueous humour, but have no effect on the outflow. If the intraocular pressure is lowered too far, the eye becomes soft, and corneal sectioning becomes both difficult and inaccurate. The intraocular pressure may be measured with a tonometer, and the aim should be to reduce pressure, by means of inhibitors, to within the range of 15 to 20 mm Hg.

The sudden constriction of the pupil during surgery may be due to histamine release from traumatized ocular tissue. Histamine is a potent miotic drug, causing constriction of the pupil by a direct action on the smooth muscle of the iris sphincter. This miosis is produced by histamine even after the iris sphincter has been paralysed by a cycloplegic agent such as atropine. Histamine, or a histamine-like substance, may be liberated by injured tissue cells, and it is possible that the incision for a cataract extraction produces sufficient tissue damage to release histamine-like substances. The administration of antihistamine agents, preoperatively, either by mouth or topically, may reduce the incidence of miosis during surgery.

The preoperative preparation of the site has been described in a previous chapter, and every effort should be made to produce an operational area that is free from debris and loose hair. The area should be draped so that as much as possible of the surrounding skin is covered, leaving only sufficient room for a canthotomy incision.

The installation of a few drops of 1:1000 adrenaline solution, just prior to surgery, is helpful in limiting haemorrhage from the conjunctiva during the preparation of a flap. Alternatively, adrenaline may be given subconjunctivally, or, preferably, mydricaine solution may be used. The latter has the advantage that it will assist in maintaining mydriasis, and in the prevention of fibrin production in the secondary aqueous, as well as controlling

18

haemorrhage from the conjunctiva and helping, mechanically, in the preparation of the flap.

The control of infection

Intraocular infection, following surgery, is uncommon in the dog; as far as intraocular surgery is concerned, the dog's eye appears resistant to infection. The precautions normally taken, in the selection of cases, the sterilization of instruments and materials, and the preoperative preparation and postoperative management of the patient are normally sufficient to prevent sepsis following cataract surgery.

The preoperative control of any conjunctival or corneal infection that may be present is imperative. The routine use of antibiotic preparations is advocated, and the operation should be postponed until any infection has been adequately controlled.

SURGICAL APPROACH FOR CATARACT SURGERY

The anatomical features that render intraocular surgery in the dog difficult to perform have already been described. The surgical approach can, nevertheless, be improved upon by the adoption of various preliminary procedures.

Positioning of the patient. The suitable placing of the patient on the operating table, so that access to the eye is improved, has been described in a previous chapter. The use of a tilting table, to produce postural hypotension as well as to elevate the dog's head, will be found advantageous (Fig. 33, p. 55).

Exposure of the globe. The small palpebral fissure of the dog renders the approach difficult, and, with the exception of some brachycephalic dogs exhibiting some degree of proptosis, the opening must be enlarged. This may be accomplished by performing a lateral canthotomy (Fig. 209). The incision is made in the horizontal plane, for approximately 2 to 3 cm using pointed scissors. Tension is applied to the skin at the lateral canthus by the surgeon's forefinger, and one blade of the scissors is passed into the conjunctival sac. Haemorrhage is often profuse, and must be controlled completely before the operation is continued. Digital pressure over gauze is sometimes sufficient, but, because of the difficulty that is sometimes experienced in obtaining good healing of a canthotomy incision, the use of haemostatic pressure along the line of incision, before this is carried out, is not recommended. Infiltration of the line of incision with adrenaline may be used, or the haemorrhage may be controlled simply and speedily by the use of coagulation diathermy, or electrocautery.

Lid retraction. It is essential that the position of the lids be controlled, and that they be widely retracted in order to assist the adequate exposure of the eyeball. The conventional type of lid speculum is quite unsuitable for cataract surgery. However constructed, a speculum is an embarrassment to some of the surgical manoeuvres and, in the dog, tends to move in position during the operation and to slip off the lids. In addition, such an appliance is not easily adjusted during the operation and may cause pressure against the

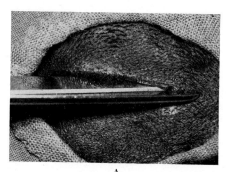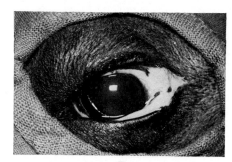

A   B

FIG. 209. *Lateral canthotomy for cataract surgery.* A *stage 1,* B *stage 2.*

globe, interfering with the accuracy of the incision into the eye and making the escape of the intraocular structures more likely.

Castroviejo's lid screw-clamps, whilst having certain advantages in effecting lid retraction, are not entirely satisfactory (Fig. 210). Once again, they slip very easily from the lids, the screw tops cause some mechanical interference, particulary with the fine sutures; and the attached sutures, which have to be fixed to the drapes, are liable to move in position during the operation.

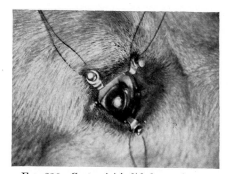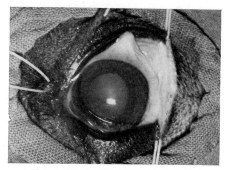

FIG. 210. *Castroviejo's lid clamps in use.*   FIG. 211. *Application of lid sutures.*

Lid sutures produce satisfactory lid retraction, without mechanical interference to instrumentation. Three sutures are used, one being passed through the skin of the lower lid, just below the centre of the lid margin, and two through the upper lid. Those in the upper lid are passed transversely through the skin of the lid, just above the margin, one in the centre of the medial half, and one in the centre of the lateral half. The three sutures are drawn taut, so as to retract the lids, and are secured to the drapes with pressure forceps.

As with screw-clamps, lid sutures (Fig. 211) are liable to move in position if, for any reason, the drapes are moved during the operation. Vierheller's spring eyelid retractor will be found very useful during intraocular surgery (Fig. 212).

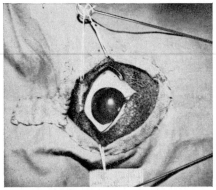

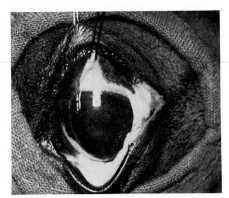

FIG. 212. *Application of Vierheller's eyelid retractor.*

FIG. 213. *Application of stay suture.*

Immobilization of the globe. At times during the operation it may be desirable to alter the position of the globe, or to control its movements. Such manoeuvres are best carried out by an assistant with the help of stay sutures (Fig. 213). Normally two such sutures, of fine thread, are used and these are passed through the bulbar conjunctiva and episcleral tissue, about

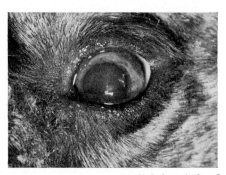

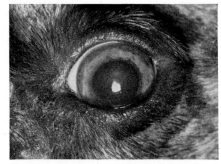

FIG. 214. *Position of eyeball before induced proptosis.*

FIG. 215. *Position of eyeball after induced proptosis.*

4 mm from the limbus, one lateral and one medial to the horizontal meridian. Each suture is held with small cross-action artery forceps, and may be clipped to the drapes if required. Where a fornix-based flap is fashioned, these sutures may be placed in the connective tissue underneath the flap.

Induced proptosis. Even following canthotomy and adequate lid retraction, the degree of rotation and retraction of the eye will often render surgical interference hazardous. These movements may, to some extent, be controlled by the stay sutures, but any undue traction upon the eyeball is liable to distort the globe, increase intraocular pressure and make accurate corneal incision difficult.

The retrobulbar injection of air will induce proptosis of a degree sufficient to prevent rotation and retraction of the eyeball, and bring the eye into a suitable position for surgery (Figs. 214, 215).

The air is sterilized by autoclaving a suitable syringe with its plunger withdrawn to its full extent. The needle is inserted into the retrobulbar space, and the air is discharged slowly until an adequate degree of proptosis is obtained. It is important that the induced proptosis is not too marked, and care must be taken that subconjunctival emphysema is not produced that might complicate the subsequent surgical procedures. Retrobulbar injection of air does not raise intraocular pressure, but it is possible that this technique makes vitreous loss more likely to occur.

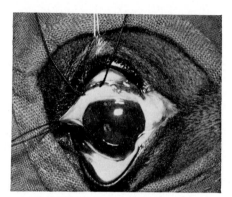 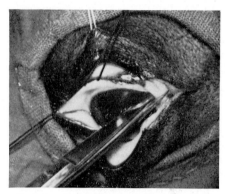

FIG. 216. *Control of the nictitating membrane.*   FIG. 217. *Control of the bulbar conjunctiva.*

The needle enters the conjunctiva close to the ventro-lateral rim of the orbit, between the insertions of the lateral and inferior rectus muscles, and is passed through until its point lies within the cone formed by the recti muscles, anterior to the apex. A needle of $1\frac{1}{2}$ in. length, 26 S.W.G. is used, and some deflection of the eye towards the needle is to be expected as the needle punctures Tenon's capsule.

Control of the nictitating membrane. If adequate proptosis is obtained, the position of the nictitating membrane will usually be such that it does not interfere with the approach to the eye. If necessary, however, it may be secured with a stay suture or its attachment may be partly severed (Fig. 216).

Control of the bulbar conjunctiva. The creeping of the bulbar conjunctiva across the corneo-sclera junction may be controlled by making small incisions into the conjunctiva on either side in the horizontal meridian (Fig. 217). When making a corneal incision, it is essential that no part of the limbus is obscured by overlying conjunctiva.

OPENING THE ANTERIOR CHAMBER

Any incision of the anterior chamber to remove the lens must, of necessity, be large enough to allow the easy removal of the lens without injury to the structures of the eye. The volume of the canine lens is comparatively large, the average diameter being about 9 to 11 mm and the antero-posterior thickness 7 mm. Any incision to remove the lens must involve from two-fifths to one-half of the corneal circumference, and attempts to remove the lens through an incision smaller than this will inevitably result in failure.

The line of incision. During the development of canine cataract surgery, which has closely followed advances in human ophthalmic techniques, various methods of opening the anterior chamber have been recommended, using many different instruments.

Incisions into the sclera, approximately 1 mm posterior to the limbus and parallel to it will be accompanied by haemorrhage, often severe, from the wound and into the anterior chamber. Control of this haemorrhage is often extremely difficult, and in most cases impossible. The value of adrenaline drops, and gentle pressure from swabs, is very limited in the control of the haemorrhage and in most cases the anterior chamber rapidly fills with blood. Attempts may be made to remove the blood by irrigation of the anterior chamber with warm normal saline, and to remove clots from the anterior chamber with forceps. The excessive intraocular instrumentation necessary, however, is likely to cause further intraocular damage, and continuing haemorrhage from the incision may often mean the abandonment of the operation. Where the haemorrhage is finally controlled satisfactorily, blood clots are likely to remain in the anterior chamber or a hyphaema may result, leading to a spastic iritis, excessive pupillary adhesions or synechiae.

Any incision in the dog, into the sclera, is likely to cause damage to the root of the iris and subsequent haemorrhage. It is not possible to avoid such damage by alterations in the angle at which the incision is made.

The transitional zone between the cornea and the sclera—the limbus—is the area in which the blood vessels which nourish the cornea—the marginal venous plexus—are found. For this reason, any incision involving the scleral side of the limbus is likely to be accompanied by haemorrhage. Any incision exactly through the limbus, whether made by the cataract knife or by the keratome and scissors technique, may be accompanied by haemorrhage, and extreme accuracy in the placement of the incision is required. The use of hypotensive anaesthetic techniques may lessen the degree of blood loss experienced, but the ideal of a bloodless field will be rarely achieved if there is any encroachment upon the sclera.

An incision into the cornea, 1 to 2 mm anterior to and parallel with the limbus, is made entirely through tissues which are avascular. Such an incision is therefore not accompanied by any haemorrhage, provided that no damage is inflicted on the iris during the sectioning. On the other hand, corneal section will lead to excessive scarring in some cases, sometimes accompanied by neovascularization and corneal oedema. Adequate corneal suturing and wound protection will limit the amount of scar formation, but corneal incision will always be followed by some degree of corneal opacity around the line of incision; this does not, in itself, necessarily detract from the value of this technique.

The two major complications arising during or after corneal sectioning are, therefore, haemorrhage and scarring. Both these complications may be avoided by making the incision just anterior to the limbus, in corneal tissue —a corneo-limbal incision. By this method, all haemorrhage may be avoided, and, provided the incision is exactly at the corneo-limbal junction, wound healing with the minimum of scar formation is obtained. Extreme accuracy of the incision is essential, for the avoidance of all haemorrhage is imperative if a successful intracapsular cataract extraction is to be completed. A good cosmetic result, with the avoidance of corneal vascularization, is also desirable, and this will depend largely on accurate apposition of the wound edges at the completion of the operation.

The method of incision

Many variations in the technique used for corneal sectioning have been described. These fall mainly into two categories, section with a knife, and section using a keratome and scissors.

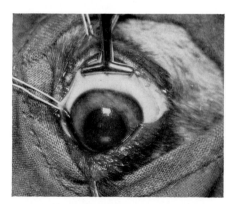

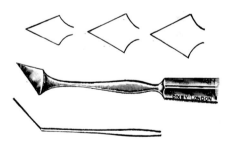

FIG. 218. *Application of fixation forceps.*   FIG. 219. *Keratome.*

Accuracy of the incision, and minimal damage to the corneal tissue, is essential if satisfactory healing of the wound is to be obtained. This will depend largely on the avoidance of any distortion of the globe whilst the incision is being made. Upward traction by stay sutures, or fixation forceps, is likely to distort the globe and make accurate incision impossible. The immobilization and control of the globe during surgery has already been described; if the suggested methods are applied, it is possible to avoid any distortion of the eyeball, using fixation forceps merely to steady the globe and control its position during sectioning.

The loose nature of the conjunctiva in the dog makes control of the globe with forceps somewhat difficult. The use of forceps with large jaws, exerting their effect over a considerable area of conjunctiva, is satisfactory; for this purpose, the forceps of Barraquer-Llovera, with a wide base and spaced settings of sharp teeth, are useful. A firm grip should be taken with the forceps, and their position should not be altered until the sectioning is completed (Fig. 218). Any backward pressure on the forceps is likely to distort the globe, encourage the rapid loss of aqueous, and make the folding of the iris over the knife more likely; for these reasons, the forceps must be kept in a forward-facing position.

Keratome and scissors incision. This is likely to produce a more even cut than that obtained by other methods. In the dog, any opening of the anterior chamber will be accompanied by rapid loss of aqueous, but with this technique the anterior chamber is better preserved throughout the section and there is less risk of the iris folding over the instruments. Again, if preplaced sutures are employed, it is easier to effect the passage of the keratome between the loops of the sutures than is the case with the cataract knife. It is impossible, however, to make the incision large enough with the keratome alone and the wound must be enlarged with scissors. The squeezing effect of scissors may influence the healing of the wound or interfere with the angle of filtration.

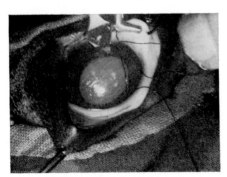

FIG. 220. *Keratome incision.*

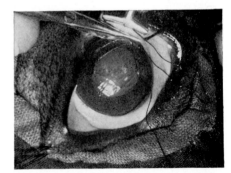

FIG. 222. *Enlargement of the keratome incision with scissors.*

A keratome incision is best made in the 12 o'clock position. The tip of the keratome (Fig. 219) is placed perpendicularly, just anterior to the limbus, and is made to enter the anterior chamber, with the handle of the instrument depressed towards the operator as entry is effected (Fig. 220). Great care must be taken to avoid injury to the iris, lens or corneal endothelium. The keratome is directed towards one side, as it is withdrawn, to enlarge the incision. Withdrawal of the instrument is accompanied by loss of aqueous and reduction in the depth of the anterior chamber.

Aqueous loss can be avoided to some extent by careful positioning of the fixation forceps, but the loss of the anterior chamber may sometimes make the insertion of the blade of the scissors difficult. Great care must be taken at this stage to avoid damage to the iris, which would result in haemorrhage. The incision is enlarged, in both directions, towards the 3 and 9 o'clock positions, and, for this purpose, curved corneal scissors are the most satisfactory (Fig. 221A). Scissors incorporating a stop (Fig. 221B), so that the closure of the jaws cannot be completed, avoid the constant repositioning of the scissors within the wound, and allow the incision to be completed with the minimum of trauma. The scissors must be placed well up in the angle, small successive bites being taken so as to enlarge the incision to the desired degree (Fig. 222).

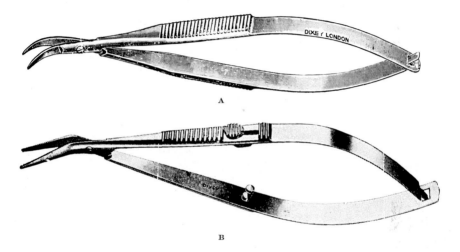

FIG. 221. A *Castroviejo's curved corneal scissors*, B *Barraquer's incision-enlarging scissors with sliding butt.*

The cornea of the dog, at the corneo-limbal area, is a remarkably tough structure, and even with scissors that are exquisitely sharp, considerable pressure must be exerted to complete the incision. Again, the progressive loss of aqueous, and lessening of the depth of the anterior chamber, as sectioning progresses, will occasionally make the accurate completion of the incision difficult. A scissors incision is a relatively slow procedure and, before it is completed, it may be found that the loss of aqueous, associated with the great depth of the anterior chamber and curvature of the cornea in the dog, allows considerable wrinkling of the cornea; this, in turn, will often lead to an inaccurate incision in the terminal stages, either encroaching too far on to the cornea, or causing damage to the iris.

The squeezing effect of scissors and consequent damage to the corneal endothelium, might lead to a higher incidence of complications such as keratitis, delayed formation of the anterior chamber, gaping of the wound, iris prolapse, peripheral synechiae and complicated glaucoma. These complications are more likely to follow a vertically placed incision that is liable to gape in its deep aspect, particularly if the incision is large. In the dog, large incisions are of course necessary, and it is not possible to produce a bevelled incision with scissors. Vertical incisions produce greater destruction of Descemet's membrane, and the retraction of this elastic structure is likely to produce greater gaping in the deeper parts of the wound.

A keratome-scissors incision is far more likely to be traumatic, and where no conjunctival flap, or a fornix-based flap, is employed, is likely to be followed by a greater number of postoperative complications than a knife incision: for example, failure of healing, iris prolapse, epithelialization of the anterior chamber and glaucoma. The use of a limbal-based flap will largely overcome these objections.

Cataract knife incision. A knife incision produces a cleaner cut with less trauma and the section tends to be more oblique. Damage to the corneal

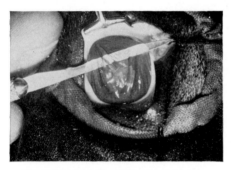

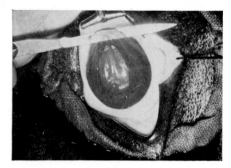

Fig. 223. *Insertion of the cataract knife.*   Fig. 224. *Completion of the cataract knife incision.*

endothelium and to Descemet's membrane is likely to be less severe, and suturing is more likely to effect accurate closure of the deep parts of the wound. The main disadvantage is the immediate loss of aqueous and the tendency for the knife to become engaged with the iris, as this structure comes forward with the loss of the anterior chamber. Any damage to the iris must, at all costs, be avoided, or subsequent haemorrhage may jeopardize the result of the operation.

When a cataract knife is used, care must be taken to see that the cutting edge is uppermost before insertion. Failure to ensure this will mean that the knife has to be withdrawn and reinserted, with the subsequent further loss of aqueous, which must, for a successful sectioning to be completed, be avoided as far as is possible.

The knife is inserted into the cornea from the temporal side, at the 3 or 9 o'clock position, depending on the eye involved, just anterior to the limbus, whilst a gentle counter-movement is made by the fixation forceps to prevent rotation of the globe (Fig. 223). The plane of the knife must be flat antero-posteriorly, and tangential with the iris. On entry into the anterior chamber, the blade is passed transversely across the chamber; at this stage, it is important not to make any upward or downward movement of the handle; such movements cause the incision at the point of entry to gape and lead to further loss of aqueous. The site of the counter-puncture should be level with and opposite to the point of entry, once again just anterior to the limbus. The refraction of the cornea is misleading, and the point of the knife should be aimed at a site about 2 mm from the limbus in the anterior direction; if this is accurately judged, it will be found that the point of the knife will emerge in the desired position. As the counter-puncture is made, the fixation forceps should, once again, be slightly moved to prevent any rotation of the eye, and the knife passed through until the full breadth of the blade is engaged. Great care must be taken that the knife is held in the correct plane, so as to avoid either splitting of the cornea or injury to the iris.

The section is completed by a smooth upward sweep of the knife, keeping the blade in the same plane until the incision is completed (Fig. 224). Two such sweeps, one towards the nasal side and one towards the temporal side, may be necessary to complete the section. On completion of the section all aqueous humour escapes and the anterior chamber is lost. There is little or no haemorrhage, but any there is is gently removed by swabbing, and any blood in the anterior chamber is removed by irrigation. The iris, if it has prolapsed through the incision, is replaced with a repositor.

Excessive or rapid loss of aqueous whilst the section is performed will cause the iris to come forward and this may engage on the knife, making incision difficult whilst avoiding damage to the iris. This may be avoided, to a large extent, by making sure that the fixation forceps controlling the globe are held well forward and by avoiding any pressure on the posterior part of the eye. It is essential to complete the section decisively and without hesitation; when these conditions are fulfilled, it is possible to complete an accurate and trauma-free section in nearly every case. Adequate dilatation of the pupil will lessen the risk of the iris folding over the advancing knife. Where it is apparent, after partial completion of the section, that the iris will become damaged by the knife, it is necessary to withdraw the knife and complete the incision with scissors.

Wound healing following cataract knife section is usually perfect, and the incidence of postoperative complications is low. Scar formation will generally be less than will follow an incision made with scissors.

Following the completion of the section, the length of the incision is tested by sweeping the wound with a spatula. If it is found to be too small, enlargement is made with scissors.

Conjunctival flaps

The use of conjunctival flaps to protect the wound and to help in the apposition of the wound edges is to be recommended in canine cataract surgery. Such flaps may be either based on the limbus or may be based on the conjunctival fornix. If the latter, they may be prepared either before or after the corneal section.

Limbus-based flaps. A flap of this type may be fashioned by grasping the conjunctiva with toothed forceps, and incising this membrane, in the 12 o'clock position, about 3 to 4 mm from the limbus. This incision is continued parallel to the limbus to the 3 and 9 o'clock positions (Fig. 225A). This flap of conjunctiva is then dissected down to the limbus, just on to the corneal margin, using a Tooke's knife (Fig. 195). Some haemorrhage is usually encountered, but it may be controlled easily by the use of electrocautery.

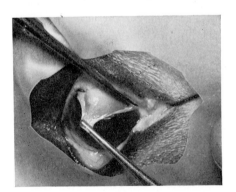
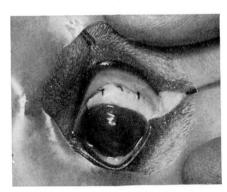

A   B

FIG. 225. *The limbus-based flap.* A *formation,* B *replacement.*

The flap is then turned down over the cornea and the limbus is identified. Puncture of the limbus is made with a keratome, 2 to 3 mm above the horizontal diameter, either medially or laterally, whichever is most convenient. It is important that no damage is caused to the iris, and the keratome must be inserted carefully so that direct entry is made to the anterior chamber. Withdrawal of the keratome is followed by loss of aqueous and a reduction in the depth of the anterior chamber. The limbal incision is then continued with scissors. Again, care must be taken, when inserting the scissors into the anterior chamber and continuing the incision, that no damage is inflicted upon the iris. Should the incision be made too posterior to the limbus, haemorrhage is likely, even if hypotensive conditions are applied; this haemorrhage may be sufficient to cause embarrassment, and, on occasion, may fill the anterior chamber. Under these conditions, it may be necessary to irrigate the anterior chamber with warm normal saline, and to remove blood clots with forceps; care must be taken not to cause further intraocular haemorrhage from damage to the iris, or to injure the corneal endothelium.

The incision should be continued for rather less than half the corneal circumference, and must be sufficiently large to allow the passage of the lens without undue manipulation. Following the suturing of the limbal wound, the conjunctival flap is replaced and maintained with about 4 or 5 interrupted silk sutures (Fig. 225B). The flap thus covers the limbal wound and supports it during the healing period.

Fornix-based flaps. A flap of this type may be made by incising the conjunctiva parallel to and about 2 to 3 mm from, the limbus, and extending this incision to approximately two-fifths of the circumference of the cornea, from the 10 to 2 o'clock positions. The conjunctiva is then undermined towards the fornix, so that it may be drawn over the limbus (Fig. 226A). Such a flap may be used with either preplaced or postplaced sutures, so that, when the sutures are tied, the conjunctival flap is brought down over the wound. Alternatively, a hooded conjunctival flap may be fashioned in the

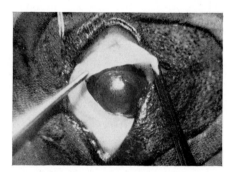 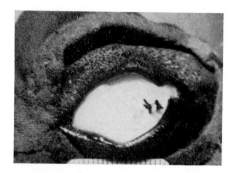

A   B

FIG. 226. *The fornix-based flap.* A *formation,* B *replacement.*

same way, involving about three-fifths of the circumference of the globe in its upper part. On completion of wound suturing, the flap is brought over the cornea and sutured to the lower part of the incised conjunctiva, so that the upper half or upper third of the cornea is covered. Using the above techniques, however, it may be found that the fixation of the flaps is insufficient to withstand postoperative movements and interference; in this case, the flap may become detached from its position and fail to provide the protection required.

The use of full, fornix-based flaps is preferable, when this technique is employed. The flap is formed by incising the conjunctiva just posterior to the limbus, and continuing this incision around the circumference of the globe to the 10 and 2 o'clock positions. This flap is then undermined, and, at either end, an incision is made at right angles to the original incision, and extending towards the fornix for a distance of about 1 cm. The flap must be dissected well away from the eyeball, so that it may be drawn completely over the cornea, and sutured to the bulbar conjunctiva of the lower lid (Fig. 226B). The flap must be of sufficient length to fit over the cornea without pressure.

Any pressure exerted on the cornea will tend to increase the loss of aqueous, and to cause unwanted pressures and tensions on the sutures in the incision. For this reason, a flap made from the nictitating membrane is usually unsuitable in cataract surgery.

To avoid haemorrhage prior to the corneal sectioning, the flap is best formed after the operation has been completed. Any undue haemorrhage may be controlled with adrenaline.

Such a flap affords good wound protection, even if postoperative inter-ference by the patient should be experienced. In most cases, however, the flap is well tolerated, and the use of a conjunctival flap will reduce the incidence of postoperative irritation or discomfort. The corneal wound will heal well under the flap. This is partly due, no doubt, to the protection offered, and partly to plasma oozing from the cut surface of the conjunctiva into the corneal incision and assisting healing.

The disadvantage of the full conjunctival flap is that it will prevent inspection of the eye whilst it remains in place. It is rarely necessary, however, to leave the flap in position for more than five days, after which time the sutures may be removed, allowing inspection of the wound and of the remainder of the eye. Once released, the conjunctival flap rapidly heals into its original position without further treatment.

Of the methods available, the limbus-based flap is to be preferred. Using this method, healing is normally excellent and postoperative scarring minimal; the incidence of delayed healing is extremely low; and iris prolapse is unlikely to occur. The incidence of delayed healing and iris prolapse is greater when a fornix-based flap is used, and scarring is likely to be more marked. However, greater accuracy of incision will be required when a limbus-based flap is used, in order to avoid haemorrhage, than will be required when a straight corneolimbal incision is made, to be covered later with a fornix-based flap.

IRIDECTOMY AND CATARACT SURGERY

The purpose of iridectomy, as a preliminary to cataract extraction, is to prevent the postoperative complication of iris incarceration and subse-quent possible hydrophthalmos. A peripheral iridectomy may be performed to effect communication between the anterior and posterior chambers, to reduce the risk of iris prolapse; a pupillary iridectomy may be performed to enlarge the access to the lens; a sphincterectomy may be performed to prevent a drawn-up pupil.

The iris in the dog is a highly vascular structure that bleeds freely if damaged. Excision of part of the iris, be it large or small, or be it peripheral or pupillary, will result in severe haemorrhage, which is always extremely difficult, and sometimes impossible, to control. The application of adrenaline to the cut iris, after it is drawn out of the corneal wound, is of little value; and the use of the electrocautery to control haemorrhage involves difficult instrumentation, and is unlikely to be successful.

The control of haemorrhage during cataract surgery is essential. The difficulty in controlling haemorrhage from the iris, the intraocular interference required in its control, and the difficulty experienced in removing blood clots from the anterior chamber, adherent to the iris, are considered to be strong contraindications for the use of iridectomy as a means of preventing iris prolapse. Any foreign matter, such as a blood clot, left in the anterior chamber, is likely to cause pupillary adhesions and occlusion; in an intracapsular operation it is essential that this be avoided.

The use of a small sphincterectomy, in the 6 o'clock position, is of value in preventing a drawn-up pupil, and will help in the performance of a

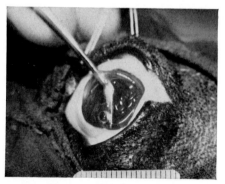

Fig. 227. *Sphincterectomy.*

satisfactory round-pupil extraction (Fig. 227). The incision is best made with de Wecker's scissors (Fig. 199), and providing the iris is not incised for more than one-half its width, no great haemorrhage is likely to be experienced.

In those cases in which a small amount of haemorrhage is met, this may usually be controlled satisfactorily by soaking up the blood with small cellulose-sponge swabs held over the corneal incision, separating the lips of the wound slightly so that the blood be attracted to the swab. The capillary attraction of the swab will usually be sufficient, aided if necessary by gentle pressure over the cornea with a lens expressor. This should be followed by irrigation of the anterior chamber with warm normal saline. Any haemorrhage must be controlled before proceeding with any further steps in the operation.

INTRACAPSULAR EXTRACTION

Intracapsular extraction requires that the lens should be separated from the suspensory ligament, and then delivered, contained within its capsule, through the corneal incision. The delivery must be accomplished without rupture of the lens capsule, without damage to the iris or ciliary body, and without loss of vitreous humour.

Methods that have been described include the use of forceps to grasp the lens capsule; suction, applied by means of an erisiphake; diathermocoagulation; and cryoextraction.

Rupture of the zonular fibres may be accomplished in various ways: by grasping the lens at the lower pole, tumbling the lens and applying pressure externally with a lens expressor; rocking motions and push-and-pull manoeuvres; by grasping the lens in the central pupillary area and applying traction; by grasping the lens at the superior equator and applying traction simultaneously with external pressure; or by grasping the lens and stripping the zonule with a blunt instrument.

Forceps delivery

Tumbling method. Capsule forceps are introduced into the anterior chamber, with the blades closed, and are positioned in the 6 o'clock position just

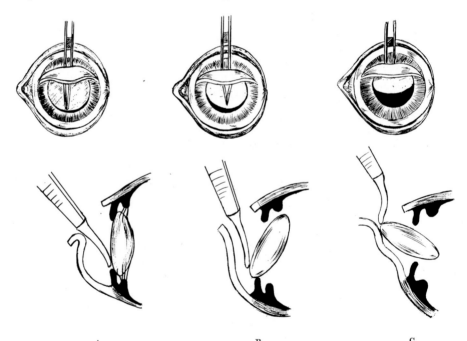

A   B   C

FIG. 228. *Extraction of the lens by tumbling.* A *1st stage,* B *2nd stage,* C *3rd stage.*

under the iris. The blades are then slightly opened, slight pressure is exerted upon the capsule and the blades are closed (Fig. 228A). Moderate pressure is applied externally with a lens expressor (Fig. 229), just below the limbus at 6 o'clock.

By slightly depressing the handle of the capsule forceps, the tip of the forceps holding the capsule is elevated. At the same time, gentle pressure is applied to the limbus by moving the expressor from side to side (Fig. 228B).

The lower pole of the lens is thus dislocated and slow upward traction is made with the forceps, at the same time applying counter-pressure with the expressor, following the lens through the anterior chamber, until it emerges from the wound (Fig. 228C). As the lens is tumbled, the zonule is broken. In cases where the zonule is resistant, side to side motions are made with the forceps to assist its rupture.

It is often impossible to deliver the canine lens by tumbling. The excessive traction required will often result in rupture of the lens capsule, and it is often impossible to dislocate the lower pole of the lens by a combination of traction and external pressure. Excessive pressure applied by the lens expressor in an attempt to rupture the zonule may result in the escape of vitreous into the anterior chamber. Attempts to rupture the zonule by rocking motions or push-and-pull manoeuvres will invariably result in rupture of the lens capsule.

Sliding method. In cases where the zonule is weak, the forceps are applied to the lens capsule in the central pupillary area, and the lens is removed with gentle traction, with little or no external pressure. However, except in those cases in which the cataractous lens is luxated, it is not usually possible to apply this technique to the dog. In cases of hypermature cataract it may be possible to grasp the capsule with ease; in most other cases, the pressure of the forceps in the central area of the lens capsule is likely to result in rupture of that capsule. In those cases where it is possible to attach the forceps satisfactorily, any traction to deliver the lens, or side-to-side movements to rupture the zonule, will often result in immediate rupture of the capsule.

Application of the capsule forceps superiorly, at the equator, is facilitated by applying pressure over the cornea below, and thus slightly tilting the lens. The forceps are applied, and moved from side to side, the external pressure with an expressor following the upward passage of the lens. As the lens dislocates and enters the wound, external pressure is directed upwards and the cornea is kept in contact with the lens. In the absence of an iridectomy, some difficulty in applying the forceps to the equator may be experienced. It is usually possible, however, to grasp the capsule, as near as possible to the equator, without capsular rupture, provided that no undue pressure is applied with the forceps (Fig. 233).

Two types of forceps are commonly used to grasp the capsule. Arruga's capsule forceps (Fig. 230) have rounded and bevelled ends and upper edges, to prevent damage to the iris when the forceps are opened and closed beneath this structure. The edge of the forceps applied to the capsule—the lower edge—is clean cut but not sharp, and must fit perfectly along the entire edge. It may be found preferable to use Castroviejo's capsule forceps

19

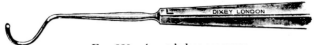

Fig. 229. *Arruga's lens expressor.*

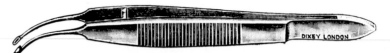

Fig. 230. *Arruga's capsule forceps.*

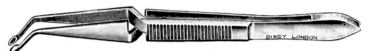

Fig. 231. *Castroviejo's capsule forceps.*

Fig. 232. *Snellen's vectis.*

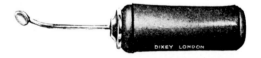

Fig. 235. *Hand erisiphake.*

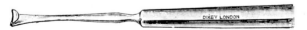

Fig. 240. *Rubinstein's iris retractor.*

(Fig. 231), where the pressure is controlled mechanically by the cross-action of the forceps, rather than Arruga's forceps, where the pressure is controlled manually. With the former, as no pressure needs to be applied, the operator is able to concentrate on the delivery of the lens. Once again, however, any traction applied to the lens, or side-to-side movements to rupture the zonule, may result in rupture of the lens capsule.

Stripping method. The lens is slightly tilted by external pressure, and the capsule is grasped by applying the forceps tangentially just below the equator at the 12 o'clock position. The iris is displaced by sliding the forceps under it to grasp the lens. By applying very gentle traction, the lens is lifted slightly and rotated to one side. A blunt instrument, such as a Snellen's

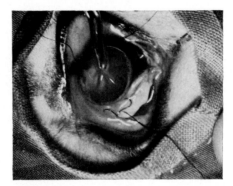

FIG. 233. *Delivery of the lens with forceps.*

vectis (Fig. 232), or a blunt curved hook, is insinuated under the iris, towards the equator, and a delicate stripping motion is applied at the insertion of the zonule. This is continued along the equator, as far as is possible, the lens is then rotated towards the other side, and the procedure is repeated, so that the whole circumference is covered. At this stage, the lens is completely, or largely, separated from its zonular attachments. The upper border of the iris is then retracted with a blunt hook (Fig. 58, p. 64), and by gentle traction, and pressure applied inferiorly with an expressor, the lens may be delivered through the wound.

Rupture of the capsule, due to excessive pressure from forceps or excessive traction following incomplete separation of the zonule, may occur in some cases. In other cases, haemorrhage from the iris or ciliary body may be experienced, due to damage to these structures by the stripping instrument; this haemorrhage may, on occasion, be severe, and interfere with the completion of the operation. The resistance of the fibres, in some cases, may be so great that undue pressure from the stripping instrument is required to complete their rupture. In such cases, the risk of damage to the ciliary body is great, and delivery of the lens may be accompanied by marked loss of vitreous.

Erisiphake extraction

The use of suction to grasp the capsule of the lens is a technique worthy of consideration. The erisiphake consists of a hollow, circular spoon, through which suction is applied, either mechanically from an electrical suction apparatus (Fig. 234), or manually through a rubber bulb (Fig. 235). The cup

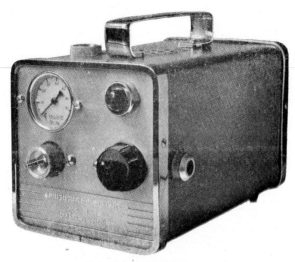

Fig. 234. *Erisiphake pump.*

is applied to the anterior surface of the lens, and the lens capsule is drawn into the cup and held there by suction (Fig. 236). Once the capsule has been firmly grasped by the instrument, rupture of the zonular fibres may be accomplished by any of the methods that have already been described.

The standard model of erisiphake used in human ophthalmology has a 4 mm internal cup diameter; and it will be found difficult to obtain an adequate

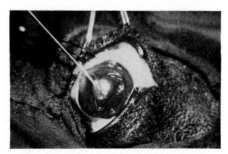

Fig. 236. *Application of the erisiphake.*

grasp of the capsule of the dog's lens with this instrument. The volume of the lens in the human is around 0·2 ml and the volume of the cup in the erisiphake is around 0·25 ml. As the volume of the lens in the dog is approximately 0·5 ml a cup of larger dimensions is required.

An erisiphake allows tension to be applied evenly all round the zonule, and allows a thin capsule to be held firmly. On the other hand, any excessive negative pressure is likely to rupture the capsule or even aspirate vitreous humour. Even using an erisiphake, traction and counter-pressure may result in rupture of the capsule. When using this instrument in the dog, it is imperative to produce rupture of the zonule by stripping in the same way as with capsular forceps. On occasion, it may be found difficult to maintain sufficient hold on the lens whilst this stripping is accomplished; in such cases, the reapplication of the erisiphake may be both difficult and hazardous.

Diathermocoagulation extraction

Coagulation of the lens substance by passing into it a diathermy current has been a suggested method of intracapsular lens extraction. A double-pronged platinum-iridium needle, sliding out of two acrylic plastic tubes set in a diathermy terminal, is passed into the lens substance, and a diathermy current of 20 to 30 mA is passed through for from 2 to 3 seconds. The lens coagulates and adheres to the needle. The lens may thus be held by the needle whilst the zonule is ruptured, and then lifted from the eye.

Some difficulty may be experienced in causing the needle to penetrate the lens capsule without undue pressure and subsequent trauma to the surrounding structures. Even following successful coagulation of the lens tissues, the adhesion of the needle is unlikely to be sufficient to permit any degree of traction without rupture of the lens capsule.

Cryoextraction

Cryoextraction signifies the extraction of the cataractous lens by application of low temperature.

The Krwawicz cryoextractor (Fig. 239A) is a pencil-shaped ball-tipped instrument, made of copper and nickel-plated. Before use, it is placed in a vacuum flask containing a mixture of dry ice and methyl alcohol, and, in this environment, assumes a temperature of about $-79°C$ ($-100°F$). The copper head is mounted in a plastic handle, to facilitate manipulation and protect the surgeon's hands; no other form of protection is necessary. The copper stem of the cryoextractor is placed in a container of ethyl alcohol to ensure sterility, and this alcohol is removed by wiping with a sterile swab before use. The whole instrument may be sterilized by boiling before it is placed in the vacuum flask, and an additional precaution may be taken by the surgeon wearing a sterile cotton glove, and discarding this when the extraction has been completed.

The instrument is removed from the flask and any alcohol is removed from the tip by swabbing. The tip is dipped in sterile water, so that a thin coating of ice forms on the metal The lens is tilted slightly, by applying pressure to the lower part of the cornea, and the ice-coated tip of the cryoextractor is applied to the lens capsule near the equator at the 12 o'clock position (Fig. 237). The capsule and subcapsular tissues, over an area about twice the size of the tip of the instrument, immediately freeze and attach themselves firmly to the cold metal. The surface of the lens should not be too wet and any excess of aqueous should be removed before the instrument is applied; neither should it be too dry from long exposure. With the lens firmly attached (Fig. 238), delivery may be effected by any of the methods already described.

A firm attachment between the instrument and the lens is formed, even though the refrigeration is limited to a relatively small part of the lens. It

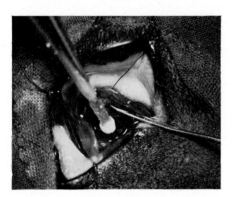

FIG. 237. *Introduction of the cryoextractor.*

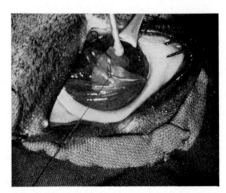

FIG. 238. *Extraction of the lens with the cryoextractor.*

is usually possible to perform rotating movements to break the zonule, without rupture of the lens capsule, to a far greater degree than is possible with any other method. Rupture of the lens capsule will occur when undue forces are applied, and a combination of lens rotation and a minimum of mechanical rupture of the zonular fibres with a vectis is usually the most satisfactory method of extraction. Apart from traction that is applied, rupture of the lens capsule may, on occasion, be due to excessive shrinking of the capsule caused by the refrigeration. However, even in those cases where rupture occurs, the lens capsule will remain firmly attached to the instrument and easily removed in its entirety.

The partial freezing of the lens does not appear to have any harmful effect on the other ocular structures. If the cornea or iris is accidentally touched by the instrument, it immediately adheres firmly to the cold metal; it is possible, in such cases, to detach the adhesion by sliding a spatula along the cryoextractor. No harm to the cornea or iris appears to result provided the adhesion is dealt with promptly.

In cases where the lens capsule has been damaged by any other instrument, the extractor may be applied to the point of injury, thus sealing the break, and the instrument used in the usual way.

Apart from the simple instrument described, many other types of cryo-extractor are now available. These range from those employing carbon dioxide snow in the handle, such as the Pierse cryoextractor (Fig. 239B), to advanced cryosurgical units operating with liquid nitrogen. The latter have the advantage that the temperature of the tip of the instrument can be

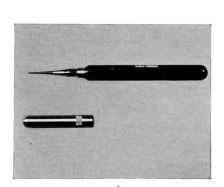 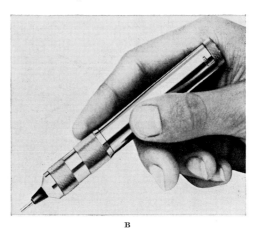

A   B

FIG. 239. A *Krwawicz cryoextractor*, B *Pierse cryoextractor*.

instantly controlled and monitored, through the range of +37°C (+99°F) to −160°C (−256°F). Sterile, disposable units have recently become available, and may eventually prove to be the instrument of choice in veterinary practice.

Complications of cryoextraction

Experience with the technique has shown that operative complications, other than those previously recognized in cataract surgery, may be met with this method.

Failure of freezing. Using the Krwawicz instrument, cases are occasionally met in which the tip of the probe fails to freeze to the lens capsule, or produces a union which is broken when attempts are made to break the zonule or remove the lens. In the dog, considerable instrumentation is often required to produce rupture of the zonular fibres, and a firm bond between lens and probe is essential. The possible reasons for this failure of freezing have been detailed by K. Rubinstein, and may be summarized thus:

(1) Any instrument that is cooled by direct immersion tends to warm rapidly on removal from the coolant. For this reason, there must be no undue delay in applying the instrument to the lens.

(2) The ethyl alcohol in the inner container must be sufficient to cover

about three-quarters of the instrument shaft. A lower level results in slow cooling.

(3) Any alcohol left on the instrument shaft, even in minute quantities, will prevent freezing. All alcohol on the shaft must be wiped away thoroughly, but small quantities may penetrate into the handle of the instrument, through the nut head, and may subsequently seep down the shaft.

(4) It is essential to dip the tip of the probe into water, forming a thin covering of ice, before application to the lens. If this is not done, the dry cold metal will not adhere to the lens capsule.

(5) Aqueous collecting on the surface of the lens will prevent efficient freezing, and this must be removed, using a brush, immediately before the application of the probe.

(6) The time taken for an effective bond to be formed between the instrument and the lens, in the case of intumescent or hypermature cataract, is appreciably greater than in the case of senile cataract.

(7) The tip of the instrument must be applied firmly to the lens in order to secure a good bond. Tilting the upper pole of the lens forward, by depression of the lower pole with an expressor, helps to achieve this.

(8) In the case of a subluxated or luxated lens, movements of the lens may make the firm application of the instrument to the lens difficult.

Accidental freezing of ocular structures. Contact between the extractor and any of the ocular structures will result in an immediate adhesion of the metal to the tissues. Very careful techniques, with a limbal flap held well away from the instrument by a suture, will normally avoid contact between probe and cornea. When adhesion does occur, involving either cornea or sclera, this may be freed by dropping saline onto the bond, at room temperature, and rapid de-freezing is produced by directing a fine jet of saline onto the adherent structures.

The iris, also, will rapidly freeze to the instrument tip, and this is often difficult to avoid in the dog, where an iridectomy is not normally performed. The normal type of iris retractor, in the form of a hook, exposes only a minimal area of the upper pole of the lens, where contact is required, and it is often difficult to prevent the instrument tip from touching the iris. Rubinstein's iris retractor (Fig. 240) helps to avoid this complication by having a wide, solid base which protects the iris from the probe, and produces a maximum area of exposure by making the sides of the pupil almost parallel. Contact of the probe with the retractor has no effect on the iris.

Adhesion of the iris to the lens may be produced by the ice spreading over the surface of the lens until it reaches the edge of the iris. This may be avoided by slightly lifting the lens above the level of the iris as soon as a firm contact is made between probe and lens.

Adhesion of the iris to either probe or lens may be reversed by the use of a jet of saline. No damage is likely to result, provided the complication is dealt with promptly.

In cases of accidental freezing of cornea, sclera or iris, the release of the bond will, in most cases, break the adhesion between instrument and lens. On occasion, it is possible to reposition the probe on the lens before it has warmed; in other cases, the probe will have to be immersed again in the coolant before the operation can proceed. For this reason, it is wise to have a spare instrument already cooled. Successive applications of the probe to the lens do not effect the lens capsule or the effectiveness of the bond.

Rupture of the lens capsule. The incidence of accidental rupture would appear to be far less with cryoextraction than with any other technique. A firm attachment between instrument and lens is formed, even though the refrigeration is limited to a relatively small part of the lens. Nevertheless, the zonule, in the dog, is often difficult to break. It is usually possible to perform rotating movements to break the zonule, without rupture of the lens capsule, to a far greater degree than is possible with any other method. Rupture of the lens capsule will occur when undue forces are applied, and a combination of lens rotation and a minimum of mechanical rupture of the zonular fibres with a vectis is usually the most satisfactory method of extraction.

Apart from the traction that is applied, rupture of the lens capsule may, on occasion, be due to excessive shrinking of the capsule caused by refrigeration.

It has been noted that intumescent cataracts freeze slowly in depth. In the case of the Krwawicz probe, where warming proceeds fairly rapidly once it is removed from the coolant, insufficient time may be available to produce effective bonding of the capsule to the lens material. In such cases, traction is likely to result in rupture.

Other instrumentation within the eye, particularly movements of an iris retractor over the anterior face of the lens, or movements of a vectis used to assist zonular rupture, may result in capsular damage.

Where capsular rupture occurs, the capsule normally remains firmly adherent to the probe, and may be removed in its entirety. The remaining lens material must subsequently be removed by irrigation. In cases where the lens capsule has been damaged by other instrumentation, the extractor may sometimes be applied to the point of injury, thus sealing the break, and the operation continued in the normal way.

The choice of method of lens delivery

Two conditions are essential for a smooth intracapsular extraction— rupture of the zonular fibres, and the successful maintenance of a hold on the lens capsule. Even if the resistance of the zonule can be abolished or interrupted, an intracapsular operation may fail because of a failure to grasp the lens capsule without rupture. The capsule may be thinned by degenerative changes, or may be, as is often found in the dog, excessively thin. In such instances, the grasping of the capsule, even if possible at all, is likely to be followed by rupture.

Due to the resistance of the zonule, and the friability of the capsule, in the dog, the methods commonly adopted in human practice are not applicable. Irrespective of the tension or friability of the lens capsule, cryo-extraction eliminates, or at least greatly reduces, the risk of rupture of the lens capsule during extraction.

Low temperature cataract extraction may be combined with enzymatic zonulolysis. The combined use of zonulolysis and the cryoextractor helps to guard against accidents which cause a planned intracapsular extraction to become an extracapsular operation, with the risk of leaving capsular fragments or cortical mass in the anterior chamber.

Cryoextraction would appear to be a safe procedure. Complications may arise, but can normally be avoided by careful technique; those complications that do arise can usually be overcome effectively without damage to the eye. In the absence of an iridectomy, however, it is not normally possible to carry out the operation single-handed—an assistant will be required to manage the iris retractor and corneal suture, allowing the surgeon to manipulate the cryoextractor, depressor or vectis.

Enzymatic zonulolysis

Enzymatic zonulolysis implies the nontraumatic detachment of the crystalline lens from its suspensory ligament, using the selective action of an enzyme upon its zonule. Zonulotomy is possible by chemical means, using the lytic action on the lens zonule of the proteolytic enzyme, a-chymotrypsin. Alpha-chymotrypsin (ACT) is an endopeptidase, having fibrinolytic and proteolytic action similar to trypsin, but differing in its action and having its own specificity.

This enzyme has a selective action on the lens zonule, and, when injected into the anterior chamber, in the human subject, causes subluxation of the lens within a few minutes of irrigation. Despite its action on the zonule, the enzyme appears to have no adverse effect on the other intraocular structures.

Cases have been reported, however, in which it would appear that the incidence of complications such as delayed wound healing, striate keratitis, loss of vitreous and secondary glaucoma is greater following the use of ACT. Degeneration of the retina and inflammatory changes in the vitreous may occur if this enzyme comes into contact with those structures.

The advantages of enzymatic zonulolysis are great, enabling the intracapsular method of extraction to be employed without the necessity of mechanical zonulotomy and its inherent disadvantages.

Alpha-chymotrypsin is obtained from its inactive precursor, a-chymotrypsinogen, which is extracted from the bovine pancreas. It is purified by crystallization and is supplied in sterile, freeze-dried packs. It will remain stable in a dry form, but will rapidly lose its activity when in solution. Solutions must be freshly prepared just prior to use, and it is important that all syringes and instruments used are free from alcohol or other chemicals likely to inactivate the enzyme. It is recommended that all-glass syringes be used, and that any contact between the solution and metallic surfaces be kept to the minimum. The enzyme is dissolved for use in normal saline.

Operative technique. Following the opening of the anterior chamber, the enzyme solution is slowly injected, using a fine lacrimal needle, carefully inserted beneath the iris, between the iris and the lens, so that all parts of the periphery of the posterior chamber are thoroughly flooded with the solution (Fig. 241). The wound is then held closed for a timed period, after which the enzyme solution is washed away by irrigation of the anterior chamber and subiritic angles with saline. If zonulolysis has been effected, the lens will be subluxated or lying free, the suspensory ligament having been digested by the enzyme, and may be removed by any of the techniques already described. If the zonulolysis is complete, the lens may be removed by expression.

The strength of solution. In the human subject, the concentration of α-chymotrypsin needed to produce zonulolysis is $1:5000$; this concentration will produce luxation of the lens within 3 minutes.

In the dog, solutions of this strength will have little or no effect on the zonule. Concentrations as high as $1:500$ will invariably produce partial or complete zonulolysis within 4 to 5 minutes. There is some evidence, however, that where the enzyme is used in such high concentration, a high incidence of postoperative pupillary adhesions and glaucoma will follow.

Used in a strength of $1:2500$, left in contact for 10 minutes, the enzyme will, in most cases, weaken the zonule to such an extent that the extraction of the lens may be performed without rupture of the lens capsule and with little or no use of any instrument to break the zonular fibres. At this strength, postoperative complications which could be attributed to the enzyme are unlikely to be noted.

The difference in behaviour of the human zonule and that of the dog, to the action of α-chymotrypsin, has not been elucidated. The zonular fibres have been shown to be surrounded by protective substances with properties of acid mucopolysaccharides, which must be broken by mechanical alteration, such as tension, before zonulolytic agents can be effective. The greater effect of zonulolytic enzymes in cases of senile cataract may be due to a deficiency of the protective substances. Conversely, the limited effect of zonulolysis in the dog, particularly the young animal, may be due to the high quality of these protective mucopolysaccharides.

The intravitreal injection of ACT. P. Papadopoulos and C. Formston have reported on the use of intravitreal injections of ACT, with the object of producing zonulolysis and reclination of the lens into the vitreous. This is suggested as a possible alternative to lens extraction, thus eliminating the hazards of cataract surgery in the dog, and improving vision by the production of an adequate aphakic crescent or even complete aphakia.

A fine needle, 0·5 mm x 13 mm, is inserted into the anterior vitreous through the sclera at a distance of approximately 5 mm from the limbus, to avoid the ciliary body, and in the 12 o'clock position. An injection of 0·2 ml of a 1:1000 solution of ACT is then injected as near as possible to the lens equator at the 10, 12 and 2 o'clock positions. The tissues around the needle are grasped with forceps as the needle is withdrawn, to prevent return of the solution.

A few hours after the operation, slight blepharospasm and increased lacrimation are exhibited, and, in some cases, slight cloudiness of the cornea.

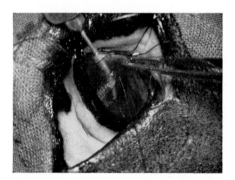

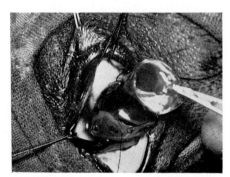

Fig. 241. *Irrigation of the posterior chamber.*   Fig. 242. *Adhesion of the vitreous to the posterior lens capsule.*

The cornea becomes more opaque within the following 24 hours, together with a bulbar conjunctivitis and evidence of an anterior uveitis. The visible inflammatory signs subside in 3 to 6 days, and by this time, posterior luxation of the lens may have commenced. The degree of dislocation, which may continue to advance over the next few days, varies from a narrow aphakic zone to complete dislocation, with the lens lying on the floor of the vitreous; in some cases, no effect on the zonule is apparent.

Postoperatively, the vitreous is likely to show marked haziness, due to uveal exudation, but the transparency is re-established within 3 to 5 days. There is also evidence that this technique may result in retinal degenerative changes in some cases, and severe reactions, even necessitating the enucleation of the eye, may follow if the enzyme is injected into the ciliary body.

Successful results following this technique were more readily obtained in young animals up to the age of 6 years, where there would appear to be a reasonable chance of success. In the old dog, results obtained were not so favourable, and the use of this technique in such animals is not recommended.

HYALOID RUPTURE AND VITREOUS LOSS

In theory, the posterior capsule of the lens and the hyaloid membrane form two distinct and separate structures. It would appear, however, that, particularly in older animals or where there are inflammatory changes within the ciliary region, these two membranes coalesce and become continuous with one another. Only very rarely will the hyaloid membrane be found to exist, intact, as a separate membrane. In most cases, except in a very few where the cataractous lens is found to be completely dislocated from its zonule, vitreous will be found to be adherent to the posterior capsule of the lens (Fig. 242). In some cases of luxated cataract, the vitreous will be found to be liquefied, with no apparent hyaloid membrane.

Vitreous loss. The removal of a lens to which the vitreous humour is attached will result in some loss of vitreous. It would appear that a small loss is not serious, but that loss of vitreous in any quantity will result in distortion of the pupil, low intraocular pressure, retinal detachment or iridocyclitis. In many cases in which marked loss of vitreous is experienced, wound healing will be found to be defective, pupillary occlusion is likely to occur and, sometimes, the globe will ultimately become shrunken.

Factors that may be responsible for excessive loss include pressure on the eye during operation, excessive traction from forceps, inadequate anaesthesia with insufficient relaxation, excessive irrigation of the anterior chamber and instrumental rupture of the suspensory ligament. In the dog, however, the main factor is the attachment of the vitreous face to the posterior lens capsule that is invariably found. In most cases, therefore, some small loss will be experienced. Steps must be taken to limit the amount lost as far as is possible.

Methods of preventing vitreous loss. Anaesthesia, exposure of the globe, lid retraction and immobilization of the eyeball have already been described; and the adoption of suitable techniques are factors which will limit the loss of vitreous. Extreme care in the use of instruments to initiate breakdown of

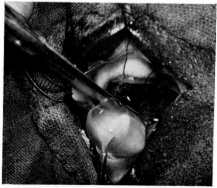

FIG. 243. *Cutting the vitreous from the lens surface.*

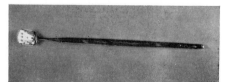

FIG. 244. *Vitreous guard.*

the zonule is also essential, for any excessive force will cause further damage to the hyaloid membrane, should it exist intact. Similarly, undue pressure applied to the outside of the globe with lens expressors will also have the effect of forcing vitreous through the pupil and into the anterior chamber.

The use of enzymatic zonulolysis to weaken the zonule, and the use of a method of lens extraction with the minimum of mechanical zonulotomy, are two factors which will greatly assist in the prevention of vitreous loss. Nevertheless, however carefully the lens is delivered from the eye, some vitreous will normally be found attached to the posterior surface of the lens.

Whatever method is used to grasp the lens, it is essential, before the lens is delivered from the eye, that it be lifted gently whilst still in the anterior chamber, and the adherent vitreous cut away with scissors (Fig. 243). Finally, as the lens is delivered through the incision, the incision should be closed by means of a preplaced suture.

The use of a vitreous guard. This instrument, which guards the anterior face of the vitreous during the final stages of lens delivery, is carried on an angulated handle, and has a spade-shaped blade, of a size to correspond with the diameter of the canine lens, and curved to the convexity of the posterior surface of the lens. The ventral border of the blade is tapered and fine, but not sharp, and the lateral edges have a slightly raised border, so that the lens will fit easily on to the instrument. The blade is perforated with several holes so that an irrigating fluid may be used whilst the instrument is in position (Fig. 244).

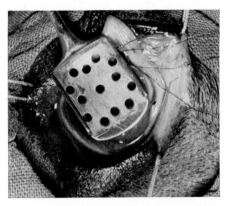

FIG. 245. *Introduction of the vitreous guard.*

In use, the instrument is introduced under the edge of the pupil, in the 12 o'clock position, and carefully slid over the posterior surface of the lens so that the whole of the lens comes to rest within the blade of the guard (Fig. 245). Any mechanical zonulotomy that may be required is carried out before the instrument is introduced, but, in many cases, following enzymatic zonulolysis, the introduction of the guard will be sufficient to break down any zonular fibres remaining intact. When in position, the guard is maintained in front of the pupil until the delivery of the lens has been completed.

The use of acetylcholine. Acetylcholine is a parasympathomimetic drug, and may be used to produce miosis at the end of an intracapsular extraction. Used as a 1:100 solution, it is injected into the anterior chamber through a fine cannula. It may be used whilst a vitreous guard is in position. Contraction of the pupil will be effected in a high proportion of cases, and will assist in the prevention of vitreous loss. Single-dose containers providing a 1:100 solution in 5% mannitol (Miochol; Smith, Miller & Patch) are available, and eliminate the difficulties associated with the preparation and sterilization of unstable solutions.

In those cases in which miosis is not obtained, the rapid closure of the incision by means of a preplaced suture, directly the lens is delivered from the wound, will help to prevent any serious loss.

CORNEAL SUTURING

The healing of the wound following cataract surgery is a most important factor in the success of the operation. With the great tendency of the iris to prolapse following cataract surgery in the dog, and with the ever present

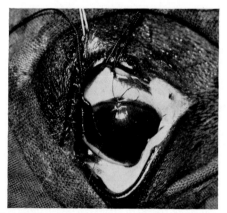

FIG. 246. *Application of a single preplaced suture.*

risk of postoperative interference by the patient, careful suturing of the cornea, with accurate apposition of the wound edges, is essential in this animal.

Sutures may be either preplaced—that is, placed in position before the corneal section is made; or may be postplaced—that is, placed in position after corneal sectioning; or a combination of the two may be used.

Preplaced sutures

(1) *Without a limbal groove.* Using this technique, two or more sutures are placed vertically through the cornea in the line of the proposed incision

(Fig. 246). The section is made by passing the knife between the needle holes, after the suture has been looped out of the way. It is difficult to place the sutures accurately, so that good wound apposition is provided, and also to direct the knife accurately so that it emerges in the exact area between the arms of the sutures.

(2) *With a limbal groove.* A corneal groove is made with a knife, through half the corneal thickness, along the line of the proposed incision (Fig. 247). The groove, which is made on the corneal side of the limbus, may be made at the 10 o'clock and 2 o'clock positions, or may be enlarged to extend from 3 o'clock to 9 o'clock. The suture is passed through the superior lip of the groove from above, so that the point of the needle is visible in the groove. It is then continued through the lower lip of the groove and emerges through

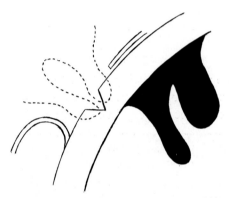

Fig. 247. *Section to show position of preplaced suture within a limbal groove.*

the cornea. The suture within the groove is withdrawn to form a loop, and reflected so that it will not interfere with the completion of the section. The section is completed, using either a knife or scissors, making the incision so that it passes between the loops of the sutures. Either a fornix-based or a limbus-based flap may be used, and incorporated in the sutures.

As the corneal incision necessary in the dog must normally be from the 3 to 9 o'clock positions, it is usually impossible, due to the limited exposure of the globe possible in this species, to fashion a groove over the whole of the distance with sufficient accuracy. It is not normally possible, therefore, to use only preplaced sutures.

Postplaced sutures

Postplaced appositional sutures are applied directly after the corneal incision has been made, and the lens delivered.

Unless it is intended to use only two or three corneal sutures, some postplaced sutures will be required. It is possible to fashion corneal grooves at 10, 12 and 2 o'clock positions, each long enough to accommodate one suture; other sutures will have to be postplaced.

The advantage of preplaced sutures is that the depth and distance from the wound can be more accurately judged, and, consequently, the apposition of the wound edges is more secure. They are easier to apply, for the eyeball is firmer before it is incised. In addition, the incision may be quickly and effectively closed at any time during the operation should this become necessary, and, finally, the risk of sutures penetrating the depth of the cornea is eliminated. The main disadvantage of the method is the possibility that the sutures may be cut in the process of completing the incision, and need replacement.

The most satisfactory results, in wound healing and freedom from iris prolapse follow the use of multiple corneal sutures (Fig. 248). The majority of these have, of necessity, to be postplaced. It is advantageous, nevertheless,

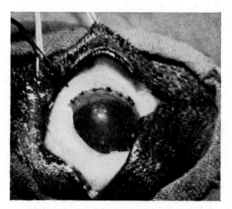

FIG. 248. *Corneal incision sutured.*

to employ one or two preplaced sutures, either at 12 o'clock or at the 10 and 2 o'clock positions. This is firstly to allow rapid closure of the wound should this be required, secondly to allow manipulation of the corneal flap during the extraction of the lens, and thirdly, to assist in the accurate alignment of the two lips of the wound.

Suturing technique

Precise coaptation of the wound edges is essential, and any lack of accuracy is likely to lead to overriding of the section, with the subsequent risk of aqueous leakage, iris prolapse, excessive scar formation or epithelial invasion of the anterior chamber.

The optimum conditions for wound healing, free from complications, follow the use of multiple sutures of very fine material. In the normal 9 to 3 o'clock incision, a minimum of seven and a maximum of nine sutures is normally employed, using either Kalt's silk or Barraquer's pure silk. In

20

the majority of cases, one preplaced suture at the 12 o'clock position will be employed, together with three or four postplaced sutures on either side of the horizontal meridian.

The use of such fine suturing material necessitates the employment of fine needles, and either Grieshaber's or Vogt's 7 mm corneal needles are suitable (Fig. 64). Small needles of this type must be matched to suitable needle holders and suturing forceps; Barraquer needle holders (Fig. 53) and Jayle's forceps (Fig. 44) are satisfactory for this purpose. Fine instruments are essential to reduce the trauma inflicted upon the edges of the incision to the minimum.

Damage to the corneal wound edges can be further limited by grasping the cornea by the epithelial surface only, never by its full thickness, and by

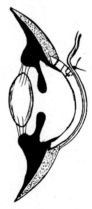

FIG. 249. *Section to show position of corneal suture and limbal-based flap.*

ensuring that the sectioned surface is held only by the single-toothed blade of the forceps.

In order to avoid damage to the cutting surface, the needle should be held with the holder as close as possible to its eye, and introduced sufficiently far through the tissues to allow it to be handled again without damage to the point or edge. It is then introduced into the epithelial surface of the cornea, very close to the holding forceps, and approximately 1 mm from the wound edge. It emerges roughly in the centre of the corneal thickness. The needle is then introduced into the opposite lip of the wound, again in the centre of the sectioned surface, and is brought through to the epithelial surface of the cornea, about 1 mm from the wound edge (Fig. 249). The lip of the wound is again held with forceps to support the passage of the needle. All sutures should be tied just sufficiently tight to ensure good coaptation of the wound, but not so tightly that any deformity of the cornea will result. In order to minimize postoperative irritation, the sutures are cut so that ends of approximately 1 to 2 mm are left.

Penetration of Descemet's membrane, and the subsequent entry of the suture into the anterior chamber, must be avoided; any suture that penetrates too deeply should be removed and reinserted. Accurate apposition of the wound edges will not be possible if too large a bridge of tissue is taken, and the sutures should be kept to within 1 mm of the wound edges.

In those cases in which only postplaced sutures are used, there may be some difficulty in ensuring accurate alignment of the wound edges. The use of one or two preplaced sutures, which are tied before further sutures are inserted, overcomes this difficulty.

Final steps in the operation

Wound toilet. Before suturing is completed, any blood clots remaining in the anterior chamber should, if possible, be removed. Irrigation of the anterior chamber, using warm saline, will be sufficient on most occasions. In a few cases, clots may have to be removed with forceps. It is important, however, that intraocular instrumentation be avoided as far as possible, and that great care is taken not to damage the wound edges or corneal endothelium during this procedure.

Injection of air. The injection of sterile air into the anterior chamber when wound closure is completed prevents delayed reformation of the

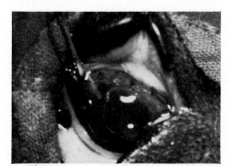

Fig. 251. *Introduction of air into the anterior chamber.*

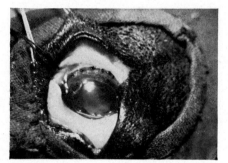

Fig. 252. *Air bubble in the anterior chamber.*

chamber and the adhesion of the vitreous face and iris to the posterior surface on the cornea.

The air is injected through a fine cannula (Fig. 250), introduced between the lips of the wound on the temporal side, and enough air to fill the anterior chamber is introduced (Fig. 251). A number of small bubbles will coalesce to form a large one, and the absorption of all air from the anterior chamber is completed within about five days (Fig. 252).

It is sometimes helpful to inject air into the anterior chamber prior to suturing; this will temporarily restore the contour of the eye and assist the apposition of the wound edges. Most of the air is lost during the suturing process, and a fresh injection should be made when the closure is complete.

Replacement of the conjunctival flap. In those cases where a fornix-based flap is fashioned, this is brought down over the eye and maintained in position by several sutures of fine silk, passed through the edge of the flap, and secured to the bulbar conjunctiva in the lower quadrant. The nictitating membrane is not involved in these sutures, but is allowed to remain free, anterior to the flap.

Closure of the canthotomy. The canthotomy wound is closed by a single row of two or three interrupted fine braided nylon sutures. It is important that this closure be made accurately; failure to ensure this will result in breakdown of the wound.

Application of antibiotic. The operation is completed by the installation of chloramphenicol drops into the conjunctival sac.

The use of lid sutures. The technique of suturing the lids, in order to protect the eye, will often lead to postoperative discomfort and interference by the patient.

Protection of the wound by suturing the nictitating membrane to the superior bulbar conjunctiva, whilst not apparently causing discomfort, would appear to cause, in some cases, pressure upon the eyeball. This, in turn, may well lead to escape of aqueous from the incision, and faulty wound healing.

Postoperative management

In order to keep movement and excitement to the minimum, it is preferable, in most cases, for the animal to be housed in kennels during the immediate postoperative period. This will also ensure that any postoperative treatment required will be carried out efficiently.

Daily cleansing of the lids is performed, to remove any accumulated discharges, and chloramphenicol eye drops are applied three times daily. The incidence of postoperative infection is extremely low. Antibiotic dressings are continued for five days, after which time a combined antibiotic-corticosteroid preparation is used; this is continued until the corneal sutures are removed.

The use of eye bandages is often most unsatisfactory. The application of bandages to the eye of the dog is, for anatomical reasons, extremely difficult. Much will depend on the conformation of the animal's head, which differs greatly in different breeds. However, unless the dressing can be applied so that it is both firm and comfortable, attempts by the patient to remove the bandages are likely to lead to damage to the eye. In the majority of the cases in which a conjunctival flap is used, covering the corneal sutures, very little postoperative irritation is exhibited. The conjunctival flap is well tolerated, and in only a few cases is there any evidence of irritation or discomfort.

Postoperative sedation will be required in some cases for a period of 24 or 48 hours. For this purpose, pethidine is the best analgesic, and may be given in full dosage for this period. By the third day, the eye appears to be no longer sensitive, and the production of self-inflicted damage is no longer likely.

The sutures are removed from a fornix-based flap at the end of one week; this can generally be carried out under topical anaesthesia. In those cases where a limbus-based flap is used, the sutures holding this in position may also be removed at the end of the first week.

Many of the corneal sutures cut out spontaneously and disappear. Where a fornix-based flap is used any remaining sutures are removed on the twelfth day. In order to avoid damage to the wound, and possible separation of the wound edges, this procedure should be carried out under general anaesthesia. It is essential that full aseptic technique should be adopted, and that instruments are used that will allow the removal of the sutures without further damage to the cornea. Identification of the sutures, where pure silk is used, can be assisted by the application of fluorescein to stain the silk. Corneal sutures covered by a limbus-based flap are left in position, but most of them will be eventually extruded.

At the time of suture removal, it is beneficial to carry out a subconjunctival injection of hydrocortisone, to reduce inflammation and prevent vascularization of the cornea. In some cases, it will be found necessary to repeat this procedure after 7 days.

Postoperative complications

(1) *Failure of corneal healing.* Faulty healing of the corneal wound is invariably due to insufficient and defective coaptation of the wound edges. The use of multiple sutures and a flap technique will largely eliminate this complication.

(2) *Iris prolapse.* Interference with the wound by the patient, or postoperative vomiting causing a rise in intraocular pressure, may cause the iris to become incarcerated in the wound before this has become firmly closed. A prolapse is particularly likely to occur where closure of the wound is delayed by imperfect suturing; and the incidence would probably be lower if it were possible to perform an iridectomy in the dog. In the very earliest and mildest of cases, it may be possible to cause the iris to be drawn back by the application of miotic drugs; in other cases, it may be possible to reposition the iris with a repositor. In yet other cases, it may be necessary to perform an abscission of the protruding part, followed by repositioning and firm suturing of the wound, together with the use of an air bubble to prevent vitreous

synechia to the incision. In all cases in which the iris is cut, however, haemorrhage, often severe in nature, will be experienced. In most cases, therefore, it is wiser to leave the iris incarcerated in the wound if this is at all possible.

(3) *Hyphaema*. Small hyphaemata may be present after the operation, and these are of no significance. Haemorrhage into the anterior chamber of such an extent as to warrant the abandonment of the operation may be experienced in cases where an iridectomy is performed. Further haemorrhage may be initiated by damage to the sclera, iris or ciliary body. Haemorrhage from the wound, a few days after the operation, may result from self-inflicted damage. Hyphaemata are normally absorbed without complication; on occasion, however, deposits in the pupillary opening may result in adhesions or after-cataract.

(4) *Persistent corneal opacity*. In a few cases, the cornea will become opaque following the operation, and will fail to clear at a later date. This is usually due to excessive instrumentation, and damage to the cornea by handling and manipulation during the operation. It is most likely to follow damage to the corneal endothelium during the extraction of the lens.

(5) *Epithelialization of the anterior chamber*. A downgrowth of conjunctival epithelial cells into the wound, so that they ultimately line the anterior chamber, is a rare complication. It is due to faulty suturing of the wound, and great care must be taken not to include the edge of the conjunctiva within the wound.

(6) *Pupillary adhesion*. Marked postoperative pupillary adhesions are likely to be due to the inadequate removal of all lens substance from within the eye. Other cases may follow hyphaema formation. There is some evidence, also, that the use of alpha-chymotrypsin in high concentrations may be responsible for adhesion formation.

(7) *Endophthalmitis*. Infection within the eye, following cataract surgery, is rare. It is difficult to assess how much this is due to adequate aseptic precautions and the use of antibiotics, and how much due the resistance of the dog to this type of infection. It is felt, however, that a natural immunity must, in part at least, be responsible.

(8) *Glaucoma*. Postoperative complicated glaucoma is a regular cause of failure. Peripheral synechiae, capsule fragments in the wound, epithelialization of the filtration angle, and herniation of the vitreous into the anterior chamber are all possible factors in the development of this condition. In some cases, however, it is not possible to demonstrate any of these factors, and the origin of the glaucoma remains obscure. Preoperative hypertension is present in some of those cases which exhibit a postoperative glaucoma, but this is not always so.

(9) *Excess vitreous loss*. Loss of vitreous to such an extent as to cause ultimate shrinking of the globe is occasionally encountered.

(10) *Postoperative interference*. Self-mutilation by the patient, resulting

in the ultimate loss of the eye, is an ever-present hazard. Such interference, if excessive, results in rupture of the sutured wound, leading either to an iris prolapse or, in bad examples, to loss of intraocular structures. Other results can be hyphaema, corneal ulceration or detachment of the retina.

(11) *Uveitis.* A mild inflammatory reaction may follow manipulation of the iris. More severe reaction may follow irritation from residual soft lens material. In cases where the uveitis is marked, the cornea will become hazy and the pupil constricted. Treatment is best carried out with the use of atropine and corticosteroids administered locally and systemically.

(12) *Displacement of iris pigment.* The detachment of pigment from the iris will often occur during an intracapsular operation, but rarely to any serious degree. The pigment will enter the anterior chamber and may be washed out. On rare occasions, pigment will become deposited on the posterior surface of the cornea.

(13) *Retinal detachment.* Complete or partial detachment of the retina may be associated with excessive vitreous loss. In a few cases, however, detachment occurs as a later sequel.

EXTRACAPSULAR EXTRACTION

Extracapsular extraction leaves the posterior lens capsule intact, and this minimizes the risk of vitreous loss. The zonule is also left intact and, as the operation is, therefore, less traumatic than the intracapsular operation, there is less risk of damage to the iris and ciliary body. The disadvantages of this method are complications such as iridocapsular synechia formation, secondary cataract, iridocyclitis due to irritation from lens fragments left in the anterior chamber, and, often, a poor visual result.

The initial stages of the operation, up to and including the opening of the anterior chamber, are identical with those in the intracapsular operation. The extraction is then performed by removal of the anterior lens capsule and expressing the lens material.

The anterior capsulotomy is performed with toothed capsule forceps (Fig. 253). The forceps are introduced into the anterior chamber and positioned against the anterior lens capsule, taking care that the forceps do not touch the iris. The forceps are then opened for about 3 mm and the teeth pressed gently backwards to engage upon the capsule (Fig. 254). The forceps are then closed, drawn forwards, and then up and out of the wound, thus removing a large part of the anterior lens capsule. It is unwise to manipulate the forceps whilst they are positioned on the capsule; too vigorous movements are liable to damage the zonule or iris.

Alternatively, the capsule may be cut with a cystitome, in a circular motion about 2 mm anterior to the equator. The cut capsule is then removed with toothed forceps. The use of a cystitome allows a wider opening in the capsule without the same risk of injuring the zonule or of tearing the capsule at or just behind the equator. Any tear in the posterior capsule will expose the vitreous face, and nullify the benefits of the extracapsular operation. It

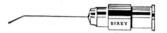

FIG. 250. *Air injection cannula.*

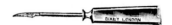

FIG. 255. *Ziegler's capsulotomy knife.*

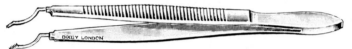

FIG. 253. *Vogt's extra-capsular forceps.*

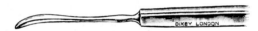

FIG. 259. *Moorfield's curette.*

is important that sufficient of the lens capsule be removed; anterior capsule epithelial cells left behind are liable to proliferate and form a dense after-cataract.

The lens nucleus is removed by pressure applied to the cornea in the 4 to 8 o'clock meridian. An Arruga's lens expressor (Fig. 229) is used for this purpose, and as the pressure is applied gently upwards, the upper part of the lens is tipped forward through the opening in the lens capsule, and presents itself at the corneal wound. The lens is followed up with the expressor, and, if the iris interferes with the passage of the lens, it is hooked out of the way with a blunt iris hook. On occasions, a vectis may be required to assist the passage of the lens nucleus through the anterior chamber. Undue pressure must not be applied to the eye, and an adequate corneal section is essential to avoid this. When the lens presents itself through the wound, it may be grasped with fine toothed forceps, or it may be held with a sharp hook or a cystitome, and so delivered from the eye.

As the lens leaves the eye, the incision should be closed with a preplaced suture. The anterior chamber is then irrigated, removing as much as possible of the soft cortical lens material. The tip of an anterior chamber irrigator is carefully introduced into the wound, care being taken that no damage is inflicted on the corneal endothelium, and the chamber washed out with warm, sterile normal saline. Particles of lens material adhering to the iris may be dislodged by gentle pressure and massage on the cornea towards the pupil. Too great a fluid pressure may damage the posterior capsule or suspensory ligament, and cause a risk of vitreous prolapse.

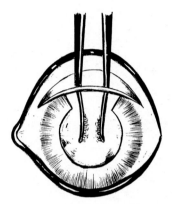

FIG. 254. *Extracapsular extraction.*

The iris is then reposited, using an iris repositor (Fig. 173), taking care that it is disengaged from the wound, where it is usually floated by the irrigation. The corneal wound is then repaired, and the operation completed, in the same way as with an intracapsular operation.

CAPSULOTOMY

In some cases, following extracapsular extraction or discission, the posterior capsule of the lens is smooth and transparent; in such cases, a satisfactory return of vision might be expected. In other cases, where the posterior capsule is thickened or opaque, or where dense after-cataract forms, the posterior capsule must be opened. Such an operation should not be performed until the eye is white, and all absorption of soft lens material has ceased, and there is no postoperative uveitis. This will usually be 4 to 6 weeks after the original operation. The success of the operation will depend to some extent on a good original anterior capsulectomy; where there is dense organized tissue in the pupil, the operation may prove difficult, and in some cases it is impossible to make an adequate opening.

The opening in the posterior capsule, which need not be large provided it is placed along the central axis of the eye, may usually be made by inserting a capsulotomy knife (Fig. 255) in the horizontal meridian under a small conjunctival flap at the limbus, and cutting a small vertical slit; the edges of the slit will open and retract to form a small hole. In other cases, a Ziegler's knife may be used to form a triangular flap, with the apex uppermost so that it falls down by gravity (Fig. 256). In cases of dense after-cataract, it may be

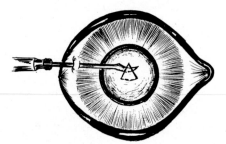

FIG. 256. *Capsulotomy with Zeigler's knife.*

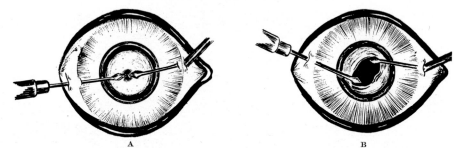

A   B

FIG. 257. *Capsulotomy with two needles.* A *stage 1*, B *stage 2*.

necessary to insert two needles, both transfixing the central point; an opening is then made by levering the two needles apart (Fig. 257).

After a capsulotomy, atropine and corticosteroids should be applied until the eye becomes white.

CAPSULECTOMY

The removal or part or the whole of the posterior lens capsule may become necessary where there is a mass of dense tissue which will not retract on simple incision.

In such cases, a corneolimbal incision will have to be made to allow the necessary instrumentation. A sharp hook is introduced into the anterior chamber and engaged upon the posterior capsule, which is then withdrawn through the wound. The capsule is cut with de Wecker's scissors. Some vitreous prolapse is likely, and some may have to be removed. A gentle injection of cold saline into the anterior chamber may help to bring about the retraction of the vitreous. In those cases where it is not possible to bring the capsule into the corneal wound, de Wecker's scissors may be inserted into the anterior chamber, and three incisions made into the capsule, to remove a triangular piece of capsule which may then be removed from the chamber with forceps.

DISCISSION

Discission is the breaking up of the lens cortex and nucleus by the use of a needle. It is of value in the treatment of congenital cataract.

A widely dilated pupil is desirable, and steps should be taken pre-operatively to achieve this as far as is possible. A Bowman's needle (Fig. 128, p. 143) is used and this is inserted into the anterior chamber at the limbus and a cruciate incision made through the anterior lens capsule, extending each incision as far as possible. The needle is then introduced into the lens substance, the lens contents stirred up to allow the free entry of aqueous, and the needle is withdrawn (Fig. 258).

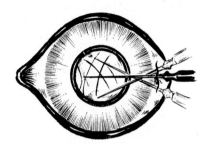

FIG. 258. *Discission technique.*

The operation may need to be repeated, or may need to be followed by a curette evacuation during the next few days. When the lens cortex is found to be hardened and not easily broken up, saline may be injected into the lens to float lens material forward into the anterior chamber. Should lens material remain in the anterior chamber causing obstruction to the drainage, and, therefore, congestion and tension, it should be removed through a keratome incision.

LINEAR (CURETTE) EXTRACTION

Linear or curette extraction is a technique for extracting a developmental cataract by means of a keratome incision, through which the opaque lens material is expressed into a curette, the residue in the anterior chamber being washed out with an irrigator.

The corneal incision is made in the usual way, and an anterior capsulectomy performed. An expressor is placed on the cornea in the 4 to 8 o'clock position and the tip of the curette (Fig. 259) introduced into the wound at the 12 o'clock position. The opaque lens material flows along the groove in the curette and out of the wound, and is swabbed away. It may be necessary to remove a hard nucleus with a spoon. The remaining lens matter is removed by irrigation and gentle pressure; or a two-way syringe, to provide both irrigation and suction, may be used.

The removal of all lens material by this technique is sometimes difficult; material left adhering to the underside of the iris is liable to form a dense after-cataract. The removal of all lens material may be assisted by suction, using a double-barrelled irrigating suction cannula.

RECLINATION

Reclination, or couching, the displacement of the lens into the vitreous humour, has very little indication. It may, however, be used in some cases of posterior luxation of the lens, where the lens is occupying part of the pupil. Some such cases may be accompanied by a rise of intraocular pressure, or even hydrophthalmos. Where the patient involved is very old, and unable to withstand major surgery, or in cases where the lens cannot be persuaded

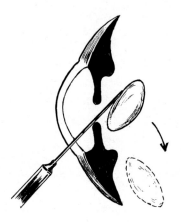

FIG. 260. *Reclination technique.*

to adopt a more forward-facing position, and extraction of the lens may result in considerable vitreous loss, the operation of reclination is justifiable.

The operation may be performed using sharp-pointed and blunt-ended Lang's knives. The point of insertion will depend on the position of the lens to be moved. The sharp-pointed instrument is passed through the cornea, just anterior to the limbus, and across the anterior chamber until it is level with the upper edge of the luxated lens. This instrument is then quickly removed, without loss of aqueous, and the blunt-ended one is inserted. The instrument is positioned against the anterior surface of the lens, the handle is raised and the instrument and the lens are forced backwards into the vitreous (Fig. 260). On withdrawal of the instrument, it is rotated to disengage any strands of vitreous and removed from the eye.

The reclination of the lens by means of the intravitreal injection of α-chymotrypsin has already been discussed.

INTRAOCULAR PLASTIC LENS IMPLANTATION

The use of this technique was first described, in human ophthalmology, to overcome the visual defect in cases of aphakia, by means of an acrylic lens inserted behind the iris and in front of an intact posterior lens capsule. H. D. Simpson has recorded the use of a plastic lens in the dog, and has described both intracapsular and extracapsular methods of implantation. The lens used in all cases was of 11 dioptres, that for the intracapsular operation being of 11 mm diameter and, for the extracapsular operation, 14 mm.

In the intracapsular implantation, a broad 11 to 13 mm iridectomy is performed just anterior to the base of the iris, parallel to the corneal section. After control of the haemorrhage has been effected, the lens capsule is incised at the equator through the dorsal third of its circumference. The lens substance is expressed and the capsule irrigated to remove all lens particles. The plastic lens is then inserted into the capsule, the iris smoothed into position, and the lens centered behind the pupil.

Extracapsular implantation is also preceded by a small peripheral iridectomy. Following this, an equatorial capsulotomy is performed, opening approximately the dorsal third of the capsule, and the anterior capsule is removed. The lens material is expressed by irrigation, and the plastic lens pushed into the pupil. The iris is pulled out from behind the lens so that it assumes its normal position, and the operation is completed in the usual way.

Plastic lens implantation is followed by an intense iritis, which subsides in 2 to 4 months. Recorded complications are iris prolapse, hyphaema, endophthalmitis and, rarely, panophthalmitis. Corticosteroids are recommended for the treatment of complications, whilst, to assist the absorption of blood clot, the injection of 20 to 50 units of hyaluronidase subconjunctivally is suggested.

ANTERIOR CHAMBER IMPLANT

Patients in which the posterior lens capsule has been divided or removed, are not eligible for an acrylic plastic lens implant, and, in human ophthalmology, an implant has been evolved that is placed in front of the iris and behind the cornea, with feet wedged in the anterior chamber angles, and carrying a central optical portion. The operation is carried out not less than 6 weeks after the cataract extraction, on a miotic eye, and the implant must be a tight fit to prevent it moving, irritating the iris and ciliary body, and causing secondary glaucoma. The length of the implant inserted is 1 mm longer than the 3 to 9 o'clock measurement white to white, and the insertion is performed through an 8 mm incision made temporally 1 mm on the corneal side of the limbus. Although no cases of this technique have been recorded yet in the dog, this procedure has been carried out in this animal using a Strampelli type implant. It may prove of use in improving the visual results of cataract extraction, but, it must be admitted, aphakic vision in the dog is usually adequate in most cases.

NUCLEAR SCLEROSIS OF THE LENS

As new lens fibres are formed throughout life, and the lens remains the same size throughout adult life, the older fibres become compressed towards the centre of the lens, forming the nucleus. The increasing compression of the lens fibres in the centre of the lens, coupled with a gradual loss of water, results in an increasing density of the lens nucleus as the animal becomes older. The formation of this dense, hard nucleus is termed nuclear sclerosis (Plate V, Fig. 8, facing p. 224).

Some degree of nuclear sclerosis occurs in most dogs from the age of 6 to 7 years and upwards, and, since this condition is frequently mistaken for cataract formation, it is important to differentiate between the two changes.

As a result of sclerosis, some rays of light are reflected instead of being refracted, and this gives a blue-grey discoloration of the pupil. The sclerotic lens, however, remains translucent, vision is not seriously impaired, and surgical interference is not indicated. The differentiation of nuclear sclerosis and cataract formation may be made by ophthalmoscopic examination. In many cases of sclerosis, the lens nucleus may be seen completely within the pupillary margin, surrounded by clear lens substance; in all cases, apart from slight aberrations that might be caused by the changes in the lens substance, the fundus is clearly visible.

LUXATION OF THE LENS

Luxation of the crystalline lens signifies that the lens has left its normal position, and is lying either in the anterior chamber, in front of the iris, or is lying behind the iris but not within the hyaloid fossa. This dislocation, therefore, due to rupture of the suspensory ligament, may occur anteriorly or posteriorly. The latter is not common and accounts for only about 5% of all cases.

Subluxation is said to have occurred when the zonule is not completely disrupted, and only partial movement of the lens takes place.

This condition is known to occur most frequently in the Sealyham, Smooth-haired Fox Terrier, Wire-haired Fox Terrier, Jack Russell Terrier or crossbreds of these breeds. Other cases have been reported in many other breeds, including the Cocker Spaniel, Labrador Retriever, French Bulldog and Scottish Terrier.

The average age of incidence is between the years of 3 and 6, but most commonly when the dog is 5 or 6 years old. There would appear to be a higher incidence in bitches than in dogs. The condition is usually bilateral, but will not necessarily occur in both eyes at the same time.

It is not known for certain whether luxation of the lens is a primary condition, arising from defects in the lens, or whether it is secondary to other ocular factors elsewhere than in the lens. All the evidence points to the fact that it is an inherited condition, in which inherited organic defects terminate in a defective zonule. The actual luxation may be precipitated by trauma, but it is unlikely that trauma, unless violent, is the primary cause.

The course of the disease

Luxation of the lens leaves the iris without support, and the resulting iridodenesis, or trembling of the iris, leads to an anterior uveitis, giving rise to an increase in the protein content of the aqueous, a consequent rise in intraocular pressure, and secondary glaucoma. The pressure on branches of the oculomotor nerve supplying the sphincter iridis causes dilatation of the pupil which interferes further with aqueous filtration. Full dilatation of the iris will cause blocking of the filtration angle.

The rise in intraocular pressure causes further breakdown of the zonule, although the lens may not escape from the hyaloid fossa immediately due to adhesions to the hyaloid membrane. The final luxation may be due to disruption of the vitreous or to external stimuli. Secondary cataract and hydrophthalmos will ultimately develop.

The hydrophthalmic eye (Plate V, Fig. 7, facing p. 224) is accompanied by marked proptosis, the eyeball fills the orbit, and its movements are markedly restricted. The cornea is flattened peripherally and bulges centrally. There is a marked scleral congestion, and a blue discoloration of the sclera in the ciliary region, as uveal pigment shows through the ectatic sclera. The central part of the cornea becomes dry, and a diffuse keratitis develops. At this stage the intraocular pressure is low, due to stretching of the sclera, and the eye is blind. Posterior luxation, into the vitreous, usually causes no trouble, although there may be marked iridodenesis and total aphakia. Changes in retina or vitreous body may develop at a later stage. Subluxation is likely to produce the same sequence of events, even in those cases in which the lens remains behind the iris; in some of these cases, however, no rise of intraocular pressure is detected, or the pressure may fluctuate from day to day.

Clinical signs

There are usually signs of transient pain, lacrimation and blepharospasm, with some visual loss, for 24 to 36 hours before the luxation is first noticed; commonly, however, as these signs are transient, they are dismissed by the owner as of no consequence, until the onset of scleral congestion and pupillary dilatation.

Iridodenesis is often the first positive sign. This is due to the lack of support afforded to the iris by the lens when the latter is in its normal position, and is exhibited as a tremulous state of the iris, which is particularly noticeable when the head is moved. In other cases, a slight trembling of the lens may be noticed on ophthalmoscopic examination. Occasionally, at the same time, fibrinous filaments may be found protruding from below the iris on to the anterior lens capsule. These fragments, which arise from the ruptured zonule, may be evident before iridodenesis is apparent. In cases of subluxation of a small degree, iridodenesis may be the only sign, but must always be regarded as evidence of impending dislocation.

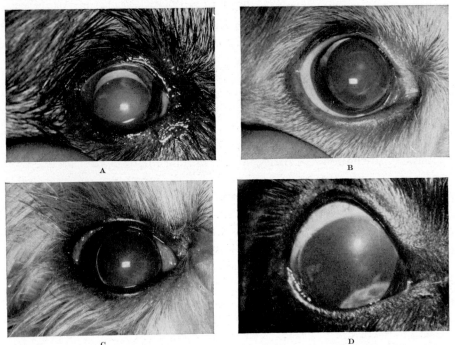

Fig. 261. *Lens luxation*. A *aphakic crescent*, B *complete anterior*, C *aphakic penumbra*, D *complete posterior*.

As luxation proceeds, congestion of the bulbar conjunctiva will appear, together with a dilatation of the pupil and lack of pupillary reflex, loss of corneal lustre and, sometimes, slight epiphora; these changes, of course, represent the early signs of secondary glaucoma.

Dislocation of the lens normally continues ventrally, and, as the lens moves in position, the aphakic crescent begins to appear. This normally shows between the upper border of the lens and the pupil as a sharply-defined luminous thin crescentic zone, representing the colourful tapetum as it is reflected over the upper border of the displaced lens (Fig. 261A).

If the lens continues to move ventrally, behind the iris, it may disappear completely from view, leaving complete aphakia. In other cases, the upper border of the lens may remain visible through the pupil (Fig. 261D). More commonly, however, the displacement of the lens continues anteriorly, into the pupil and the anterior chamber, thus reducing the depth of the chamber (Fig. 261B). Sometimes the lens will move into the pupil and be held there, giving a bright, narrow zone completely encircling the lens, the so-called aphakic penumbra (Fig. 261c). More often, the lens will pass completely into the anterior chamber, where it is normally easily recognizable; in some cases, a characteristic cuffing of the iris behind the lens is noticeable. In this position, the lens may rest against the endothelium of the cornea, producing a posterior keratitis, exhibited as a partial clouding of the corneal tissues. Other changes in the cornea may result from the increasing loss of vision and subsequent trauma. In cases where the diagnosis of luxation is in doubt, confirmation may be obtained by examination under a Wood's glass, when the lens appears opaque and may be easily detected.

Whatever the position of the lens, once it is luxated or subluxated, a progressive rise of intraocular tension is likely. This secondary glaucoma may be delayed, or may not be so noticeable, in those cases in which the lens is situated behind the pupil. However, in all cases of luxation or subluxation, some rise in tension is likely due to interference with the filtration angle. In the early stages of glaucoma, the rise in pressure may be detected by digital examination. As it develops, the appearance of the eye is sufficient indication of the existence of secondary glaucoma, and, as the pressure increases, some degree of hydrophthalmos will develop as the wall of the eyeball yields to the increasing pressure. The time taken for hydrophthalmos to be apparent and the rate at which it develops will be variable, depending upon the position of the lens. The rise in intraocular pressure will ultimately lead to retinal degenerative changes, and the eye will progress to the stage of absolute glaucoma and complete loss of vision.

In a very few unexplained cases the lens may remain subluxated within the pupil, or even totally dislocated into the anterior chamber, without any rise of intraocular pressure being detectable; and in some instances, this situation may continue indefinitely, although, of course, vision will be greatly impaired.

Treatment

It is essential that the earliest signs of lens luxation be recognized; successful treatment depends, almost always, on the early removal of the luxated or subluxated lens, before the inevitable complications of secondary glaucoma and hydrophthalmos have developed. In the majority of cases, a lendectomy should be performed as soon as the condition is diagnosed. Unfortunately, many cases are seen only when the signs of increasing intraocular tension are apparent, and, in these, the chances of successful surgery being performed are diminished. In those breeds in particular, which are

21

known to be predisposed to lens luxation, any information from the owner that the animal is suffering from an ocular complaint should be promptly investigated. In cases that are seen in the very early stages only a mild iridodenesis may be noticed; this is usually sufficient indication that surgery is warranted.

The prognosis in those cases exhibiting advanced scleral congestion, enlargement of the bulb, inhibition of the pupillary reflex or fundal changes, is necessarily poor; and, on some occasions, enucleation may be advisable. It is most important that, when presented with luxation in one eye, the other, often apparently normal, eye be examined; very often, the early signs of luxation may be present, and surgery may be indicated on the 'normal' eye rather than on the eye in the more advanced stages. Where a definite rise in intraocular pressure is apparent, or even an established mild hydrophthalmos, it is possible, in some cases, to control the hypertensive condition medically prior to surgery.

Medical preoperative treatment

In cases in which a lendectomy cannot be performed immediately, for one reason or another, and those in which the rise in intraocular pressure constitutes a contraindication to immediate surgery, the intraocular pressure should be controlled by the administration of carbonic anhydrase inhibitors, such as dichlorphenamide or acetazolamide, together with the application of miotic drops in the form of DFP (di-isopropyl fluorophosphonate 0·1% solution in arachis oil). It is sometimes possible to control the hypertensive signs for long periods, until the conditions for surgery become more favourable. It is emphasized, however, that success will ultimately depend on the removal of the dislocated lens from the eye.

Surgical treatment

The performance of a lendectomy for the removal of a luxated or subluxated lens is, in the main, identical to the operation for cataract. Where the lens is completely detached from its zonule and is lying free, either within the pupillary area or in the anterior chamber, the lens can be extracted by expression or sliding, and, quite often, little or no intraocular instrumentation is required (Fig. 262A). However, dislocation of the lens is invariably accompanied by rupture of the hyaloid membrane, and delivery of the lens is often accompanied by some vitreous prolapse. In nearly all cases, vitreous will be found adherent to the posterior lens capsule, and delivery of the lens from the incision must be accomplished carefully to avoid any serious vitreous loss. It is sometimes of value to retract the upper border of the iris with a blunt hook, to make the passage of the lens easier and to grasp the lens with lens forceps (Fig. 262B) or a cryoextractor (Fig. 262C) as it emerges from the wound. It may then be gently extracted from the eye, cutting any vitreous attachments before the lens is delivered too far from the incision, and keeping the incision closed with a preplaced suture.

In other cases, a vitreous guard may be of value in preventing vitreous loss. This instrument, adapted from a Rycroft's corneal graft shovel, has been described in connection with cataract extraction. In use, with forceps or cryoextractor in position on the lens, the guard may be introduced so that

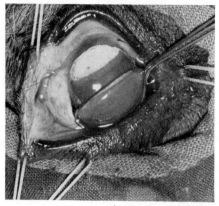

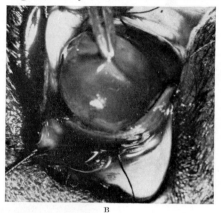

A   B

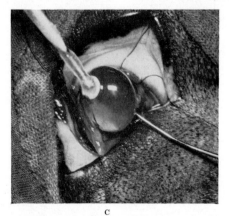

C

FIG. 262. *Extraction of the luxated lens, A by expression, B with forceps, C with a cryoextractor.*

the whole of the lens comes to rest within the blade (Fig. 263A). Where a few zonular fibres may still be intact, the introduction of the guard will be sufficient to release the lens completely (Fig. 263B). With the guard in front of the vitreous, the lens may be delivered, and if desired, acetylcholine solution may be introduced to try to effect miosis. In such cases, it is possible to remove the guard with little or no loss of vitreous humour. If miosis is not obtained, careful withdrawal of the guard, and immediate closure of the wound behind the guard, by means of a preplaced suture, will prevent serious vitreous loss. Failure to ensure that these precautions are taken may result in serious loss of vitreous and consequent failure of the operation.

The ease with which the lens can be removed depends entirely upon its position within the eye. In some cases, where the lens is posterior to the iris, it may be necessary to grasp the lens with capsule or fixation forceps, whilst enlarging the pupillary opening by retracting the iris with a hook. Great care must be taken to avoid damage to the iris, and consequent haemorrhage, and to avoid vitreous loss to any degree. Difficulties may be

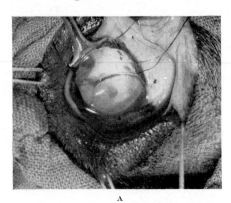 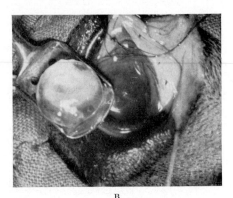

A   B

Fig. 263. *Vitreous guard* A *introduced behind luxated lens,* B *lens contained on vitreous guard.*

encountered in grasping the lens with forceps in this position; in such cases, it may be necessary to use a lens spoon or vectis, passed behind the lens, to assist its removal. As the lens is brought forward by the vectis (Fig. 264) it may be grasped with forceps, again taking great care to keep vitreous loss to the minimum. In view of the nature of the vitreous body and the hyaloid membrane in the dog, however, such manoeuvres are likely to be accompanied by heavy vitreous loss. Such loss may often be avoided by the use

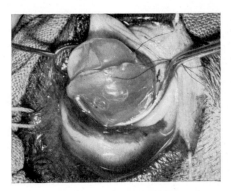 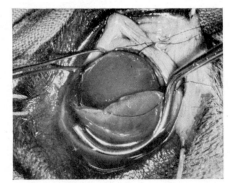

Fig. 264. *Extraction of the luxated lens with a vectis.*

of a Beer's cataract needle or similar instrument. This is introduced into the anterior chamber, at the limbus, in the 3 or 9 o'clock position, before the corneal section is made (Fig. 265A). It is passed through the chamber towards the lens, and is made to penetrate the capsule so that it enters well into the lens cortex. It is then possible to draw the lens forward into the anterior chamber, where it is held while corneal sectioning is accomplished (Fig. 265B). Following sectioning, the vitreous guard is introduced and the lens delivered (Fig. 265c). If zonular fibres remain intact, these may be broken by manipulation of the lens with the transfixing needle.

Alternatively, Lopez-Lacarrere's double-pronged diathermy needle may be employed. With the prongs retracted into the insulated glass sleeve, the instrument is introduced into the anterior chamber and its end made to impinge upon the lens capsule. The prongs are then slid forward to enter the lens, and a diathermy current of 20 to 30 mA is applied for 3 seconds. The

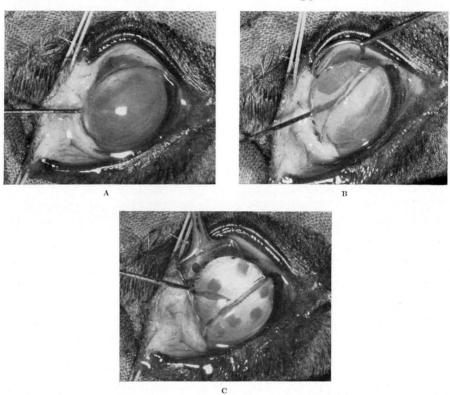

FIG. 265. A *Introduction of a Beer's cataract needle,* B *shows extraction of the luxated lens with the needle,* C *extraction of the luxated lens with a Beer's needle and vitreous guard.*

lens capsule and cortex become coagulated onto the prongs and may be lifted from the eye. In some cases, the capsule ruptures and will have to be removed separately with forceps. Alternatively, a cryoextractor may be employed for the same purpose.

Dislocations of the lens into the vitreous body are particularly difficult to treat successfully. If the capsule is intact, the lens may be tolerated in this position for many years, and, if the eye is quiet, the lens is best left alone. If, on the other hand, uveitis or secondary glaucoma develop, or if the capsule is ruptured and the nucleus loose in the vitreous, then extraction is indicated. The operation becomes justifiable, for failure to remove the lens in such cases will mean loss of the eye.

Blind searching for the lens with a vectis is likely to end in excessive vitreous loss, damage to the retina or damage to the iris and ciliary body. Occasionally, where the vitreous is fluid, the lens may be removed by irrigation. In this procedure, a balanced solution is forced into the eye towards the ciliary body, so that the lens is forced out on the other side, into the anterior chamber (Fig. 266).

In cases in which the lens is free and completely detached from all zonular attachments, it may sometimes be induced to settle anterior to the pupil by placing the patient, under anaesthesia, in a prone position. If this is accomplished, it is sometimes possible to trap the lens in the anterior chamber by

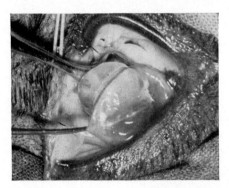

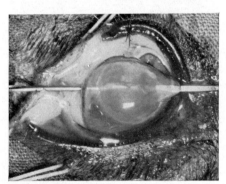

Fig. 266. *Extraction of the luxated lens by irrigation.*

Fig. 267. *Transfixion of the luxated lens with a needle.*

the use of miotics; in other cases, miotics fail to produce satisfactory constriction of the pupil, either due to a rise of intraocular pressure being present, or because vitreous in the anterior chamber prevents the lens from having complete access to the chamber.

If the lens can be induced into the anterior chamber by posture, it is possible to trap the lens in this position by the use of Barraquer's double needle technique. In this procedure, a double needle, with the prongs about 4 mm apart, is passed through the cornea at the limbus, through the anterior chamber posterior to the floating lens, to emerge at the limbus on the opposite side. With the needle in position, the head of the patient is then turned into the normal position, and the lens removed in the normal way. Alternatively, it may be possible to trap the lens in this position by use of a needle, passed through the cornea at the limbus, so that it emerges at the limbus on the far side, either passing posterior to or impaling the lens, and holding it in position (Fig. 267).

A common complication of all operations, where attempts are made to remove the dislocated lens from the vitreous, is excessive vitreous loss, and subsequent retinal detachment and phthisis bulbi. Such attempts are indicated only where the loss of the eye is, in any case, inevitable.

Reclination—displacement of the lens into the vitreous—has been described, and may be of value in certain selected cases.

Dislocation of the cataractous lens

Spontaneous rupture of the suspensory ligament, and subsequent luxation or subluxation of the lens, is not uncommonly met in cases of cataract formation (Fig. 268). Such dislocation is most commonly met in cases of hypermature and Morgagnian cataract.

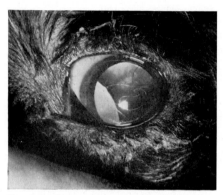

FIG. 268. *Luxation of a cataractous lens.*

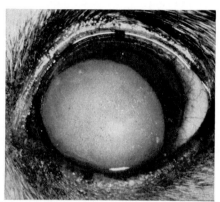

FIG. 269. *Complete anterior luxation of a cataractous lens.*

In some instances, the result of luxation will be identical to that experienced in most cases of dislocated lens. In others, particularly with hypermature cataracts, where the lens becomes smaller, little interference with aqueous drainage is shown, and the intraocular pressure may remain normal. On occasion, the cataractous lens will lie entirely anterior to the iris (Fig. 269), and wholly within the anterior chamber, with little ill-effect other than a mild posterior keratitis.

In all cases in which the dislocated cataractous lens gives rise to an increase in intraocular pressure, or where the removal of the cataractous mass from the pupillary opening would restore some vision to the patient, the extraction of the lens is indicated. Where there is no interference with drainage, and retinal changes prevent the restoration of vision, there would seem to be little indication for removing the lens.

16

THE VITREOUS HUMOUR

The vitreous body, or vitreous humour, is the jelly-like, transparent substance, that fills the posterior four-fifths of the eyeball, posterior to the lens. It is enclosed by the retina, ciliary epithelium, zonule and lens. It is bounded by the so-called hyaloid membrane, formed by condensation of the vitreous on its surface. Anteriorly, the hyaloid membrane helps to form the zonule and, on its anterior surface, forms an indentation to contain the posterior surface of the lens—the patella fossa. It is weakly attached to the optic disc, and rather more strongly attached to the ciliary epithelium.

The absorption of the hyaloid artery in the foetus—the artery responsible for the development of the vitreous—leaves a narrow canal running through the centre of the vitreous, from the optic disc to the pole of the lens. This canal, which is not visible by ordinary methods of examination, has small expansions at either end.

The vitreous body is composed of a homogeneous collagen gel. This gel is supported by a framework of collagen filaments, the spaces between the filaments being occupied by molecules of hyaluronic acid, which is responsible for the viscosity of the body.

Liquefaction of the vitreous body may take place, as the result of enzyme action or disease. Following liquefaction, or loss of vitreous through surgery, however, regeneration never takes place. Liquefaction or loss of aqueous may result in hypotony, or the vitreous may be replaced by a fluid similar to aqueous humour.

DISEASES OF THE VITREOUS

Vitreous haemorrhages

Haemorrhage in the vitreous body is rare in the dog. Occasional cases may be met associated with trauma or where there is retinal detachment, the haemorrhage resulting from massive bleeding from the retina or choroid. In such cases, which are likely to be accompanied by other ocular damage, the fundus may be excluded from view, and a uniform black reflex will be obtained on ophthalmoscopy.

Providing that the haemorrhage is not massive, it will tend to clear in time, although this process may be very slow. In cases of massive haemorrhage, reabsorption may extend over years, and irregular opacities may persist permanently. In other cases, the haemorrhage will become organized by the ingrowth of fibrous tissue, producing a *retinitis proliferans*, showing bands of white fibrous tissue extending across the retina. No treatment is of value.

Spontaneous haemorrhage has been reported in the Beagle, producing blood spots in the ventronasal quadrant of the vitreous, due to ruptured veins in the ganglionic layer of the retina, close to the ora ciliaris.

Liquefaction of the vitreous

Degenerative changes may lead to a liquefaction of the vitreous, and, apart from the aged animal, this change will most often be encountered in cases where the lens is cataractous, or where the lens has become dislocated. Other cases may result from inflammatory changes within the eye. In all cases, intraocular tension may be lowered, and cataractous lenses are likely to become detached from the zonule, due to lytic changes in this structure.

Vitreous opacities

Opacities may arise as primary defects of the vitreous, or may be secondary to other changes in the retina or choroid. Known generally as 'vitreous floaters', the larger ones are visible with the ophthalmoscope; smaller bodies may only be detected with the use of a slit-lamp beam.

Persistent capillary remnants of the primary vitreous, or remnants of the hyaloid artery, may occasionally be observed, floating in the vitreous humour with gentle oscillation as the vitreous is jelly-like. The so-called *muscae volitantes* occur as fine filaments or dots, but are not apparent objectively.

Exudates may result from vitreous haemorrhage, showing as strands of fibrinous residue by ophthalmoscopy.

Asteroid bodies occur as small, round, white bodies suspended in a random fashion throughout the vitreous. Composed of calcium salts, birefringent in plane-polarized light, they are often uniocular and will occur mainly in aged animals. They are not associated with liquefaction of the vitreous, and thus tend to oscillate but remain fixed in position, and do not settle when the eyes are still. They produce no effects, the vitreous remains normal and there is no treatment. There would appear to be no breed or sex predisposition, and they do not appear to be associated with concurrent ocular disease.

Synchisis scintillans is a condition similar to the above, but here the bodies are composed of cholesterol, and, therefore, are irregular in shape and tend to glisten. They occur in degenerate eyes in which synchisis—liquefaction of the vitreous—has occurred. They tend to gravitate to the bottom of of the vitreous, therefore, and are stirred up with movements of the eye. This condition is rare in the dog, but has been reported and tends to be bilateral. Again, it is symptomless and no treatment is either required or possible.

Hyalitis

Inflammation of the vitreous body is rare in the dog, and when it does occur is usually associated with an intraocular foreign body. Complications may be haemorrhage and infection leading to an endophthalmitis. Cases not complicated by infection may lead to liquefaction of the vitreous.

17

THE RETINA AND OPTIC NERVE

THE RETINA

The retina, which, when detached from its pigment epithelium, is a thin delicate transparent membrane, forms the inner coat of the eyeball, adjacent to the choroid. It is, in fact, an extension of the brain, to which it is connected by the optic nerve (2nd cranial), which passes through the choroid and sclera to enter the orbit. In the anterior direction, it extends forward and becomes continuous with the epithelium overlying the inner surface of the ciliary body. This scalloped anterior border is known as the ora serrata.

Embryologically, the retina arises from the two layers of the ectoderm which forms the optic cup. The outer layer of this ectoderm gives rise to the pigment epithelium; the remainder of the retina arises from the inner layer. The inner layer of the retina is only loosely attached to the underlying choroid, except in two places—the ora serrata, and the optic disc, where the nerve fibres pass through the wall of the bulb to form the optic nerve.

The retina contains two forms of light-sensitive cells, the rods and the cones. The rods are highly sensitive and used for vision during low illumination and at night. The cones function only at higher levels of illumination, and are thought to be also responsible for colour vision. These receptor cells connect with nerve fibres which eventually collect to form the optic nerve.

The retina, which in the dog, is 0·24 mm thick in the area of the tapetum, tapering to a thickness of 0·12 mm at the periphery (Prince), consists of 10 layers, which are designated as follows, from without inwards (Fig. 270):

(1) Pigment epithelium.   (6) Inner nuclear layer.
(2) Layer of rods and cones.   (7) Inner plexiform layer.
(3) External limiting membrane.   (8) Ganglion layer.
(4) Outer nuclear layer.   (9) Nerve fibre layer.
(5) Outer plexiform layer.   (10) Internal limiting membrane.

Pigment epithelium. Consists of a single layer of cells, the outer part of which contains the nuclei, and the inner part the dark granules of the pigment fuscin. That part of the pigment epithelium overlying the choroidal

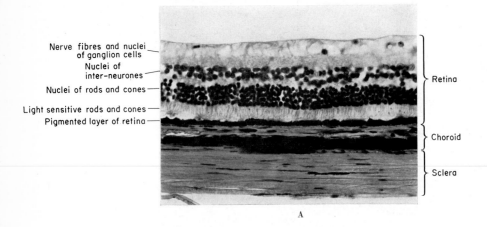

Nerve fibres and nuclei of ganglion cells
Nuclei of inter-neurones
Nuclei of rods and cones
Light sensitive rods and cones
Pigmented layer of retina

Retina

Choroid

Sclera

A

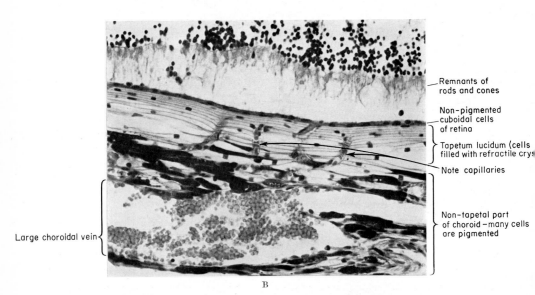

Remnants of rods and cones

Non-pigmented cuboidal cells of retina

Tapetum lucidum (cells filled with refractile cry≋

Note capillaries

Non-tapetal part of choroid—many cells are pigmented

Large choroidal vein

B

FIG. 270. *Transverse section of the retina of a greyhound.* A *The peripheral non-tapetal layer,* B *the tapetal area.*

tapetum contains no pigment, but an abundance of pigment appears in the lower half of the retina.

Layer of rods and cones. This area contains the outer, light-sensitive portions of the rod and cone visual cells, which are arranged in parallel fashion, perpendicular to the surface. In the dog, rods predominate, the proportion of cones totalling only about 5% of the receptor cells. No part of the retina is entirely free of rods, and there is no definite fovea in the retina, as in man. There is, however, a macular area of greatest sensitivity—the area centralis—situated about 3 mm lateral to the optic nerve head, which may be recognized by its freedom from the larger blood vessels (Prince).

The rods appear as long, slender, cylindrical elements, approximately 40 to 60μ in length, and 2μ in diameter. Each consists of two parts, an inner, thicker segment, and an outer, thinner segment. The outer end of the inner segment shows a longitudinal arrangement of fibres—the ellipsoid. From its inner end passes a slender filament—the rod fibre—which continues through the external limiting membrane to the outer nuclear layer. In this area, it enlarges, forming the rod nucleus and continues, as a fibre, into the outer plexiform layer, terminating as the end bulb.

In the fresh retina, the appearance is of a purplish-red coloration that fades in light. This coloration is produced by the substance visual purple— rhodopsin—which is present in the outer segment of the rods, and is intimately concerned with the function of these structures.

The cones, which show great variations in form, and, where they occur in the dog tend to be collected in groups or clusters, are more bottle-shaped. Again, inner and outer segments are exhibited, the former being bulbous and the latter conical. The inner segment is continuous with the cone nucleus, which passes through the inner limiting membrane. Just under this membrane, the cone granule appears, which continues as a fibre, and terminates in a cone foot.

External limiting membrane. A thin membrane, formed by the supporting elements of the retina—Muller's fibres.

Outer nuclear layer. This comprises 12 to 15 rows of nuclei from the receptor cells, surrounded by a delicate cytoplasm. The rod nuclei tend to be small and round; the cone nuclei larger and oval.

Outer plexiform layer. A meshwork formed by the terminal fibres of the rods and cones. Connection is made by these fibres to the bipolar cells of the inner nuclear layer. In the case of the rods, several fibres may be related to one bipolar cell, whereas single cone fibres travel to each bipolar cell.

Inner nuclear layer. This layer contains the nuclei of the bipolar cells, and the nuclei of Muller's fibres, together with the associated neurons— amacrine cells and horizontal cells—which interconnect the various regions of the retina. The layer consists of 4 or 5 rows or nuclei.

Inner plexiform layer contains the dendrites of the ganglion cells, the processes of the amacrine cells and the axons of the bipolar cells.

Ganglion cell layer. A single layer of typical ganglion cells, in 1 or 2 rows, together with a capillary network.

Nerve fibre layer. This contains the axons of the ganglion cells, which are nonmedullated and arranged in bundles. These bundles run parallel to the retinal surface and converge at the optic disc. This layer is richly vascular, containing the retinal blood vessels.

Inner limiting membrane. A thin, hyaline membrane, separating the retina from the vitreous.

The fundus

The appearance of the retina in the living animal, when viewed with an ophthalmoscope, is known as the fundus oculi. The fundus may be divided into two main parts: the tapetal fundus in the dorsal quadrants, behind which is the reflective tapetum lucidum, and the non-tapetal fundus, in the ventral quadrants, behind which is the heavily pigmented choroid (Fig. 271).

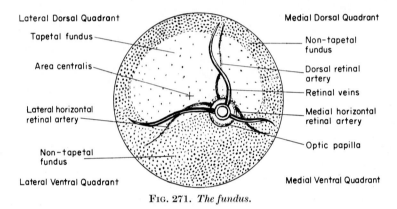

Lateral Dorsal Quadrant

Tapetal fundus

Area centralis

Lateral horizontal retinal artery

Non-tapetal fundus

Lateral Ventral Quadrant

Medial Dorsal Quadrant

Non-tapetal fundus

Dorsal retinal artery

Retinal veins

Medial horizontal retinal artery

Optic papilla

Medial Ventral Quadrant

FIG. 271. *The fundus.*

The tapetal fundus occupies the majority of the dorsal quadrants of the fundus, but does not extend to the periphery. This area is half-moon shaped, and, at the periphery, is surrounded by a narrow zone of non-tapetal fundus. Similar areas, free of tapetum, occur irregularly in the mid-tapetal fundus.

The retina overlying the tapetal fundus is translucent and flat, and exhibits a texture of fine granular beading, which appears rather coarser towards the periphery. The granular appearance is rather more marked in adolescence. Situated between the beading is a reticulum composed of dark triangular spaces—the stars of Winslow.

The central retinal artery and vein, arising from the optic nerve head, give rise to between 4 and 8 large vessels, which, leaving the optic papilla, bifurcate freely. In addition, several smaller vessels radiate from the papilla, so that the whole retina is supplied with a rich capillary network as far as its periphery. Other, small, vessels arise from the choroidal vessels to supply the retina.

The blood vessels of the retina do not anastomose, but give off smaller branches, especially near the periphery of the fundus. They are usually well spaced and distinct. The arteries, which are bright red, are normally arranged as three main trunks, in the form of an inverted 'T', forming the dorsal retinal artery, and the lateral and medial horizontal retinal arteries. The arteries arise independently in the substance of the papilla near its centre. The smaller subsidiary arteries arise within the substance of the papilla, at the junction of the peripheral and central areas, and are normally 10 to 15 in number. The veins, which are slightly darker, arise from a circular vessel which in turn arises from the central retinal vein. It is often difficult to distinguish between arteries and veins except from their calibre. The retinal vessels, which are thin-walled and sharply defined, lie on or just within the superficial layers of the retina.

The non-tapetal fundus, occupying the ventral area of the fundus, is normally deep brown in colour, and the granular texture is not so marked as in the tapetal fundus. The blood vessels supplying this area arise from the medial and lateral horizontal retinal vessels, and are very numerous. The pigment in the non-tapetal fundus usually completely obscures the choroidal blood vessels.

The optic papilla is that part of the fundus through which fibres of the optic nerve pass before being distributed to the retina. It is normally placed about 1 to 3 mm medially from the centre line, and may be present either in the tapetal fundus, or in the non-tapetal fundus, or midway between the two. There is, sometimes, a tapetal-free zone around the papilla. The optic papilla is usually circular, but may be elliptical, triangular or oval. It normally lies flat against the retina, but is sometimes slightly elevated; there may be a slight depression in the centre, 1 to 2 dioptres deep—the so-called 'physiological cupping'. The margins of the papilla are normally well demarcated, but may, sometimes, have a slightly ragged appearance. In colour, it is normally pinkish white, but considerable variation may occur, related to the calibre of the vessels present.

There is no true *macula* in the dog, as in man. The *area centralis* is detectable only by a slight reduction in the number of blood vessels over an area of the tapetal fundus, dorsal and temporal to the disc.

The upper part of the tapetum—the *tapetum lucidum*—may occupy a large part of the fundus, or may take up only a small area. The shape is usually triangular, with the base horizontally placed. The apex is normally rounded, extending rather more than half-way to the periphery. The tapetum lucidum varies greatly in colour, usually in the range of from gold to pale green, sometimes blue or orange-red, shading off to mauves and browns below. In the pup it is grey, becoming yellow by the age of 2 months.

The *tapetum nigrum* occupies the lower part of the tapetal fundus and is pigmented with melanin. It is usually chocolate in colour, but may show masses of black pigment. There is usually a distinct outline from the tapetum lucidum by the difference in colour. In albinos, it may be pink or almost white. In some dogs, particularly the brown Poodle and the liver-and-white Springer, the pigment epithelium may be absent, so that the choroidal vessels are visible—the so-called *tigroid fundus* (Plate VI, Fig. 2, facing p. 328). The choroidal vessels appear orange-red, broad and ribbon-like, forming an ill-defined network. The tigroid fundus is seen also in blue merle Collies and harlequin Great Danes and may be associated with hetero-chromic changes in the iris (Plate VI, Fig. 5, facing p. 328).

The fundus of the dog shows considerable variation in pattern, colour and vascular arrangement; there may even be variation in the two eyes of one dog. Familiarity with these normal variations is important, in order to be able to recognize the abnormal (Plate VI, Figs. 1 to 5, facing p. 328).

Development of the retina. Sight is not apparent in the pup until about the age of 6 weeks, before which the media are not clear and the retina not fully differentiated. The retina of the new-born pup is essentially nonvas-cular, although hyaloid vessels may be seen travelling from the disc to the posterior surface of the lens. Vessels first appear at about 17 to 20 days, and at this time a pupillary light reflex is demonstrable. At first, the tape-tum is grey and shows a fine granular texture; at 4 weeks, the tapetum appears violet-grey and reflective, and blood vessels are well marked (Plate VI, Fig. 6, facing p. 328). The colour of the reflex changes gradually over the next few weeks, and the adult colour is usually apparent by the age of 8 weeks.

Congenital abnormalities

Although rare in the dog, various congenital defects of the retina have been recorded from time to time.

Congenital hypoplasia, of the optic nerve and retina, has been described in blue merle Collies (L. Z. Saunders). These pups, which appear blind, exhibit a grossly normal vascular pattern of the fundus, but histological examination reveals involvement of the ganglion cell layer. The condition is thought to be hereditary in origin—linked to coat colour—but may be due to avitaminosis.

Microphthalmia, associated with lens opacities and blindness, where no definite optic disc has been present, and an optic nerve hypoplasia has been confirmed histologically, has been recorded in the Collie and Miniature Poodle.

Posterior scleral ectasia, resulting in degenerative changes in the retina and intraocular haemorrhage, has been demonstrated in the Collie. Simil-arly, in the Coonhound, a case of *atypical coloboma of the choroid*, in which the retina was disorganized, has been described (L. F. Rubin).

Cases of congenital retinal detachment, possibly due to a recessive factor, have been recorded in the Bedlington Terrier (L. F. Rubin). These pups showed blindness, relatively small eyes, entropion, and complete detach-ment. Histologically, changes were demonstrated in the central portions of the inner retinal layer and the outer layer of rods and cones.

PLATE VI

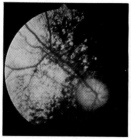 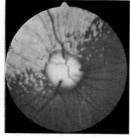 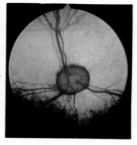 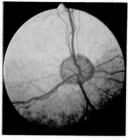

1. Normal fundus (Miniature Poodle, black)

2. Normal fundus (Miniature Poodle, brown, showing tigroid tapetum nigrum)

3. Normal fundus (Labrador Retriever, black)

4. Normal fundus (Labrador Retriever, yellow)

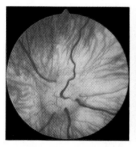 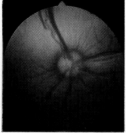 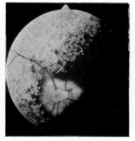 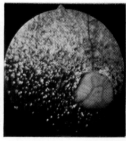

5. Normal fundus (semi-albinotic, Shetland Sheepdog, blue merle)

6. Normal fundus (puppy, 6 weeks)

7. Generalized progressive retinal atrophy (Miniature Poodle, silver)

8. Generalized progressive retinal atrophy (Miniature Poodle, black)

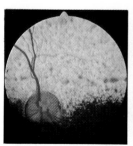 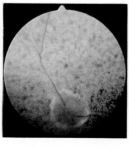 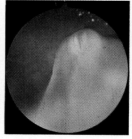 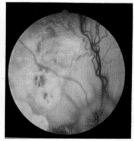

9. Central progressive retinal atrophy (Labrador Retriever, black)

10. Central progressive retinal atrophy (Border Collie)

11. Retinal detachment (total)

12. Retinochoroiditis

The existence of preretinal anteriolar loops has been described in the Beagle. (L. F. Rubin). The cases, which were unilateral and produced no visual signs, were confined to one retinal arteriole. Both limbs of the loop arose from within the retinal structure, extending with the vitreous, in the peripapillary tapetal zone. It is thought that such loops may arise from a membrana vasculosa retinae in the early stages of ocular development.

Retinal haemorrhage

This, also, is a rare condition in the dog, probably because arteriosclerosis is rarely encountered in this species. Haemorrhage into the retina may occasionally be associated with trauma, and may rarely be seen in the terminal stages of nephritis, septicaemia, hypertensive conditions, leptospirosis, diabetes and phosphorus poisoning.

Cases have been reported in India of retinal haemorrhage and detachment associated with cysticercus infestation. In these, cysts occurred on the surface of the brain, retinal damage being produced by pressure on the ophthalmic veins.

The signs exhibited will be impaired vision, oedema of the retina, and discernible haemorrhages within the retina. The haemorrhage may be either preretinal, in which case it is usually completely absorbed, or intraretinal, leading to permanent damage. Treatment is dependent upon the use of rest, atropine, and enzyme therapy.

Retinitis

True inflammation does not occur in the retina, but inflammatory cells may become deposited on the surface of the retina, and there may be infiltration around the vessels. Otherwise, retinitis occurs only as an extension of a choroiditis (Plate VI, Fig. 12, facing p. 328).

The presence of a tapetum in the dog makes a diagnosis of retinitis difficult. In some instances, the tapetum will appear dull due to a greyish exudate, which may conceal the retinal vessels. In others, the fundus may show grey or yellowish patches and, sometimes, a pigmentary degeneration will give a striped appearance. Tuberculous retinitis and anaemic retinitis have been recorded in the dog.

Retinitis may occur in cases of leukaemia in the dog. In such cases, the fundus may have a yellowish appearance, with dilated veins surrounded by tumour cells. In such instances, retinal haemorrhage may also be present, related to the associated anaemia, and, on rare occasions, papilloedema may be exhibited.

Some breeds show marked melanin pigmentation in the retina, which sometimes hides the tapetum and may even involve the papilla.

22

Detachment of the retina

Retinal detachment, recorded regularly in the cat, is uncommon in the dog (Plate VI, Fig. 11, facing p. 328). Essentially, it consists of a separation of the retina from the underlying choroid, and this separation may be partial or complete. In this last example, attachment remains at the ora serrata and at the optic papilla. The cause may be congenital, or due to disease or trauma. Congenital detachment is reported in the Collie and Bedlington Terrier. Some cases of progressive retinal atrophy, particularly in the Miniature and Toy Poodle, exhibit detachment as a late complication.

The retina may come forward due to propulsion from behind, where there is considerable exudate, as in acute choroiditis, retinal haemorrhages, or choroidal neoplasia. In these circumstances, the exudate or new tissue forms between the retina and the pigment epithelium.

The retina may come forward due to traction from within, in cases where there is liquefaction or loss of vitreous. Loss of vitreous, in turn, may be due either to perforating injuries or to surgical interference. In such cases, the loss of the support of the vitreous, which normally keeps the retina in close contact with the choroid, may result in detachment. Similarly, the retina may be brought forward by the shrinking of fibrous bands, formed during intraocular infections, or from intraocular haemorrhages. Luxation of the lens may allow vitreous to enter the anterior chamber, and so reduce its supportive power, or if the lens is luxated posteriorly, the resultant cyclitis may lead to the formation of fibrous attachments to the retina; in both these cases, detachment of the retina may result. Liquefaction of the vitreous may take place where there is degenerative change in this body, and result in a detachment.

The retina may also come forward where retinal tears are present. In these circumstances, the vitreous, particularly if it is fluid, may herniate through into the subretinal space, and produce a detachment. Such tears, in the dog, are most likely to be traumatic in origin, although systemic or metabolic diseases may be responsible in a few cases. Cases of retinal atrophy are occasionally associated with detachment.

Small areas of detachment are likely to go unnoticed in the dog, and cases will normally be presented for examination only when the detachment has progressed to an advanced degree, or where detachment is sudden and complete. In most cases, diagnosis is easily made by ophthalmoscopy, but, in some cases, opacity of the media makes diagnosis difficult or impossible.

Cases are normally presented with a history of failing vision, or sudden loss of vision. The intraocular tension is usually reduced, and the pupillary reflex is weak or absent. The appearance on ophthalmoscopic examination varies according to the degree of detachment present. *Radiating detachment* shows as large, round, undulating folds; *total detachment* appears funnel-shaped, the 'funnel' being anchored at its smaller end at the papilla and opening out into a cloud-like structure at the larger end.

The vitreous is often cloudy and floating opacities may be seen. The retinal blood vessels are tortuous and undulate with the folds of the retina. Once detachment has occurred, a progressive and fairly rapid atrophy will take place, and the normal retinal pattern will be lost. Later complications may include secondary glaucoma, secondary cataract, intraocular haemorrhage or phthisis bulbi.

The prognosis in these cases must always be doubtful, for the surgical procedures that are adopted for its relief in man, operations designed to localize the retinal hole and seal it, do not appear to be applicable to the dog. If a case were diagnosed in the early stages, it might be possible to adopt one of the recognized procedures such as perforating diathermy or cryocoagulation, but postoperative care would present great problems. Most of the cases that are presented in the dog, however, are complete, or at least very extensive, and surgical interference is not feasible.

W. G. Magrane, however, reports success in cases of obscure spontaneous detachment, using ACTH at intervals of 48 hours, Chymar injections 12-hourly for 5 to 7 days, followed by oral maintenance, and Diuril tablets at 12-hourly intervals, the whole procedure being continued for 10 to 14 days. In some cases, this treatment has been followed by absorption of the sub-retinal fluid, reattachment of the retina, and return of vision.

Complete or incomplete retinal breaks, without detachments, have been reported as occurring in a large percentage of senile dogs.

Retinal neoplasia

Neoplasia of the retina is rare in the dog, but melanotic sarcomata, involving the retina, have been seen. Such tumours are normally secondary to uveal neoplasia. Retinoblastoma, or so-called 'glioma', has been recorded as a congenital tumour arising from the nuclear layer of the retina, and also as affecting the ciliary portion of the retina, and extending into the vitreous and the anterior chamber.

Retinal granuloma

Cases have been recorded (Rubin and Saunders) of intraocular larva migrans in the dog. The lesions, containing *Toxacara* larvae, appear as granulomata, visible by ophthalmoscopy—small, raised, greyish nodules, from a quarter to a sixth of the diameter of the optic disc, visible on the surface of the retina.

Retinopathy

The various changes that take place in the retina, as a result of disease, have not been intensively studied in the dog, although many isolated case reports are available.

Ischaemia of the retinal vessels, in which these vessels become kinked, with marked variations in calibre, has been reported as occurring, following excessive doses of quinine, phenobarbitone and nicotine. It may also occur in leptospiral infections, due to arteriosclerosis of the choroidoretinal vessels.

Diabetic retinopathy would appear to be rare in the dog, possibly due to the fact that it will only occur after the disease has been in existence for a long time. In some experimental reports, however, some cases have shown retinal changes when the diabetes has been in existence for more than 4 years. Other cases have been maintained in a diabetic state for 8 years without retinal change. In this condition, oedema and haemorrhage around the optic papilla has been described, giving a 'cotton-wool' appearance, together with yellowish-white spots in the retina and sometimes glistening crystals of cholesterol. The retina may show micro-aneurysms and haemorrhages.

Glaucoma will ultimately produce blindness, associated with atrophy of the optic disc, which becomes greyish-white and ischaemic, together with cupping, and atrophy of the retina.

Vitamin A deficiency can result in blindness, although it is unlikely that such a deficiency will occur under natural conditions. There is little evidence that vitamin A deficiency occurs spontaneously in the dog, but, experimentally, such a deficiency will produce papilloedema and degeneration of the layers of the retina, commencing with the layer of rods and cones, and extending as far as the inner nuclear layer. Blindness due to vitamin A deficiency is reversible in the adult, but irreversible changes take place in young animals, due to pressure effects upon the optic nerve and blood vessels, resulting from retardation of skull growth.

Canine distemper infection may be followed by retinal degeneration, when complete atrophy and blindness may develop rapidly. Such atrophies are associated with necrosis of the ganglion cells, whereas hereditary retinal atrophy is rarely associated with such necrosis, even though the retina be otherwise completely atrophic. Differences in the layers of the retina affected in viral and hereditary cases may be explained by differences in blood supply. The central retinal artery supplies the inner retinal layers, and these layers will be involved in primary retinitis or inflammation of the inner retinal layers associated with virus infections. The rods and cones have no vessels, being nourished by the choroidal vessels, and the outer layers will be involved in retinochoroiditis and progressive retinal atrophy (P.R.A.). These changes may, or may not, be associated with brain lesions, but many cases of blindness associated with distemper are due to lesions of the visual apparatus central to the retina. In cases where the brain is involved, a retrograde degeneration of the retinal ganglion cells may occur via the optic nerve. In such cases, the histological changes found may include, in addition: oedema of the retina, perivascular cuffing of retinal blood vessels, eosinophilic inclusion bodies in glial cells, pigment epithelium proliferation, atrophy of all retinal layers and loss of organization, focal gliosis and pigment deposits.

The differential diagnosis of retinal atrophy associated with virus infection, and progressive retinal atrophy of hereditary origin, is difficult. Diagnosis might be based on history, the onset of sudden blindness and the existence of other neurological signs, but, in most cases, it is possible to differentiate the two types only by histological examination. However, in some cases of retinal atrophy, associated with the distemper virus, retinal changes may occur as a late sequel 1 or 2 years after the primary infection. It is always possible, of course, that a virus infection will hasten the development of atrophic changes of hereditary origin.

Toxoplasmosis. Retinal atrophy may be caused by toxoplasmosis, producing a focal retinochoroiditis. Viewed with an ophthalmoscope, the lesions appear as circular or oval patches, usually in the tapetum lucidum, where an increased reflectivity is shown, and usually a change in colour from green to orange. These areas may have a pigmented edge and are usually one to three times the size of the optic disc.

Senile retinal atrophy. Cystoid degeneration of the retina, in the area of the ora serrata, is common and may be regarded as a normal ageing process. Retinal breaks in senile animals have also been reported as occurring commonly.

Toxic retinopathy. Many drugs may produce blindness, either from optic atrophy or by their effect on retinal cells. Among those that may be of clinical importance are filix mas, lead, cobalt, phosphorus, naphthalene, quinine and quinoline.

Lipodystrophy. Cases of lipodystrophy of the central nervous system, resulting in blindness, have been described in the dog. Degenerative changes have been noted in the midbrain, pons and cerebellum, with massive lipocarbohydrate deposits in the nerve cells, and associated optic disc atrophy or retinal atrophy. These changes have been likened to Tay-Sachs disease in the human, an hereditary central retinal degenerative disorder.

The lipid dystrophic changes may also affect the ganglion cells of the retina, and it would appear that this rare metabolic anomaly may be familial in the English Setter.

PROGRESSIVE RETINAL ATROPHY

The most common disease of the retina in the dog is progressive retinal atrophy of hereditary origin. This form of atrophy has been reported in many breeds, particularly the Gordon Setter, Irish Setter, Miniature and Toy Poodles, Labrador Retriever, Golden Retriever, Cocker Spaniel and Border Collie. Other cases have been noted in the Flat-coated Retriever, English Springer Spaniel, Rough Collie, Boxer, Alsatian, Pembroke Corgi, Standard Poodle, Cairn Terrier, Elkhound, Greyhound, Dachshund, Irish Terrier, Sealyham, Wire-haired Fox Terrier, Smooth-haired Fox Terrier, Airedale, Whippet, Pekingese, Beagle and Yorkshire Terrier. It has not been possible, in all cases, to show that the disease is hereditary in origin, but the ophthalmoscopic findings have been similar in most cases. Cases have also been reported in a variety of crossbreeds and mongrels.

It is often impossible to differentiate, on clinical findings, atrophy of hereditary origin and that caused by virus infections. In the former case, however, the history of vaccination and lack of evidence of any previous disease that might have been of viral origin, the gradual loss of vision noticed by the owner, the history of increased tapetal reflectivity and the onset of 'night blindness', and the absence of any other neurological signs, are all indications that hereditary factors may be involved.

Types of progressive retinal atrophy (P.R.A.)

Two distinct forms of primary tapetoretinal degeneration, of hereditary origin, are currently recognized in the dog. The first, which is termed *generalized progressive retinal atrophy* is associated with overall retinal function loss. Cases are bilateral, although, in the early stages, one eye may be at a more advanced stage than the other; progressive; and end in total blindness. The age of onset and the progressive rate vary between breeds and individuals. An early sign is night blindness, which is progressive until day vision is also affected. Early loss of peripheral vision is often noted, resulting in 'tunnel vision' where only objects immediately in front of the animal are recognized. There is no evidence of pigment migration in the tapetal fundus in this type. Breeds showing generalized P.R.A. include the Irish Setter, Miniature and Toy Poodles, Cocker Spaniel, Miniature Long-haired Dachshund, Cairn Terrier and Elkhound.

The second form is termed *central progressive retinal atrophy*, and is also bilateral and progressive. In this there is early loss of central vision, but peripheral vision may be retained for several years. The early and main change in this type of atrophy is the formation of brown pigment foci throughout the tapetal fundus. Night blindness is not so commonly noticed, but a central scotoma (blank spot in the visual field) is the main sign. Affected dogs may see moving objects until the atrophy is far advanced, but collide with stationary objects in their path. Distance vision is poor. Breeds showing central P.R.A. include the Labrador Retriever, Border Collie, English Springer Spaniel and Rough Collie.

The Irish Setter

The condition of generalized progressive retinal atrophy in the Irish Setter is noted clinically by defective vision, first at night and later in daylight, and is associated with atrophy of the receptor cells of the retina and reduction of the retinal blood vessels. It has been concluded that the condition is hereditary, probably a simple Mendelian autosomal recessive factor.

First signs are seen when the pups are 6 to 8 weeks old, at which age vision at dusk and in daylight is normal, but there is an increased reflection from the tapetum, which appears green rather than the normal yellow-orange-green colour. There is a progressive loss of vision, at first in dusk or at night, over months or even years, until there is complete night blindness and, at a later stage, day blindness as well. The pupillary reflex is usually retained, although there is some increase in pupil size, both pupils remaining equal.

The remainder of affected eyes is normal, but some cases develop anterior subcapsular cataracts, occasionally as early as 4 months old. Sexual abnormalities are common in affected dogs. Tests for defective vision are best made in dusk light.

In the early stages, there is little or no change in the fundus, although the tapetum is found to be highly reflective, and the green colour more prominent. In the second stage, the tapetum has a marked green colouration, and a 'crystalline' appearance. The optic disc appears more pallid and, although the larger vessels are not affected, the small vessels, both of the tapetal fundus and the disc, and also of the nontapetal fundus, are less numerous. In the third stage, the disc appears white and its margin irregular, the small vessels are absent, and the larger ones are reduced in size; the tapetum is highly reflective and crystalline, the fundus vessels are scanty and the nontapetal fundus shows a grey colour.

As the disease is hereditary, and due to a simple recessive factor, dogs may be either free, or carriers (that is, carrying one normal factor and one factor for blindness, but outwardly normal), or affected. K. C. Barnett lists six possible matings of these three groups:

(1) Both parents affected—all progeny affected.
(2) One parent affected, one carrier parent—50% affected, 50% carriers.
(3) One parent affected, one parent free—all progeny carriers.
(4) Both parents carriers—50% carriers, 25% free, 25% affected.
(5) One parent free, one carrier parent—50% carriers, 50% free.
(6) Both parents free—all progeny free.

Thus, both the parents and all the progeny of an affected animal must be at least carriers.

Carriers may be detected by test matings, but these animals should not, of course, be used for future breeding. In test-mating, the suspected animal is mated with a known affected animal and the pups reared to an age when the condition can be diagnosed. If the suspect is, in fact, a carrier, it is considered reasonable to expect at least one affected puppy in a litter of six, as the chances of an affected pup being produced are 1 in 2.

The Miniature and Toy Poodle (Plate VI, Figs. 7 and 8, facing p. 328).

Progressive retinal atrophy in the Poodle is generalized and may first be exhibited at any age between 6 months and 9 years; it would appear to be rather more common in the male. The history normally given by the owner is one of defective vision, particularly at night or in poor light, so that the dog appears nervous under these conditions and moves cautiously; of dilatation of the pupil and increased tapetal reflectivity; of changes in behaviour; or of limitation in the field of vision.

In all cases, pupillary dilatation is shown, which increases as the retinal atrophy develops, until, ultimately, no reaction to light is demonstrable. The pupillary reflex is inhibited and the response is slow.

Approximately two-thirds of cases show secondary cataract formation, which develops after the initial signs of atrophy, but which progresses at varying rates. In some cases, complete lens opacity is shown in a few months, in others only after years. The two lenses often show differing degrees of opacity, but the rate of development of the cataracts matches that of the retinal degeneration. In most cases, the initial changes take place in the posterior cortex, either as radiating lines from the periphery or as posterior polar cataracts. The density and the area of the opacity increases progressively, involving both anterior and posterior cortices and then the lens substance, giving a soft, granular cataract, and leading, ultimately, to a dense, diffuse, total cataract, often with a crystalline appearance and showing Y sutures on the anterior face (Fig. 272). In some cases, cataract formation is followed by lens luxation, usually posterior, and secondary glaucoma. Glaucomatous signs are not as marked as with cases of hereditary luxation in terriers.

The optic disc, which, in the Poodle, is normally a circular pinkish-grey structure, with clearly-defined edges, lying at the junction of tapetum lucidum and tapetum nigrum, becomes paler and structureless, then later very white and avascular, larger than normal and with an indefinite edge as it spreads around the roots of the main vessels. The shape varies according to the number of vessels present. Sometimes the disc appears pale, but of normal shape and size, but the shape and colour of the disc in the two eyes always forms a mirror image.

The retinal blood vessels show progressive constriction, at first in the fine vessels, later in the main ones. Different vessels are sometimes affected to different degrees. The venous circle of the disc is affected later, and finally disappears.

The tapetum lucidum in the Poodle is normally clear and mosaic-like, the colour varying with the coat colour, but usually showing orange, yellow and green. In cases of P.R.A. a progressive loss of detail is exhibited, with the changes spreading from the periphery towards the disc, together with increased reflectivity. Later stages show golden-orange splashes, and, finally, loss of colour. Pigmentation of the fundus, which is found in cases of P.R.A. in other breeds, is not present in cases in the Poodle.

The tapetum nigrum, normally dark grey-brown and homogeneous, sometimes tigroid, shows progressive loss of colour, changing to pale grey or brown, often in patches, with a scattering of dark pigment granules throughout the area.

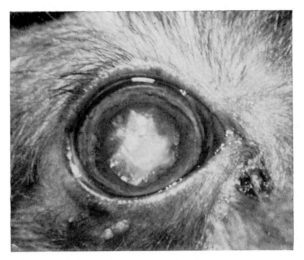

Fig. 272. *Cataract associated with progressive retinal atrophy.*

In advanced cases, retinal detachment, associated with liquefaction of the vitreous, may be exhibited, the detachment being normally complete. Occasionally, cases will exhibit synchisis scintillans.

The condition is always bilateral, progressive and nonpainful. It will always terminate in complete blindness, although, normally, one eye will be affected before the other. The rate of development varies from case to case, but, as a general rule, dogs afflicted early in life progress to blindness more rapidly than those that show signs at a later age. Similarly, the rate of cataract formation varies, but follows the progression of the retinal changes.

Although most cases are presented only when the disease is comparatively well advanced, it would probably be possible to establish a diagnosis at a much earlier stage if the fundi were to be examined. The available evidence suggests that progressive retinal atrophy in the Poodle is hereditary, involving a simple, autosomal, recessive gene.

The Labrador Retriever (Plate VI, Fig. 9, facing p. 328)

Central progresssive retinal atrophy affects both yellow and black varieties of this breed, and both sexes in approximately equal numbers. The age incidence is normally between 4 and 10 years. In this breed, it is possible that both recessive and dominant modes of inheritance are operative.

The presenting history is one of gradually failing vision, increased tapetal reflex and sometimes night blindness. Central vision is lost at an early age, but peripheral vision may be retained for several years. The rate of deterioration is variable, but the condition is always progressive, terminating in complete blindness. All cases are bilateral, but the changes are sometimes more advanced in one eye. Pupillary dilatation and slow pupillary reflexes are exhibited.

Secondary cataract formation is not so constant a feature as in the Poodle, and tends to occur later in the disease. Most cases are at first cortical, later appearing as a granular, diffuse density, progressing to complete opacity. Synchisis scintillans may be present in a few cases.

The optic disc appears very white, with an indistinct edge, often triangular, but not enlarged as in the Poodle. The changes in the two eyes are often noted to be at different stages. Retinal vessel constriction is obvious in advanced cases, but not always so in the early ones, although the smaller vessels sometimes show irregular segmentation.

The tapetal fundus in the Labrador tends to be more constant in appearance, without the mosaic pattern, than in the normal Poodle. Typically, the tapetum shows a broad green band next to the tapetum nigrum, the remainder being golden yellow. In affected dogs, the tapetum shows loss of clarity, some loss of colour and increased reflectivity. In nearly all cases, the most marked change is the presence of dark brown pigment spots, scattered on the surface of the tapetum, varying in number, size, shape and density. In a few cases, the whole tapetum appears to be covered by a faint brownish film, but the pigmentary changes are not always noticeable in advanced cases. The nontapetal fundus shows loss of colour and increased reflectivity in the advanced stages.

The Cocker Spaniel

Again, in this breed, all cases are bilateral and progressive and similar in all respects to those in the Poodle. Secondary cataract formation is commonly seen and, sometimes, lens luxation and glaucoma. Dilated pupils, poor pupillary reflexes and increased reflectivity are shown. The optic disc appears pallid, larger than normal, with an indistinct edge, and is often triangular in shape, the original disc appearing within the triangle in some cases. The retinal vessels show marked constriction, those of the optic disc being the last to show changes. The tapetum, which is normally mosaic-like, shows loss of clarity, increased reflectivity, loss of colour, but no pigmentation. The tapetum nigrum shows loss of colour and is sometimes tigroid.

The Elkhound

Hereditary retinal atrophy of the type that occurs in the Poodle, has been shown to occur in the Elkhound (Cogan and Kuwabara), and the name of photoreceptive abiotrophy of the retina has been applied. An abiotrophy is a progressive, partial or complete destruction of a tissue which has started to develop normally, the destruction being brought about by hereditary causation of premature tissue death, and not by trauma or inflammation. A recessive factor is thought to be responsible, and signs of night blindness have been exhibited at 6 to 8 months of age, associated with narrowing of the retinal vessels.

Other breeds (Plate VI, Fig. 10, facing p. 328)

Similar changes have been noted in cases in all the other breeds that have been mentioned. Synchisis scintillans and retinal detachment may occur, and pigmentation, similar to that shown by the Labrador, has been reported in the Golden Retriever, English Springer Spaniel, Rough Collie, Boxer, Alsatian and Border Collie. In the Sealyham Terrier, cases have been reported at the early age of 8 months.

The electroretinogram

As in other nervous tissue, electrical currents are generated in the retina, and a large potential exists between cornea and fundus, the former being the more positive. Light striking the retina results in rapid changes in this potential, these changes constituting the electroretinogram or E.R.G.

The electroretinogram has been studied in the normal dog and in those affected with P.R.A. (Parry, Tansley & Thomson; Barnett). It may be recorded by placing one electrode on the cornea and one on the shaved forehead, and a stimulus applied by a timed light flash. Four basic components form the E.R.G. and these are known as the a-, b-, c- and d-waves. The initial stimulation of the cornea causes this structure to become negative, producing the a-wave which originates in the photoreceptor layer. This is followed by a large positive wave—the b-wave—originating in the bipolar cell layer. In the dog, the positive b-wave is followed by a large negative wave, originating in the retina (in the human, this wave is produced by pupillary constriction). This large negative wave is obtained in the dog by virtue of the rod-dominated retina and can be abolished by light adaptation.

In cases of hereditary retinal lesions, where rods are destroyed, the negative wave, together with the b-wave, disappear. This loss of the E.R.G. may, therefore, be used experimentally as a sensitive indicator of the existence of P.R.A. In the Irish Setter, Parry and his co-workers have shown that it is possible to demonstrate loss of E.R.G. at 30 days of age, before it is possible to employ clinical tests.

There is early loss of the E.R.G. in cases of generalized progressive retinal atrophy, even where there is good day vision and a fair pupillary light reflex. In the case of central progressive retinal atrophy, however, the E.R.G. is present until late in the course of the disease, and may be obtained even when there are obvious changes in the fundus.

Histopathology of retinal atrophy

K. C. Barnett has described the histopathology of retinal atrophy in various breeds. In the Poodle, the main changes are an absence of the bacillary layer, great reduction in the width of the outer nuclear layer, and some reduction in the width of the inner nuclear layer. No evidence of inflammatory change has been noted, and the other layers of the retina, and the other structures of the eye, other than the lens, remain normal except in very advanced cases. In the Labrador, the main changes noted have been an absence of the bacillary layer, disorganization of the inner and outer fibre and nuclear layers, and hypertrophy of the pigment epithelium.

Treatment of retinal atrophy

There is no known treatment that will either slow down the atrophic process or reverse the changes that have already taken place. Clinically, however, it would seem that certain cases have improved visually, following the administration of regular large doses of vitamin A, and it would seem prudent to use this form of therapy, at least in early cases.

THE OPTIC NERVE

The nerve fibres of the retina converge at the optic disc, where they pass through the sclera, at the sieve-like lamina cribrosa, to form the optic nerve. The intraocular portion of the optic nerve—forming the optic nerve head or optic disc—is formed of nonmedullated fibres surrounded by neuroglia cells. The optic disc, which may be round, oval or triangular, is approximately 1 mm in diameter.

Immediately behind the lamina cribrosa, the nerve fibres acquire a myelin sheath, and the nerve shows a diameter of between 1·2 to 2·4 mm. The optic nerve, being an extension of the brain rather than a peripheral nerve, resembles the brain in its coverings histologically. Although the nerve fibres are myelinated, they do not possess neurilemma sheaths. In cross-section, the orbital portion of the optic nerve shows an outer dura, an inner pia and an intermediate arachnoid; these sheaths are continuous with the meninges of the brain, and, at the globe, they become continuous with the sclera. The central core of connective tissue—the central supporting tissue strand—carries the central artery and the central vein of the retina.

The orbital portion of the optic nerve, which passes from the eyeball to the optic foramen of the skull, is curved to allow for the movements of the eyeball. Passing through the optic foramina, the intracranial portions of the nerve meet, join and partly decussate (the chiasma) immediately behind the foramina, before passing on to the lateral geniculate bodies.

Congenital abnormalities

These are most commonly seen in the Collie, and include *hypoplasia of the optic nerve*, which has been noted under congenital abnormalities of the retina, and the *ectasia syndrome* (previously described as posterior scleral ectasia, excavation of the optic disc or coloboma of the optic disc).

The Collie ectasia syndrome would appear to be common in this breed in the U.S.A. and similar cases have been noted in the Collie and the Shetland Sheepdog in Great Britain. The clinical and pathological picture has been described by S. R. Roberts and his co-workers. The condition is hereditary, and, although the hereditary pattern has not yet been fully elucidated, it would seem to be associated with the gene responsible for merling. Inheritance is not sex-linked and is probably recessive. Both sexes are affected, and many minor cases may go unnoticed unless some complication such as retinal detachment or intraocular haemorrhage occurs. Mild cases, in the early stages, may show no loss of vision, but retinal degeneration may occur at a later stage.

Clinically, the signs presented vary according to the degree of involvement of the eye or eyes. The vision of affected dogs may vary from being normal to complete blindness. The common factor in all cases, recognizable by fundal examination at 6 weeks of age, is a decrease in the pigmentation of the fundus. The commonest finding is pale areas in the fundus; other changes, in order of frequency, are tortuous blood vessels, pits in the optic disc, posterior scleral ectasia, retinal detachment, retinal haemorrhage and vermiform streaks in the fundus. Central corneal opacities are exhibited by a few cases.

Five grades are recognized by Roberts and his co-workers, ranging from Grade I, showing merely focal pale areas, supratemporal to the optic disc, where choroidal vessels are visible beneath the retinal vessels, through larger pale areas, degenerative changes of the retina, detachment and haemorrhages, and excavations of the optic nerve; to Grade V, showing posterior scleral ectasia in the region of the optic nerve. Animals showing Grade I defects may produce litters exhibiting all grades.

Although obvious signs may be shown from the age of a few months, many cases are only detected by routine ophthalmoscopy. In some cases, dilatation of the pupils, increased fundal reflectivity or corneal opacities will be visible on examination.

The findings on examination of the fundus will likewise vary according to the degree of severity of the case presented. The tapetal fundus may show merely a loss of colour; or a change from yellow-green to orange-red, or may be tigroid. Those cases associated with either retinal detachment or retinal atrophy exhibit marked loss of vision. Most cases show a small eye, and many Collies exhibit microphthalmos, which, in turn, is often associated with colobomata of the optic disc, retina and choroid.

Where posterior scleral ectasia occurs, enlargement and excavation of the optic disc is shown. In some cases, the excavation may be maximal, requiring a lens of −8 to −20 dioptres to bring the floor of the disc into focus, and, in these cases, the blood vessels dip suddenly over the edge of the disc. In other cases, only part of the disc may be affected, showing a deep excavation or an avascular area, whilst the remainder of the disc appears normal. The sclera may bulge around the disc at its nasal or temporal edge. The vessels approaching the disc are, in most cases, tortuous; in others, very few vessels may be present, with no apparent underlying choroid.

Papilloedema

Oedema of the optic disc—a choked disc—may be associated with advanced choroidoretinitis, or with conditions causing a rise in intracranial pressure such as cerebral tumours, cerebral tuberculosis or hydrocephalus. A case of rhabdomyosarcoma of the orbit, producing papilloedema, has been recorded, but the condition would appear to be rare in the dog.

In cases of papilloedema, the disc shows a reddish discoloration, with blurred margins and grey oedematous streaks. The disc appears elevated above the surrounding area, and this elevation, which may be measured with an ophthalmoscope, may amount to as much as 6 dioptres. Measurement is made by noting the difference in the ophthalmoscope lenses necessary to focus first on the apex of the disc and then on the adjacent retina. The veins of the disc are engorged, and the elevation of the disc causes, in some cases, the vessels traversing the outer third of the optic disc to be lost from view. Small haemorrhages or exudates may be present in the adjacent retina.

Pseudopapilloedema, an uncommon abnormality of the optic disc, must be differentiated from papilloedema. In the pseudopapilloedema, the disc appears elevated, but, although the disc margins may be somewhat indistinct, there is no venous distention and no exudates or haemorrhages. Such cases are probably congenital in origin.

Atrophy of the optic nerve

Optic nerve atrophy may be caused by choroidoretinitis, brain trauma or intracranial haemorrhage, pressure from tumours, glaucoma, avitaminosis-A, certain poisonings, or as a result of progressive retinal atrophy. Occasional cases, normally bilateral, may be associated with encephalitis complicating distemper. Congenital cases may be associated with optic nerve hypoplasia.

The optic disc appears shrunken and pale, the vessels shrunken or absent, and there may be some yellowish discoloration or pigmentation of the papilla.

Optic nerve neoplasia

Tumours involving the optic nerve are rare in the dog, but those that have been recorded include glioma and meningioma. Metastasis of the latter to the lungs has been noted. They will be associated with loss of vision and exophthalmos, and are normally unilateral. One case has been recorded, of a malignant syncytial meningioma, affecting the ventral surface of the brain, including optic chiasma and optic nerves, in which there was blindness but no ophthalmic changes.

AMAUROSIS

Blindness (*amaurosis*) or partial blindness (*amblyopia*) without apparent cause and without organic changes is occasionally presented in the dog. In such cases, often in apparently healthy animals, there is sometimes no suggestive history, and clinical and ophthalmic findings are negative.

Some cases of amblyopia may be due to drug or chemical toxic effects, and, in some instances, the loss of vision is only transient. Other cases may be associated with *optic neuritis*, an inflammation, degeneration or demyelinization of the optic nerve. In this case, treatment has been suggested using vitamin A, vitamin B_{12}, and ACTH, but the prognosis remains doubtful in all cases.

Blindness may be due to disturbances in the media of the eye, or to disturbances of any part of the nervous portion of the visual system—retina, optic nerve, chiasma, optic tract, lateral geniculate body (in the thalamus), optic radiation (in the internal capsule) or primary visual cortex (in the occipital lobe). In general, lesions of the forebrain tend to be associated with blindness; those of the medulla and cerebellum with nystagmus.

Accurate diagnosis of blindness due to central lesions is often difficult in the dog, partly due to the inability to perform functional tests in this animal. In many cases, the cause remains obscure, or may be revealed only at a postmortem examination. It is possible, however, to detect some lesions that interfere with major areas of the central pathways.

The nerve fibres concerned with the pupillary constriction leave the optic tracts at the level of the lateral geniculate body and enter the midbrain. The existence of normal pupillary light reflexes, therefore, indicates that the visual system is intact up to the level of the lateral geniculate body. Blindness may occur in cases where the pupillary light reflexes are normal if a lesion exists in lateral geniculate body, optic radiation or occipital cortex, for disturbances here whilst preventing the perception of vision do not interfere with these reflexes.

Loss of vision in half of the visual field of each eye is termed *hemianopia*. Cases in which there is loss of vision in the temporal part of the visual field of one eye and the nasal part of the other are referred to as *homonymous hemianopia;* those in which there is loss of vision in either the temporal or the nasal parts of the visual fields of both eyes are referred to as *heteronymous hemianopia* (binasal or bitemporal).

The outer temporal part of the retina is stimulated by light rays from the nasal visual field; the inner nasal part by rays from the temporal visual field. Careful testing, therefore, may sometimes reveal the presence of a hemianopia. This examination may take the form of a carefully observed maze test; or stimulation of one half of the retina by careful focal illumination; or by testing the response to the menace reflex, from different angles, of each eye separately, the other being covered.

HEMERALOPIA

Hemeralopia, or day blindness, signifies an inability to see under conditions of bright light, although vision in conditions of decreased illumination is retained.

This condition has been reported in two breeds, the Miniature Poodle and the Alaskan Malamute. In this last breed, the condition has been reported as being hereditary in origin (Rubin & co-workers), a Mendelian autosomal recessive mode of inheritance, not sex-linked, being involved. In Malamutes affected with hemeralopia, no other eye defects are reported.

18

OPHTHALMIC SIGNS
IN INFECTIOUS DISEASE

Little study has been made, as a subject in its own right, of the ocular manifestations associated with the various infectious diseases of the dog. However, changes in the eye often appear early in the course of such diseases and, although not diagnostic in themselves, they may be a useful aid to diagnosis. The following list notes the various ocular changes that have been described in various infectious diseases; not all the signs described will appear in each and every case of any particular infection.

Blastomycosis
Exophthalmos associated with lesions of the orbital bones.
Uveitis or extensive intraocular lesions.
Hypopyon.
Subconjunctival abscesses.
Retinal detachment.
Hyalitis, retinitis, optic neuritis.

Coccidioidomycosis
Keratoconjunctivitis.
Granulomatous uveitis.

Contagious rhinotonsillitis
Ulcerative keratitis, staphyloma.
Exudative or atrophic choroidoretinitis.

Cryptococcosis
Subretinal granulomatous foci.
Retinal detachment.
Fundal colour changes.
Granulomatous orbital lesions affecting the optic nerve.

Distemper
Conjunctivitis, ranging from mucoid to purulent.
Less commonly, keratitis and corneal ulceration.
Occasionally, transient blindness.
Occasionally, retinal atrophy of varying degree.

Leishmaniasis
Depilation of eyelids.
Conjunctivitis.
Interstitial keratitis.
Iridocyclitis.
Retinitis.

Leptospirosis
Catarrhal conjunctivitis.
Occasionally, uveitis.
Icterohaemorrhagiae infection—jaundice of the sclera and petechiae under the conjunctiva.

Nosematosis (Encephalitozoonosis)
Spasmodic divergent strabismus.
Keratitis.

Rabies
Mucopurulent conjunctivitis.
Anisocoria.
Strabismus, divergent or convergent.
Protrusion of the nictitating membrane.

Tetanus
Miosis.
Prominence of the nictitating membrane.

Toxoplasmosis
Iridocyclitis.
Choroidoretinitis.
Optic neuritis.
Vitreous opacities.

Toxoplasmosis—continued

Retinal necrosis (mostly in tapetum lucidum).

Keratic precipitates (K.P.s) on the cornea.

Tropical canine pancytopaenia

Corneal opacity, associated with deposits on the endothelium.

Iris haemorrhages.

Conjunctival injection or acute purulent conjunctivitis.

Virus hepatitis

Serous conjunctivitis.

Iridocyclitis.

Corneal opacification, as a result of hypersensitivity reaction—keratitis profunda.

BIBLIOGRAPHY

Many contributions to the literature on the diseases of the canine eye cover several aspects of the whole subject. In the following list of references, articles have been included under the main item discussed, or where one particular aspect is particularly stressed. A few medical references are included where they seem particularly appropriate.

General

ARCHIBALD, J. (Ed.) (1965) *Canine Surgery*. Amer. Vet. Publ., California.
BEAMER, R. J. (1959) *Canine Ophthalmology*. Alcon Laboratories Ltd, Texas.
DALLING, T. (Ed.) (1966) *International Encyclopedia of Veterinary Medicine*. Edinburgh: Green.
GRAHAM-JONES, O. (Ed.) (1966) *Aspects of Comparative Ophthalmology*. Oxford: Pergamon.
HANSALL, P. (1957) *A System of Ophthalmic Illustration*. Springfield: Thomas.
HOSKINS, H. P. (Ed.) (1959) *Canine Medicine*. American Vet. Publ., California.
JUBB, K. V. F. & KENNEDY, P. C. (1963) *Pathology of Domestic Animals*, Vol. 2. New York & London: Academic Press.
MAGRANE, W. G. (1965) *Canine Ophthalmology*. London: Baillière.
MARCOWITZ, J. (1964) *Experimental Surgery*. London: Baillière.
MILLER, M. E., CHRISTENSEN, G. C. & EVANS, H. E. (1964) *Anatomy of the Dog*. Philadelphia: Saunders.
NICOLAS, E. (1925) *Veterinary and Comparative Ophthalmology*. London, Brown.
ORMROD, A. N. (1966) *Surgery of the Dog and Cat*. London: Baillière.
PRINCE, J. H. (1956) *Comparative Anatomy of the Eye*. Springfield: Thomas.
PRINCE, J. H., DIEMSEM, C. D., EGLITIS, I. & RUSKELL, G. L. (1960) *Anatomy and Histology of the Eye and Orbit in Domestic Animals*. Springfield: Thomas.
SMYTHE, R. H. (1958) *Veterinary Ophthalmology*. London: Baillière.
TAYLOR, J. A. (1955) *Regional and Applied Anatomy of the Domestic Animals*. Part I. Edinburgh: Oliver & Boyd.
TREVOR-ROPER, P. D. (1962) *Ophthalmology*. London: Lloyd-Luke.

The Optical Mechanism

ADLER, F. H. (1953) *Physiology of the Eye*. St. Louis: Mosby.
BRAZ, M. B. (1953) Estudo da relação entre a ontogénese dos globos oculares a seu sistema reticulo-histiocitario e a suas localizações leucósicas. (A study of the ontogeny of the globe, its reticulo-endothelial system, and local leucocytosis.) *Rev. Cienc. vet. (Lisboa)*, **48**, 65.
DANIEL, P. M. et. al. (1953) Studies of the carotid rete and its associated arteries. *Phil. Trans. B.*, **237**, 173.
HEGEDUS, S. A. & SHACKLEFORD, R. T. (1965) A comparative-anatomical study of the cranio-cervical venous systems in mammals with special reference to the dog. *Amer. J. Anat.*, **116**, 375.
KISTLER, R. (1927) Untersuchungen über die Refraktion von 105 Hunden mit Bemerkungen über senile Veränderungen des Hundeauges. (Investigations on refraction in 105 dogs, and senile changes in the eye.) *Klin. Mbl. Augenheilk.*, **80**, 181.
KRAWITZ, L. (1963) Practical anatomy and physiology of the canine eye. *J. Amer. vet. med. Ass.*, **142**, 770.

LOVE, W. G. (1940) Some diseases of the eye of animals. I. Anatomy and physiology. *J. Amer. vet. med. Ass.*, **97**, 387.

MAGRANE, W. G. (1955) Ocular physiology—clinical application. *N. Amer. Vet.*, **36**, 387.

—— (1955) Ocular physiology—clinical application. *Ibid.*, **36**, 484.

—— (1955) Ocular physiology—clinical application. *Ibid.*, **36**, 561.

NICKEL, R. & SCHWARZ, R. (1963) Vergleichende Betrachtung der Kopfartevien der Haussäugetiere. *Zbl. Vet.-Med.*, **10**, 89.

REINHARD, K. R. et al. (1962) The craniovertebral veins and sinuses of the dog. *Amer. J. Anat.*, **111**, 67.

ROBERTS, S. R. (1955) Animal vision. *J. Amer. vet. med. Ass.*, **127**, 236.

SCHAUENBURG, G. & SCHEURMANN, E. (1962) Versuche über das Erkennen von Bildern durch Hunde. (Experiments on the recognition of pictures by dogs.) *Z. Tierpsychol.*, **19**, 723.

SLOME, D. (1966) Physiological features of the eye of man and animals. *Aspects of Comparative Ophthalmology*, Oxford: Pergamon. p. 11.

Examination of the Eye

—— (1959) Ocular biomicroscopy. *Proc. Amer. soc. vet. Ophthal.*

BARNETT, K. C. (1963) A target graticule for measuring the optic disc of the dog. *Dispens. Optn.*, **18**, 272.

—— (1967) Principles of ophthalmoscopy. *Vet. Med.*, **62**, 56.

BRYAN, G. M. (1965) Tonometry in the dog and cat. *J. small Anim. Pract.*, **6**, 117.

BUNCE, D. F. M. (1955) The use of the ophthalmoscope in veterinary practice. *Vet. Med.*, **50**, 599.

CATCOTT, E. J. (1952) Ophthalmoscopy in canine practice. *J. Amer. vet. med. Ass.*, **121**, 35.

CROFT, P. G. (1962) The EEG as an aid to diagnosis of nervous diseases in the dog and cat. *J. small Anim. Pract.*, **3**, 205.

DIMIC, J. & GLIGORIVEJIĆ, J. (1952) *Foundations of Ophthalmological Diagnosis in Domestic Animals*. Belgrade: Naucna Kniga. (In Serbian.)

FISHER, C. & SMALL, E. (1967) A new look at canine ophthalmology. *Mod. vet. Pract.*, **48**, (6), 19.

FORMSTON, C. (1955) Examination of the eye with special reference to the horse and dog. *Vet. Rec.*, **68**, 984.

FOX, M. W. (1963). Postnatal ontogeny of the canine eye. *J. Amer. vet. med. Ass.*, **143**, 968.

KRAWITZ, L. (1965) Clinical examination of the canine and feline eye. *J. Amer. vet. med. Ass.*, **147**, 33.

LESCURE, F. (1967) Perspectives nouvelles en ophtalmologie canine. *Proc. XVIIIth World Vet. Congr., Paris.* p. 471.

—— & AMALRIC, P. (1961) L'angle camérulaire du chien. Étude préliminaire. Goniophotographie. (The chamber angle of the dog. Preliminary report. Goniophotography.) *Bull. Soc. Ophtal. Fr.*, **11**, 927.

LEVY, M. C. et al. (1965) Technique for preparing histological sections of dogs' and rabbits' eyes in paraffin. *Arch. Ophthal.*, **73**, 122.

MAGRANE, W. G. (1951) Tonometry in ophthalmology. *N. Amer. Vet.*, **32**, 413.

McGRATH, J. T. (1960) *Neurological Examination of the Dog*. London: Kimpton.

MICHEL, W. E. (1963) Use of the ophthalmoscope. *Missouri Vet.*, **12**, (2), 6.

PALMER, A. C. (1959) The clinical examination of the nervous system of the dog. *Brit. Small Anim. Vet. Ass. Congr. Proc.* p. 61.

ROBERTS, S. R. (1956) A system of testing vision in animals. *J. Amer. vet. med. Ass.*, **128**, 544.

RUBIN, L. F. (1960) Indirect ophthalmoscopy. *J. Amer. vet. med. Ass.*, **137**, 648.

SAUNDERS, L. Z. & JUBB, K. V. (1961) Notes on technique for post-mortem examination of the eye. *Canad. vet. J.*, **2**, 123.

SCHLOTTHAUER, C. F. (1939) Some diseases of the eyes of lower animals; methods of examination, diagnosis and treatment. *J. Amer. vet. med. Ass.*, **94**, 404.

STARTUP, F. G. (1961) The use of the ophthalmoscope. *Advances in Small Animal Practice*. Vol. 3, Oxford: Pergamon. p. 108.

SZUTTER, L. (1961) Ophthalmoskopische und Lupenspiegeluntersuchungen an Neugeborenen Haustieren. (Ophthalmoscopic and biomicroscopic examination in newborn animals.) *Acta vet. Acad. Sci. hung.*, **11**, 183.

THÉRET, M. (1961) Aspect génétique de quelques anomalies oculaires chez les animaux domestiques. (Genetic aspects of some ocular anomalies in domestic animals). *Bull. Soc. franç. Ophtal.*, **74**, 505.

TUSAK, E. A. (1935) Diagnosis and therapy in veterinary ophthalmology. *N. Amer. Vet.*, **16** (10), 20.

ÜBERREITER, O. (1954) Augenuntersuchungsmethoden. (Examination of the eye). *Wien. tierärztl. Mschr.*, **41**, 767.

—— (1956) Augenuntersuchungsmethoden mit besonderer Berücksichtigung der Mikroskopie am lebenden Tierauge. (Examination of the eye in animals, with special reference to biomicroscopy.) *Ibid.*, **43**, 1.

—— (1956) Die Mikroskopie am lebenden Tierauge. (Biomicroscopy in animals). *Ibid.*, **43**, 77.

—— (1959) Der derzeitige Stand der Augenuntersuchung und der Augenoperationen bei Tieren. (The present state of eye examination and eye surgery in animals.) *Ibid.*, **46**, 855.

—— (1959) Examination of the Eye and Eye Operations in Animals. *Advances in Veterinary Science*, Vol. 5. New York: Academic Press.

—— (1961) Tier-Augenheilkunde. (Veterinary ophthalmology.) *Wien. klin. Wschr.*, **73**, 889.

VAINISI, S. J. (1966) Ophthalmoscopy. *Proc. Amer. anim. Hosp. Ass.*, 33rd Ann. Meeting. 231.

VIERHELLER, R. C. (1966) Clinical experience with indirect ophthalmoscopy. *Mod. vet. Pract.*, **47**, (4), 41.

WHITEFORD, R. D. (1959) So you think your dog has 20-20 vision? *Auburn vet.*, **16**, 38.

WINTER, F. C. (1966) Correlation of clinical ophthalmology and ophthalmological pathology. *Proc. Amer. anim. Hosp. Ass.*, 33rd Ann. Meeting. 64.

Medical Treatment

ABBOTT, G. W. & ABBOTT, R. J. (1964) Clinical experience with a topical ophthalmic solution. *Vet. Med.*, **59**, 1024.

BLEEKER, G. M. & MAAS, E. R. (1955) The penetration of Aureomycin, Terramycin and Chloranphemicol in the ocular tissues. *Ophthalmologica (Basle)*, **130**, 1.

BREHM, –. (1951) Behandlung von Augenleiden mit Yatren-Penicillin-Puder insbesondere bei Hunden. (The use of Yatren-penicillin powder in ophthalmology, especially in the dog.) *Berl. Münch. tierärztl. Wschr.*, **64**, 41.

BUNCE, D. F. M. (1954) Use of trypsin in veterinary practice. *N. Amer. Vet.*, **35**, 526.

CARLIN, J. R. et al. (1955) Beta ray and X-ray therapy in diseases of the eye. *N. Amer. Vet.*, **36**, 295.

CATCOTT, E. J. et al. (1953) Beta ray therapy in ocular diseases of animals. *J. Amer. vet. med. Ass.*, **122**, 172.

DALTON, P. J. (1959) Radiotherapy in small animal practice. *Brit. Small Anim. Vet. Ass. Congr. Proc.* p. 12.

DAVIDSON, J. L. (1952) Neomycin sulfate in veterinary dermatology and ophthalmology. *Vet. Med.*, **47**, 239.

EASTMAN, D. A. (1932) Treatment of the diseases of the eye and accessory organs. *Vet. Med.*, **27**, 56.

—— (1932) Treatment of the diseases of the eye and accessory organs. *J. Amer. vet. med. Ass.*, **80**, 751.

EIKMEIER, H. (1955) Das Cortison in der Augenheilkunde. *Berl. Münch. tierärztl. Wschr.*, **68**, 83.

ELLIS, P. P. (1965) Ocular pharmacology and toxicology. *Arch. Ophthal.*, **74**, 96.

ESPOSITO, A. C. (1952) Therapeutics of common eye diseases of animals. *J. Amer. vet. med. Ass.*, **121**, 297.

GELATT, K. N. (1967) Postoperative subpalpebral medications in horses and dogs. *Vet. Med.*, **62**, 1165.

GLIGORIJEVIĆ, J. et al. (1954) Eksperimentalna ispitivanja delovanja na penetraciju oenicilina u oko pas. (Experiments on the influence of ultrasound on the penetration of penicillin into the dog's eye.) *Acta vet. Acad. Sci. hung.*, **4**, (3), 3.

—— (1955) Our first results in the ultrasonic treatment of eye disease in domestic animals. (In Serbo-Croat.) *Ibid.*, **5**, 3.

GRIFFITH, C. R. (1963) Basic treatment and surgical procedures for ocular disease. *Mod. vet. Pract.*, **44**, (8), 49.

HARMS, H. P. et al. (1950) Aureomycin ointment used in infections of the eye, ear and skin in dogs and cats. *J. Amer. vet. med. Ass.*, 117, 462.

HSUING, G-D. et al. (1950) Penicillin ointment in the treatment of conjunctivitis in dogs. *Cornell Vet.*, 40, 4.

JACKSON, B. (1965) Use of Penotrane in ophthalmology. *Brit. J. Ophthal.*, 49, 307.

KNOWLES, R. P. (1961) Canine ophthalmology: Useful practice facts. *Vet. Med.*, 56, 163.

LANGHAM, M. (1951) Factors affecting the penetration of antibiotics into the aqueous humour. *Brit. J. Ophthal.*, 35, 614.

LARSEN, L. H. (1958) The use of newer drugs in the treatment of eye disease in animals. *Aust. vet. J.*, 34, 238.

LYNCH, R. & RUBIN, L. F. (1965) Salivation induced in dogs by conjunctival installation of atropine. *J. Amer. vet. med. Ass.*, 147, 511.

MAGRANE, H. J. (1955) Basic treatments for common ophthalmic lesions. *Vet. Med.*, 50, 267.

MAGRANE, W. G. (1951) An evaluation of the use of antibiotics in canine ophthalmology. *N. Amer. Vet.*, 32. 169.

—— (1951) Cortisone in ophthalmology. *Ibid.*, 32, 763.

—— et al. (1953) The clinical use of Chloromycetin in canine ocular infections. *Ibid.*, 34, 39.

MANN, P. G. H. & STOCK, J. E. (1965) Sub-conjunctival antibiosis. *Vet. Rec.*, 77, 405.

MICHAELSON, S. (1954) The use of beta irradiation in veterinary ophthalmology. *Vet. Med.*, 49, 475.

MOSS, L. C. (1952) Terramycin ophthalmic preparation in small animal practice. *J. Amer. vet. med. Ass.*, 121, 89.

POLTE, K. (1951) Prontosil solubile bei äusseren Augenerkrankungen in der Hundepraxis. (Prontosil in eye diseases of dogs.) *Mh. Vet.-Med.*, 6, 191.

RECORDS, R. E. & ELLIS, P. P. (1967) The intra-ocular penetration of Amplicillin, Methacillin and Oxacillin. *Amer. J. Ophthal.*, 64, 135.

RIPPS, J. H. (1951) Cortisone for canine eye infections. *J. Amer. vet. med. Ass.*, 118, 304.

ROBERTS, S. R. (1957) Simple procedures in ophthalmology. *Proc. Amer. Anim. Hosp. Ass.*, p. 226.

——(1964) Salivation after installation of atropine into the eye. *Mod. vet. Pract.*, 45, (3),70.

RODGER, F. C. (1965) Repository corticotherapy in ophthalmic theory and practice. *Brit. J. Ophthal.*, 49, 298.

RUBIN, L. F. (1964) Review of intraocular penetration of corticosteroids. *M.S.U. Vet.*, 24, 54.

—— & GELATT, K. N. (1967) Corneal epithelial sloughing in dogs with glaucoma. *J. Amer. vet. med. Ass.*, 151, 1449.

—— & WOLFES, R. L. (1962) Mydriatics for canine ophthalmoscopy. *J. Amer. vet. med. Ass.*, 140, 137.

RYCROFT, P. V. (1966) Recent advances in drug therapy of the human eye. *Aspects of Comparative Ophthalmology*. Oxford: Pergamon. p. 243.

SCHLEITER, H. & DIETZ, O. (1957) Antibiose am und im Bulbus unter besonderer Berücksichtigung der Blut-Kammerwasser-schranke. (Antibiosis on and in the eyeball with particular consideration of the blood-aqueous barrier.) *Wien. teirärztl. Mschr.*, 44, 641.

SORSBY, A. & UNGAR, J. (1960) *Antibiotics and Sulphonamides in Ophthalmology*. London: Oxford University Press.

STARTUP, F. G. (1965) Subconjunctival injections. *J. small Anim. Pract.*, 6, 363.

STEPHENSON, H. (1930) A discussion of some diseases of the eye of the dog. *Cornell Vet.*, 20, 385.

STONE, R. M. (1956) Treatment of certain eye and ear diseases of the dog. A clinical report. *Vet. Med.*, 51, 531.

TUSAK, E. A. (1934) Surgical and medical procedure in the treatment of external diseases of the eye in veterinary practice. *J. Amer. vet. med. Ass.*, 85, 379.

UVAROV, O. (1958) Veterinary uses of cortisone and related drugs for small animals. *Brit. Small Anim. Vet. Ass. Congr. Proc.* p. 91.

—— (1959) Corticosteroids in veterinary medicine. *Vet. Rec.*, 71, 335.

VEENENDAAL, H. (1924) De locale werking van epioculaire applicaties de solutio peroxydi hydrogenii (3%) bij hond, kat en konijn. *T. Diergeneesk.*, 51, 177.

—— (1924) De locale werking van epioculaire applicaties de solutio peroxydi hydrogenii (3%) bij hond, kat en konijn. *Ibid.*, 51, 216.

Ophthalmic Surgery

BERENS, C. & KING, J. H. (1961) *An Atlas of Ophthalmic Surgery.* Philadelphia: Lippincott.

BORDET, R. (1961) Quelques particularitiés de la chirurgie oculaire vétérinaire. (Some points relevant to veterinary ocular surgery.) *Bull. Soc. franç. Ophtal.*, **74**, 460.

GRAHAM, P. A. & STANWORTH, A. (1961) Miniature ophthalmic diathermy machine. *Brit. J. Ophthal.*, **45**, 75.

KRAWITZ, L. (1959) Preparation for surgical procedures of the eye. *Proc. Amer. Soc. Vet. Ophthal.*

ORMROD, A. N. (1962) Notes on canine intra-ocular surgery. *Vet. Rec.*, **74**, 828.

PHILPS, S. & FOSTER, J. (1961) *Ophthalmic Operations.* London: Baillière.

SIBAY, T. M. et al. (1964) An operating platform for animal eye surgery. *Amer. J. Ophthal.*, **57**, 482.

SMYTHE, R. H. (1957) Some observations on the surgery of the eye in animals. *Vet. Rec.*, **69**, 322.

STALLARD, H. B. (1958) *Eye Surgery.* Bristol: Wright.

THOMAS, R. P. & TERRY, W. (1960) An eye speculum for animal surgery. *Amer. J. Ophthal.*, **50**, 660.

ÜBERREITER, O. (1939) Zur technik der Augenoperationen beim Hunde. (The technique of eye surgery in the dog.) *Arch. wiss. prakt. Tierheilk.*, **72**, 235.

Anaesthesia

DIETZ, O. (1954) Eine retrobulbäre Anästhesie beim Hund zur Erzeugung einer Mydriasis. (Retrobulbar anaesthesia in the dog to produce mydriasis.) *Berl., Münch. teirärztl. Wschr.*, **67**, 325.

FORMSTON, C. (1964) Ophthaine (Proparacaine hydrochloride): a local anaesthetic for ophthalmic surgery. *Vet. Rec.*, **76**, 385.

HALL, L. W. (1957) Bromochlorotrifluoroethane ('Fluothane') a new volatile anaesthetic agent. *Vet. Rec.*, **69**, 615.

—— (1960) The use of tranquillisers in canine practice. *Advances in Small Animal Practice.* Vol. 2. Oxford: Pergamon. p. 94.

—— (1966) Anaesthesia for surgery of the eye in animals. *Aspects of Comparative Ophthalmology.* Oxford: Pergamon. p. 259.

—— (1966) *Wright's Veterinary Anaesthesia and Analgesia.* London: Baillière.

MAGRANE, W. G. (1953) Investigational use of Ophthaine as a local anaesthetic in ophthalmology. *N. Amer. Vet.*, **34**, 568.

—— (1967) Methoxyflurane anesthesia in intraocular surgery. *Pract. Vet.*, **3**, 75.

MAKSIMOVIĆ, B. M. (1953) Akinesia of the orbicularis muscle in cattle, horses and dogs. (In Serbo-Croat.) *Vet. Fac. Belgrade Univ.*

ORMROD, A. N. (1960) An assessment of the value of Fluothane as an anaesthetic in canine surgery. *Vet. Rec.*, **72**, 96.

SIMS, F. W. (1960) Halothane anaesthesia in small-animal practice. *Vet. Rec.*, **72**, 617.

SINGLETON, W. B. (1960) The use of Fluothane in canine surgery. *J. small Anim. Pract.*, **1**, 2.

The Eyelids

ABE, K. et al. (1963) A case report on melanoma of the eyelid of a dog. *J. Japan vet. med. Ass.*, **16**, 417.

BARRON, C. M. (1962) The comparative pathology of neoplasms of the eyelids and conjunctiva with special reference to those of epithelial origin. *Acta derm.-venercol. (Stockh.)*, **42**, Supp. 51, 1.

BERNOULLI, R. (1948) Lidkrebs bei einem Hund, ausgehend von der Tarsaldrüse und einem Papillom. (Malignant tumour of the eyelid of a dog, arising from the tarsal glands and a papilloma.) *Ophthalmologica (Basle)*, **116**, 101.

BLACK, L. & FRITH, H. (1961) The correction of simultaneous entropion and ectropion by pedicle graft technique. *Vet. Rec.*, **73**, 884.

CHRISTOPH, H. J. (1957) Anwendung von Dondren beim Hund nach Anlegen eines künstlichen Ankyloblepharons und Versuche mit Dondren beim Entropium. (The application of 'Dondren' following the formation of artificial ankyloblepharon in the dog, and its use in entropion.) *Kleintier-Prax.*, **2**, 67.

DARRASPEN, E. & LESCURE, F. (1961) Le syndrome de Claude Bernard-Horner, chez les carnivores domestiques. (The Claude Bernard-Horner syndrome in domestic animals.) *Rev. Méd. Vét.*, **112**, 493.
—— et al., (1961) Le syndrome de Claude Bernard-Horner chez les carnivores domestiques. *Bull. Soc. franç. Ophtal.*, **74**, 465.
DEITRICK, L. E. (1928) Some diseases of the eye. *N. Amer. Vet.*, **10**, 54.
DIXON, A. C. (1948) Advancement flaps in entropion. *Vet. Rec.*, **60**, 665.
DOBIASZ, L. (1931) Die Wirkung der operativen Eingriffe beim Entropium. (The effect of operative interference on entropion.) *Przegl. wet.*, **44**, 88.
DREYFUS, M. (1953) A note on ectropion and entropion in dogs. (In Czech). *Čs. Oftal.*, **9**, 57.
FORMSTON, C. (1952) Observations on diseases of the eye in animals, with particular reference to the dog. *Vet. Rec.*, **64**, 47.
—— & OTTOWAY, C. W. (1937) The correction of entropion by the intrapalpebral injection of sterile liquid paraffin. *Vet. Rec.*, **49**, 1056.
FRICK, E. J. (1936) A method of treating entropion. *J. Amer. vet. med. Ass.*, **89**, 212.
HALLIWELL, W. H. (1965) Undermined skin flaps as a method of entropion correction. *Vet. Med.*, **60**, 915.
—— (1967) Surgical management of canine distichia. *J. Amer. vet. med. Ass.*, **150**, 874.
HODGMAN, S. F. J. (1964) Abnormalities and defects in pedigree dogs—I. An investigation into the existence of abnormalities in pedigree dogs in the British Isles. *Advances in Small Animal Practice*. Vol. 5. Oxford: Pergamon. p. 35.
KHUEN, E. C. (1948) Traumatic injuries of the eyelids and eye. *N. Amer. Vet.*, **29**, 715.
LENNOX, W. J. (1966) Thallium poisoning. *Canad. vet. J.*, **7**, 113.
LOVE, W. G. (1940) Some diseases of the eye of animals. *J. Amer. vet. med. Ass.*, **97**, 254.
McCUISTION, W. R. (1965) Pulmonary edema and persistent ankyloblepharon in puppies. *Vet. Med.*, **60**, 1206.
MENGES, R. W. (1946) An operation for entropion in the dog. *J. Amer. vet. med. Ass.*, **109**, 464.
MITCHELL, W. M. (1931) Entropion in the dog and its treatment by external canthotomy. *Vet. Rec.*, **11**, 410.
PULLAR, E. M. (1938) The correction of entropion by the intra-palpebral injection of sterile liquid paraffin. *Aust. vet. J.*, **14**, 121.
ROBERTS, S. R. (1964) External eye diseases. *Mod. vet. Pract.*, **45**, (6), 38.
SERGEJEV, A. (1927) Eine Vereinfachung der Operation des Ectropiums bei Hunden. (A simplified ectropion operation in dogs.) *Prakt. vet. konev.*, **10**, 57.
STARTUP, F. G. (1960) Diseases of the canine eye. Part I. *Vet. Rec.*, **72**, 653.
STEPHENSON, H. (1930) A discussion of some diseases of the eye of the dog. *Cornell Vet.*, **20**, 385.
VAINISI, S. J. (1966) Diseases and surgery of the lid. *Proc. Amer. anim. Hosp. Ass.*, 33rd Ann. Meeting. 66.
VEENENDAAL, H. (1936) Een iets gewijzigde entropium-operatie bij de hond. (Modified entropion operation in the dog.) *T. Diergeneesk.*, **63**, 299.
VERWER, M. A. J. (1961) Grepen uit de Praktijk der Oogheelkunde het Kleine Huisdier. (Facts from small-animal ophthalmology practice.) *T. Diergeneesk.*, **86**, 1612.
—— (1964) Grepen uit de Praktijk der Ooheelkunde het Kleine Huisdier. *Ibid.*, **89**, 1364.
WAARDENBURG, P. J. (1957) Hyperplasia interocularis cum Dystopia lateroversa canthi medialis, blepharophimosis, Dyschromia iridocutanea et Dysplasia auditiva. *Acta ophthal. (Kbh).*, **35**, 311.
WRIGHT, J. G. (1934) Injuries to the dog's eye. *Vet. Rec.*, **14**, 1435.
ZIETZSCHMANN, O. (1904) Vergleichend histologische Untersuchungen über den Bau der Augenlider der Haussäugetiere. (Comparative histology of the eyelids in domestic animals.) *Albrecht v. Graefes Arch. Ophthal.*, **58**, 61.
—— (1904) Zur Frage des Vorkommens eines Tarsus im Lide der Haussäugetiere. (Questions concerning the tarsal plate in the eyelid of domestic animals.) *Ibid.*, **59**, 166.

The Nictitating Membrane

AITKEN, J. (1949) Congenital protrusions of the membrana nictitans with adhesions. *Vet. Med.*, **44**, 359.

BRENNING, I. F. (1931) Surgery of the eye (canine). *J. Amer. vet. med. Ass.*, **78**, 242.

HODGMAN, S. F. J. (1957) Cauterisation of the membrana nictitans. *Vet. Rec.*, **69**, 658.

—— (1960) Cauterisation of the membrana nictitans. *Advances in Small Animal Practice.* Vol. 2. Oxford: Pergamon. p. 115.

KERPSACK, R. W. & KERPSACK, W. R. (1966) The orbital gland and tear staining in the dog. *Vet. Med.*, **61**, 121.

MAYER, K. (1952) Ablation of the third eyelid. *N. Amer. Vet.*, **33**, 697.

MILLER, M. E. & HABEL, R. E. (1951) Harder's gland in the dog. *J. Amer. vet. med. Ass.*, **118**, 155.

OJAY, E. & MILINSKY, H. C. (1964) Surgical correction of unpigmented membrana nictitans. *J. Amer. vet. med. Ass.*, **144**, 857.

TEICHERT, G. (1966) Plazmazelluläre Infiltration des dritten Augenlides beim Hund. (Plasma cell infiltration of the third eyelid in dogs.) *Berl. Münch. tierärztl. Wschr.* **79**, 449.

WERNER, H. J. & ROBERTS, J. H. (1951) The Harderian gland of the dog in chronic ectopia. *J. Amer. vet. med. Ass.*, **118**, 16.

The Orbit

BARNETT, K. C. et al. (1967) Retrobulbar and chiasmal meningioma in a dog. *J. small Anim. Pract.*, **8**, 391.

GEIB, L. W. (1966) Ossifying meningioma with extracranial metastasis in a dog. *Path. Vet.*, **3**, 247.

HARDING, H. P. & OWEN, L. N. (1956) Eosinophilic myositis in the dog. *J. comp. Path.*, **66**, 109.

MAGRANE, W. G. (1957) Diseases of the orbit. *Vet. Med.*, **52**, 449.

RUBIN, L. F. & JORTNER, B. (1965) Clinico-pathologic conference. *J. Amer. vet. med. Ass.*, **146**, 148.

WINTER, H. & STEPHENSON, E. C. (1952) A case of eosinophilic myositis in the dog. *Cornell Vet.*, **42**, 531.

The Conjunctiva

—— (1965) Ocular parasites. *Mod. vet. Pract.*, **46**, (5), 10.

ALLERTON, F. R. (1929) Worm parasites on conjunctiva in dog. *N. Amer. Vet.*, **10**, (7), 56.

CELLO, R. M. (1956) The use of conjunctival scrapings in the diagnosis and treatment of external diseases of the eye. *Gaines Vet. Symp.*

CORREA, W. M. et al. (1961) Neisseria flava II: Etiologic agent in canine conjunctivitis. *J. Amer. vet. med. Ass.*, **138**, 503.

COTCHIN, E. (1954) Further observations on neoplasms in dogs, with particular reference to site of origin and malignancy. Part II. Male genitalia, skeletal, lymphatic and other systems. *Vet. J.*, **110**, 274.

DOUGLAS, J. R. (1938) A survey of canine Thelaziasis in California. *J. Amer. vet. med. Ass.*, **93**, 382.

FAUST, E. C. (1928) Studies on Thelazia callipaeda. *J. Parasit.*, **15**, 76.

GRIFFITH, C. R. (1967) Differential diagnosis of common causes of inflamed eye. *Proc. Amer. anim. Hosp. Ass.*, 34th Ann. Meeting. p. 196.

GRUENBERG, K. (1959) Kleine Chirurgie am Auge des Hundes. (Minor surgery of the canine eye.) *Berl. Münch. tierärztl. Wschr.*, **72**, 245.

HOFMEYR, C. F. B. (1957) Operation for corneal dermoid in the dog. *Vet. Rec.*, **69**, 455.

JONES, V. G. (1955) A preliminary report of the flora in health and disease of the external ear and conjunctival sac of the dog. *J. Amer. vet. med. Ass.*, **127**, 442.

JOSHUA, J. O. (1956) Some allergic conditions in the dog and cat. *Vet. Rec.*, **68**, 682.

KNAPP, S. E. et al. (1961) Thelaziasis in cats and dogs—a case report. *J. Amer. vet. med. Ass.*, **138**, 537.

KNOWLES, R. P. (1960) The eye and its problems. *Fla. vet. Bull.*, **10**, 14.

KOIFOID, C. A. et al. (1937) Thelazia californiensis, a nematode eyeworm of dog and man, with a review of Thelazias of domestic animals. *Univ. Calif. Publ. Zoo.*, **41**, 225.

PARMALOE, W. E. et al. (1956) A survey of Thelazia californiensis, a mammalian eye worm, with new locality records. *J. Amer. vet. med. Ass.*, **129**, 325.

PERRY C. S. (1941) Dermoids of the eye in dogs. *Vet. Rec.*, **99**, 56.

PRICE, E. W. (1930) A new nematode parasite in the eyes of dogs in the United States. *J. Parasit.*, **17**, 112.

—— (1931) A note on the occurrence of eye-worms in the United States. *N. Amer. Vet.*, **12** (11), 49.

RAILLIET, A. & HENRY, A. (1910) Nouvelles observations sur les Thelazies, nematodes parasites de l'oeil. (New observations on Thelazia, nematode parasites of the eye.) *C. R. Soc. Biol. (Paris)*, **68**, 783.

SCHAUFFLER, A. C. (1966) Canine Thelaziasis in Arizona. *J. Amer. vet. med. Ass.*, **149**, 521.

VERWER, M. A. J. (1967) On the bacterial flora appearing in chronic purulent eye inflammations in dogs. *Proc. XVIIIth World Vet. Congr., Paris.* p. 483.

—— & GUNNINK, J. W. (1968) The occurrence of bacteria in chronic purulent eye discharge. *J. small Anim. Pract.*, **9**, 33.

The Eyeball

BACKGREN, A. W. (1965) Lymphatic leukosis in dogs. *Acta vet. Acad. Sci. hung.*, **6**, Supp. 1.

BARONE, R. & LESCURE, F. (1959) Heterochromie et microphtalmie chez le chien. (Heterochromia and microphthalmos in the dog.) *Rev. méd. vét.*, **110**, 769.

BEAMER, R. J. (1957) Subconjunctival ablation of the eyeball of pet animals. *J. Amer. vet. med. Ass.*, **131**, 84.

BERGE, E. (1927) Indikation und Technik des künstlichen Ankyloblepharons unter Berücksichtigung der Operation am Bulbus. (Indications and technique for artificial ankyloblepharon following removal of the eye.) *Berl. Münch. tierärztl. Wschr.*, **43**, 509.

BÖHLER, H. (1929) Ein rechtsseitiger Mikro- und Kryptophthalmus congenitus vom Hunde. (Right-sided congenital micro- and cryptophthalmos in a dog.) *Albrecht v. Graefes Arch. Ophthal.*, **121**, 715.

CHILD, E. (1906). Excision of the eyeball and substitution of a glass eye in a dog. *Vet. J.*, **13**, 366.

DISTAVE, R. F. H. (1967). Deux nouvelles possibilités de traitment du prolapsus de l'oeil chez le chien et le chat. *Proc. XVIIIth World Vet. Congr., Paris.* p. 487.

ELLINGER, F. (1935) Kunstaugen als Augenprotheses—insbesondere in der tierärztlichen Praxis. (Eye prostheses in veterinary practice). *Berl. Münch. tierärztl. Wschr.*, **51**, 273.

FOX, M. W. (1966) Canine diseases of possible hereditary origin. *Mod. vet. Pract.*, **47** (6), 51.

GREEN, R. L. (1905) Excision of the eye and insertion of a glass one in a dog. *Vet. J.*, **12** 330.

HUANG, T. C. et al. (1954) Nitrophenide and other anticoccidial studies with dogs. *J. Amer. vet. med. Ass.*, **124**, 212.

KEIL, J. H. (1960) Use of KB ocular prosthesis instead of enucleation. *Maryland Vet.*, Feb., p. 22.

—— (1960) Canine ocular prosthesis. *Mod. vet. Pract.*, **41**, (13), 27.

KILLIAN, B. S. (1940) Enucleation of the eyeball. *J. Amer. vet. med. Ass.*, **97**, 268.

KIRK, H. (1947) A lost eye. *Vet. Rec.*, **59**, 563.

KÓMÁR, G. & SCHUSTER, A. (1967) Ein seltenes ophthalmologisches Krankheitsbild (Exophthalmus pulsans) bei einem Hunde. (A rare ophthalmological disease (Exophthalmos pulsans) in a dog.) *Berl. Münch. tierärztl. Wschr.*, **80**, 359.

LANTOINE, R. (1930) De la luxation du globe oculaire chez le chien. *Dissertation, École Natl. Vét. Alfort, Paris.*

LONG, E. I. (1934) Surgical excision of the eye. *Vet. Med.*, **29**, 289.

MILKS, H. J. et al. (1929) Enucleation of eyeball. *Vet. Med.*, **24**, 168.

PALMER, A. C. (1960) Clinical and pathologic features of some tumours of the central nervous system in dogs. *Res. Vet. Sci.*, **1**, 36.

—— (1961) Clinical signs associated with intracranial tumours in dogs. *Ibid.*, **2**, 326.

PREU, E. (1936) Prolapsus bulbi beim Hund. *Dissertation, Vienna.*

RIPPETOE, C. W. (1934) Strabismus in the canine. *Vet. Med.*, **29**, 320.

ROBERTS, S. R. (1965) Surgical conditions of the canine eyeball. *Mod. vet. Pract.*, **46** (11), 59.

—— & Vainisi, S. J. (1967) Hemifacial spasm in dogs. *J. Amer. vet. med. Ass.*, **150**, 381.

Rogers, R. J. & Elder, J. K. (1967) Purulent leptomeningitis in a dog associated with an aerogenic Pasteurella multocida. *Aust. vet. J.*, **43**, 81.

Rubin, L. F. & Patterson, D. F. (1965) Arteriovenous fistula of the orbit in a dog. *Cornell Vet.*, **55**, 471.

Sigling, T. (1924) Luxatio bulbi oculi bij den hond. (Prolapse of the eyeball in the dog.) *T. Diergeneesk.*, **51**, 36.

Simpson, H. D. (1956) Reconstructive surgery of the canine eye. I. Plastic eye prostheses. *N. Amer. Vet.*, **37**, 770.

—— (1956) Reconstructive surgery of the canine eye. II. Intrascleral prostheses. *Ibid.*, **37**, 1060.

Startup, F. G. (1960) Diseases of the canine eye. Part II. *Vet. Rec.*, **72**, 675.

Sundaram, —— (1927) Few interesting clinical notes. IV. Excision of eyeball in the dog. *Indian vet. J.*, **3**, 212.

Veenendaal, H. (1936) Iets over exstirpatio bulbi de hond en het bewerkstelligen daarbij van een kunstmatig ankyloblepharon. (Extirpation of the dog's eye with the formation of an artificial ankyloblepharon.) *T. Diergeneesk*, **63**, 481.

—— (1936) Orbitaalcyste en Microphthalmus van het rechteroog, chorioideaal coloboom en cataracta zonularis van het linkeroog, bij een jonge Herdershond. (Orbital cyst and microphthalmos of the right eye, choroidal coloboma and zonular cataract of the left eye, in a young Alsation.) *Ibid.*, **63**, 557.

Wilkinson, D. E. (1935) Ablation of the eyeball and closure of the palpebral fissure; an improved technique. *Vet. J.*, **91**, 139.

The Lacrimal Apparatus

Baxter, H. (1933) Variations in the inorganic constituents of mixed and parotid gland saliva activated by reflex stimulation in the dog. *J. biol. Chem.*, **102**, 203.

Dayal, Y. (1962) Corticosteroids and Fibrolysin in the prevention of lacrimal duct obstruction. *Brit. J. Ophthal.*, **46**, 27.

Kast, A. (1957) Mikuliczscher Symptomenkomplex beim Hund. (The Mikulicz syndrome in a dog.) *Berl. Münch. tierärztl. Wschr.*, **70**, 510.

Michel, G. (1955) Beitrag zur Anatomie der Tränenorgane von Hund und Katze. (Anatomy of the lacrimal system of the dog and cat.) *Dtsch. tierärztl. Wschr.*, **62**, 347.

Milosevic, Z. (1961) Rendgensko prikazivanje suzovoda u domacih zivotinja. (Radiographic demonstration of the naso-lacrimal canal in domestic animals). *Vet. Arh. (Zagreb).*, **31**, 246.

Roberts, S. R. (1962) Abnormal tear secretion in the dog. *Mod. vet. Pract.*, **43** (6), 37.

—— & Erickson, O. F. (1962) Dog tear secretion and tear proteins. *J. small Anim. Pract.*, **3**, 1.

Rubin, L. F. et al. (1965) Clinical estimation of lacrimal function in dogs. *J. Amer. vet. med. Ass.*, **147**, 946.

Weis, J. (1956) Bösartige Geschwulst des Tränensackes beim Hund. (Malignant neoplasia of the lacrimal sac in a dog.) *Mh. Vet.-Med.*, **11**, 302.

The Cornea and Sclera

Ammann, K. (1966) Hornhauterkrankungen beim Hund. Vergleichendklinische Untersuchungen. (Keratitis in the dog. Comparative clinical investigations.) *Kleintier-Prax.*, **11**, 1.

Barnett, K. C. (1966) The corneal ulcer. VI. Surgical Treatment. *J. small Anim. Pract.*, **7**, 275.

Beamer, R. J. (1960) Keratitis pigmentosa. *Mod. vet. Pract.*, **41** (3), 34.

Bellhorn, R. W. & Henkind, P. (1966) Superficial pigmentary keratitis in the dog. *J. Amer. vet. med. Ass.*, **149**, 173.

—— —— (1967) Ocular nodular fasciitis in a dog. *Ibid.*, **150**, 213.

Belot, P. & de Ratuld, Y. (1960) Les ulcères de la cornée du chien; leur traitement par recouvrement conjonctival. (Corneal ulcers in the dog: treatment by conjunctival flaps.) *Écon. Méd. anim.*, **2**, 109.

Bernis, W. O. (1961) Partial penetrating keratoplasty in dogs. *Southwestern Vet.*, **15**, 30

Bhardwaj, K. R. et al. (1962) Trypanosomiasis in dogs. *Indian vet. J.*, **39**, 396.

Bone, J. F. (1961) New treatments of ocular lesions. *Mod. vet. Pract.*, **42** (1), 34.

Candlin, F. T. (1953) Treatment of chronic corneal lesions with beta radiation. *Proc. Amer. vet. med. Ass.*, p. 221.

—— & Levine, M. H. (1952) The use of beta radiation on corneal lesions in the dog. *N. Amer. Vet.*, **33**, 632.

Carlson, W. D. & Severin, G. J. (1960) Radiation therapy in eye diseases. *Proc. Amer. Soc. Vet. Ophthal.*

Catcott, E. J. & Griesemer, R. A. (1954) A study of corneal healing in the dog. *Amer. J. vet Res.*, **15**, 265.

Cella, F. (1961) Corneal graft in the dog. *Advances in Small Animal Practice.* Vol. 3. Oxford: Pergamon. p. 101.

—— & Dozza, G. (1957) Sull' Innèsto della cornea nel cane. (Corneal graft in the dog.) *Atti Soc. ital. Sci. vet.*, **11**, 411.

Cello, R. M. (1959) Ocular changes of leukaemia in dogs. *Proc. Amer. Soc. Vet. Ophthal.*

—— & Hutcherson, B. (1962) Ocular changes in malignant lymphoma of dogs. *Cornell Vet.*, **52**, 492.

—— & Lasmanis, J. (1958) Pseudomonas infection of the eye of the dog resulting from the use of contaminated fluorescein solution. *J. Amer. vet. med. Ass.*, **132**, 297.

Claus, C. E. (1961) A case of long standing panophthalmitis. *The Pennant.*, **32**, 6.

Dalton, P. J. (1958) Beta-ray therapy in veterinary practice. *Vet. Rec.*, **70**, 233.

Darraspen, E. et al. (1964) Esthésiometrie de la cornée du chien. (Aesthesiometry of the cornea of the dog.) *Bull. Soc. Ophtal. Fr.*, **64**, 597.

Dempster, W. J. (1959) Biological spare parts. *Vet. Rec.*, **71**, 319.

Dimic, J. M. (1957) Zur Behandlung der Korneaerkrankungen bei Haustieren. (The treatment of corneal wounds in domestic animals.) *Dtsch. tierärztl. Wschr.*, **64**, 501.

—— et al. (1961) Experimentelle Untersuchungen über die Wirkung einiger Medikamente auf Hornhauterunden. (Experimental investigations on the influence of some medicaments in the treatment of wounds of the cornea.) *Berl. Münch. tierärztl. Wschr.*, **74**, 94.

Dreyfuss, M. (1930) Symmetrische zentrale Hornhautverfettung beim Hund. (Symmetrical fat infiltration of the cornea in a dog.) *Albrecht v. Graefes Arch. Ophthal.*, **125**, 67.

Dykes, G. (1934) Splenic extract in the treatment of nonulcerative parenchymatous (interstitial) keratitis. *Vet. J.*, **90**, 383.

Emerson, J. L. (1962) Beta radiation therapy of the cornea. *Speculum*, **15**, 34.

Formston, C. (1966) Keratitis in animals. *Aspects of Comparative Ophthalmology.* Oxford: Pergamon. p. 205.

Foulds, W. S. (1961) Intra-canalicular implants in the treatment of kerato-conjunctivitis sicca. *Brit. J. Ophthal.*, **45**, 625.

Goret, P. et al. (1961) Sur l'étiologie virale de la kératite 'bleue' du chien. (Viral aetiology of 'blue' keratitis in the dog.) *Bull. Soc. franç. Ophtal.*, **74**, 482.

Grover, A. D. & Agarwac, K. C. (1961) Mycotic keratitis. *Brit. J. Ophthal.*, **45**, 824.

Heeley, D. M. (1958) Diseases of the anterior segment of the eye. *Brit. small Anim. Vet. Ass. Congr. Proc.* p. 104.

—— (1966) The corneal ulcer. IV. Causes—miscellaneous. *J. small Anim. Pract.*, **7**, 267.

—— (1966) Corneal grafting in the dog. *Aspects of Comparative Ophthalmology.* Oxford: Pergamon. p. 177.

Henderson, W. (1951) The repair of corneal injuries in the dog by conjunctival keratoplasty. *Vet. Rec.*, **63**, 240.

Hime, J. M. (1966) The corneal ulcer. II. The diagnosis of corneal ulceration. *J. small Anim. Pract.*, **7**, 257.

Hogg, A. H. (1949) Treatment of a case of keratitis with pannus formation in a dog. *Vet. Rec.*, **61**, 441.

Holt, J. R. (1957) Corneal graft in a dog. *Vet. Rec.*, **69**, 454.

—— (1966) The corneal ulcer. III. Causes—micro-organisms. *J. small Anim. Pract.*, **7**, 261.

Hübner, L. (1966) Die Abheilung von operativ gesetzten Hornhauteinschnitten unter dem Einfluss von Corticosteroiden beim Hund. (The healing of surgical incisions of the cornea in the dog under the influence of corticosteroids.) *Wien. tierärztl. Mschr.*, **53**, 75.

Hurov, L. (1961) Surgical correction of a perforating ulcer of the cornea. *Small anim. Clin.*, **1**, 201.

Jensen, E. C. (1963) Experimental corneal transplantation in the dog. *J. Amer. vet. med. Ass.*, **142**, 11.

Jovanovic, V. (1951) Influence of dressings and suturing of the eyelids on the epithelialisation of corneal wounds in dogs. Dissertation, Belgrade.

KELLER, W. F. (1966) Experimental and clinical keratoprosthesis. *Proc. Amer. anim Hosp. Ass.*, 33rd Ann. Meeting. 72.

KRAWITZ, L. (1959) Canine keratitis. *N.Y.C. Vet.*, **2**. March.

LAVIGNETTE, A. M. (1962) Lamellar keratoplasty in the dog. *Small anim. Clin.*, **2**, 183.

—— (1966) Keratoconjunctivitis sicca in a dog treated by transposition of the parotid salivary duct. *J. Amer. vet. med. Ass.*, **148**, 778.

—— (1967) Surgical relief of keratoconjunctivitis sicca by transposition of the parotid salivary duct. *Proc. Amer. anim. Hosp. Ass.*, 34th Ann. Meeting. 194.

LETTOW, E. et al. (1964) Epitheliom der Cornea bei einem Hund. (Epithelioma of the cornea of a dog.) *Berl. Münch. tierärztl. Wschr.*, **77**, 248.

LEWIS, D. G. (1958). Thermo-cautery in the treatment of excessive granulation following corneal ulceration. *Vet. Rec.*, **70**, 424.

LIVINGSTON, A. A. (1950) Conjunctival flap operation for treatment of perforated corneal ulcer. *J. Amer. vet. med. Ass.*, **116**, 103.

MAGRANE, W. G. (1948) X-ray therapy in interstitial and pigmentary keratitis. *N. Amer. Vet.*, **29**, 582.

—— (1955) Vascularisation; its significance in diseases of the cornea. *J. Amer. vet. med. Ass.*, **126**, 392.

—— (1961) Surgical procedures of the cornea. *Advances in Small Animal Practice*. Vol. 3. Oxford: Pergamon. p. 172.

—— (1964) Surgical procedures of the cornea. *Vet. Med.*, **59**, 145.

—— (1965) Globe fixation and surgical procedures of the cornea. *Proc. Amer. anim. Hosp. Ass.*, 32nd Ann. Meeting. 145.

MICHAELSON, I. C. (1952) Proliferation of limbal melanoblasts into the cornea in response to a corneal lesion. *Brit. J. Ophthal.*, **36**, 657.

MILKS, H. J. (1931) Keratitis. *Vet. Med.*, **26**, 438.

NEAME, H. (1927) Parenchymatous keratitis in trypanosomiasis in cattle, and in dogs and in man. *Brit. J. Ophthal.*, **11**, 209.

ODA, Y. & FUKUDA, S. (1962) Electron microscopic studies on the animals' cornea. *J. Electronmicroscopy*, **11**, 179.

O'NEILL, P. et al. (1967) On the preservation of corneae at −196°C. for full-thickness homografts in man and dogs. *Brit. J. Ophthal.*, **51**, 13.

PAUFIQUE, L. et al. (1948) *Les Greffes de la Cornée*. Paris: Masson.

PECK, J. G. & WEBER, W. P. (1962) Antibody therapy in chronic dermatitis and ulcerative keratitis of dogs. *Small anim. Clin.*, **2**, 261.

REIHART, O. H. (1932) Conjunctival keratoplasty. *N. Amer. Vet.*, **13** (1), 57.

RICKARDS, D.A. (1966) A new treatment for canine melanosis. *Mod.vet.Pract.*, **47** (1), 38.

ROBERTS, S. R. (1953) The conjunctival flap operation in small animals. *J. Amer. vet. med. Ass.*, **122**, 86.

—— (1954) The nature of corneal pigmentation in the dog. *Ibid.*, **124**, 208.

—— (1960) Congenital posterior ectasia of the sclera in Collie dogs. *Amer. J. Ophthal.*, **50**, 451.

—— (1961) Congenital posterior ectasia of the sclera in Collie dogs. *Vet. Excerpts*, **21**, 63.

—— (1963) A feasible technique for corneal grafting. *Mod. vet. Pract.*, **44** (4), 40.

—— (1965) Superficial indolent ulcer of the cornea in Boxer dogs. *J. small Anim. Pract.*, **6**, 111.

—— & DELLAPORTA, A. (1965) Congenital posterior ectasia of the sclera in Collie dogs. Part I. Clinical features. *Amer. J. Ophthal.*, **59**, 180.

ROBIN, V. & CHARTON, A. (1939) La lipoidose cornéenne du chien. (Corneal lipidosis in the dog.) *Rec. Méd. vét.*, **115**, 321.

ROHEN, J. (1956) Arteriovenose Anastomosen im Limbusreich des Hundes. (Arteriovenous anastomoses in the limbus of the dog.) *Albrecht v. Graefes Arch. Ophthal.*, **157**, 361.

RUBIN, L. F. & AGUIRRE, G. (1967) Clinical use of pilocarpine for keratoconjunctivitis sicca in dogs and cats. *J. Amer. vet. med. Ass.*, **151**, 313.

RYCROFT, B. W. (1955) *Corneal Grafts*. London: Butterworth.

SAXENA, O. P. et al. (1967) Bilateral corneal opacity in a dog—successful treatment with vitamin A. *Indian vet. J.*, **44**, 434.

SCHLEICH, G. (1893) Beiderseitiges angeborenes hinteres Skleralstaphylom bei Hunden. (Bilateral congenital posterior scleral staphyloma in dogs.) *Z. vergl. Augenh.*, **7**, 171.

SCHMIDT, O. (1952) Neue Wege zur Behandlung von Hornhautgeschwüren. (New ways of treating corneal ulcers.) *Berl. Münch. tierärztl. Wschr.*, **65**, 32.

SCHOCK, K. (1910) Eine noch nicht beschriebene Harnhautaffektion beim Hund. (A previously undescribed corneal lesion in a dog.) *Arch. vergl. Ophthal.*, **1**, 313.

SCHRAMM, A. W. (1967) How scleral contact lenses aid in corneal lesion therapy. *Mod. vet. Pract.*, **48** (8), 46.

SHUTTLEWORTH, A. C. (1939) An interesting conjunctival graft. *Vet. J.*, **95**, 292.

SINGH, M. M. et al. (1965) Corneal opacity in a dog. *Indian vet. J.*, **42**, 879.

SPREULL, J. S. A. (1966) The corneal ulcer. I. Anatomy and physiology of the cornea of the dog. *J. small Anim. Pract.*, **7**, 253.

STARTUP, F. G. (1963) The treatment of corneal perforation in the dog. *The Veterinary Review*, **14**, 107.

—— (1966) The corneal ulcer. V. Medical treatment. *J small Anim. Pract.*, **7**, 271.

STERN, A. J. (1950) Conjunctival flap operation. *J. Amer. vet. med. Ass.*, **117**, 44.

ÜBERREITER, O. (1961) Eine besondere Keratitisform (Keratitis superficialis chronica) beim Hund. (A peculiar form of keratitis (Chronic superficial keratitis) in dogs.) *Wien. teirärztl. Mschr.*, **48**, 65.

VEENENDAAL, H. (1928) Twee nog weinig bekende hoornvliesaandoenigen bij den hond. (Two rare corneal affections in the dog.) *T. Diergeneesk.*, **55**, 853.

—— (1928) Keratitis superficialis (Keratitis pannosa et pigmentosa) bij den hond. *Ibid.*, **55**, 1175.

—— (1936) Door een doorntje veroorzaakte, perforeerende hoornvliesverwonding bij een hond. (Perforating corneal wound from a thorn in a dog.) *Ibid.*, **63**, 483.

—— (1937) Dystrophia corneae adiposa bij den hond. (Corneal lipidosis in the dog.) *Ibid.*, **64**, 913.

—— (1953) Mededelingen uit de oogheelkundige afdeling van de kliniek voor kleine huisdieren van de Rijksuniversiteit de Utrecht. (Notes from the Ophthal. Dep. of the Small Anim. Clinic of the Univ. Utrecht.) *Ibid.*, **78**, 662.

—— (1958) Meddlingen uit de veterinair oogheelkundige afdeling. (*Commun. of the Dep. vet. Ophthal.*). *Ibid.*, **83**, 329.

VIERHELLER, R. C. (1962) Ocular surgery in the dog. *Mod. vet. Pract.*, **43** (12), 42.

VLADUTIU, O. (1960) Cercetari asupra vindecarii plagilor corneene la animale sub artiunea diferitilor factori terapeutici. (Treatment of corneal lesions in animals with different therapeutic agents.) *Lucr. Inst. Agron. Bucuresti.* Ser. C., **4**, 287.

YOUNG, M. (1948) Removal of a dermoid from the cornea. *Vet. Rec.*, **60**, 94.

ZIMMERMANN, W. (1897) Ueber angeborene Veränderungen der Cornea und Sklera eines Hundes. (Congenital changes in the cornea and sclera of the dog.) *Klin. Mbl. Augenheilk.*, **35**, 226.

The Uveal Tract

APTER, J. T. (1960) Distribution of contractile forces in the iris of cats and dogs. *Amer. J. Physiol.*, **199**, 377.

BARRON, C. N. & SAUNDERS, L. Z. (1959) Intraocular tumours in animals. II. Primary non-pigmented intraocular tumours. *Cancer Res.*, **19**, 1171.

—— et al. (1963) Intraocular tumours in animals. III. Secondary intraocular tumours. *Amer. J. vet. Res.*, **24**, 835.

—— —— (1963) Intraocular tumours in animals. V. Transmissible venereal tumour of dogs. *Ibid.*, **24**, 1263.

BLOOM, F. (1942) Melanocarcinoma of the iris in a dog. *J. Amer. vet. med. Ass.*, **100**, 439.

—— & MEYER, L. M. (1945) Malignant lymphoma (so-called leukaemia) in dogs. *Amer. J. Path.*, **21**, 683.

CARTER, J. D. (1965) Extrabulbar extension of ocular melanoma. *Vet. Med.*, **60**, 819.

COATS, G. (1914) Two instances of congenital abnormality in the dog. II. Bilateral failure in the separation of the pupillary membrane from the cornea, and partial albinism, in a Bull Terrier. *Roy. Lond. ophthal. Hosp. Rep.*, **19**, 391.

CONCEICÃO, J. M. (1939) Um caso de leucemia da iris do cão. (A case of leukaemia of the iris of the dog.) *Med. vet. (Lisboa).*, **34**, 237.

COTCHIN, E. (1959) Some tumours of dogs and cats of comparative veterinary and human interest. *Vet. Rec.*, **71**, 1040.

DARRASPEN, E. & FLORIO, R. (1937) La cholestérolémie dans quelques affections oculaires du chien. *Rev. Méd. Vét.*, **89**, 257.

—— et al. (1939) Des modifications humorales dans certaines variétés de tumeurs oculaires, cérébrales et viscérales, chez les Équidés et les carnivores domestiques. *Ibid.*, **91**, 65.

DE TOLEDO PIZA, P. (1955) Musculo ciliar no cão. Influencia dos estimulos nervoso a medicamentosa. (The ciliary muscle in the dog.) *Rev. bras. Oftal.*, **14**, 59.

HUBNER, L. (1959) Neoplasmen der iris beim Hunde. (Neoplasms of the iris in dogs.) *Wien tierärztl. Mschr.*, **46**, 121.

HUFF, R. W. (1966) Iritis. *Mod. vet. Pract.*, **47** (6), 44.

KRAWITZ, L. (1964) Diseases of the anterior uvea of the dog. *J. Amer. vet. med. Ass.*, **144**, 986.

LECALVÉ, — (1898) Persistance congénitale de la membrane pupillaire chez un chien. *Bull. Soc. centr. Méd. Vét.*, **16**, 476.

LIEBERMAN, L. O. (1956) Melanoma of eye and oral mucosa with metastases in a dog. *J. Amer. vet. med. Ass.*, **128**, 602.

LOPPNOW, H. & LINKE, E. (1961) Zur Kasuistik primärer melanotischer Augentumoren beim Hund. (A case of primary melanotic eye tumour in a dog.) *Berl. Münch. tierärztl. Wschr.*, **74**, 317.

LUCAS, D. R. (1954) Ocular associations of dappling in the coat colour of dogs. *J. comp. Path.*, **64**, 260.

MAGRANE, W. G. (1954) Cavernous haemangioma of the iris. *N. Amer. Vet.*, **35**, 516.

—— (1965) Tumours of the eye and orbit in the dog. *J. small Anim. Pract.*, **6**, 165.

MICHAEL, S. J. (1948) Melano-sarcoma of the eye with metastasis to the kidneys and ovaries. *J. Amer. vet. med. Ass.*, **113**, 253.

MONTABAUR, J. (1941) Beitrag zur Kenntnis der Membrana pupillaris persistens des Hundes. (A contribution to the knowledge on persistent pupillary membrane in the dog.) *Arch. wiss. prakt. Tierheilk.*, **76**, 219.

NORDMANN, — & HOERNER, — (1946) Neuroépithélioma du corps ciliare chez un chien. *Arch. Ophtal. (Paris)*, p. 472.

OWEN, L. N. (1964) The treatment of spontaneous tumours in dogs with Triethylene Glycol Diglycidyl Ether. *Acta. Un. int. Cancr.*, **20**, 240.

PALLASKE, G. & CHRISTOPH, H. J. (1956) Ein weiterer Beitrag zur Leukose des Hundes. *Mh. Vet.-Med.*, **4**, 74.

PIGOT, M. (1947) Sur une anomalie congénitale oculaire du chien. *Bull. Acad. vét. Fr.*, **20**, 55.

PIRIE, A. (1966) The chemistry and structure of the tapetum lucidum in animals. *Aspects of Comparative Ophthalmology*. Oxford: Pergamon. p. 57.

PURTSCHER, E. (1961) Die grossen Irisarterien beim Hunde. (The large arteries of the canine iris). *Berl. Münch. tierärztl. Wschr.*, **74**, 436.

—— & HAGAR, G. (1963) Zur anatomischen und funktionellen Struktur der Iris des Hundes. (The anatomical and functional structure of the iris of the dog.) *Zbl. Vet.-Med.*, **10**, 227.

ROBERTS, S. R. (1959) Iris-cysten beim Hund. (Iris cysts in the dog.) *Wien. tierärztl. Mschr.*, **46**, 20.

—— (1967) Three inherited ocular defects in the dog. *Mod. vet. Pract.*, **48** (2), 30.

RUBIN, L. F. (1963) Atypical coloboma of the choroid in a dog. *J. Amer. vet. med. Ass.*, **143**, 841.

SAUDERS, L. Z. & BARRON, C. N. (1958) Primary pigmented intraocular tumours in animals. *Cancer Res.*, **18**, 234.

—— —— (1964) Intraocular tumours in animals. IV. Lymphosarcoma. *Brit. vet. J.*, **120**, 25.

SCHIMMEL, — (1902) Korektonia, Dyskoria, Albinismus und Nystagmus bei einem Hunde. (Pupillary enlargement, discoria, albinism and nystagmus in a dog.) *Österr. Mschr. Tierheilk.*, **26**, 337.

SCHINDELKA, H. (1883) Ein Fall von Membrana pupillaris perseverans beim Hund. *Z. Augenheilk.*, **2**, 102.

SCHEGEL, M. (1922) Über Augentuberkulose bei Haustieren. *Arch. wiss. prakt. Tierheilk.*, **48**, 1.

SEVERIN, G. A. (1966) Anterior uveitis and associated changes. *Proc. Amer. anim. Hosp. Ass.*, 33rd Ann. Meeting. 68.

SIGRIST, K. (1960) Die Kammerwasservenen des Hundes. (Veins associated with the aqueous humour in the dog.) *Schweiz. Arch. Tierheilk.*, **102**, 308.

SODIKOFF, C. H. (1966) Use of adrenal cortical steroids in metabolic, neoplastic and infectious diseases. *J. Amer. vet. med. Ass.*, **149**, 1735.

SORSBY, A. & DAVEY, J. B. (1954) Ocular associations of dappling (or merling) in the coat colour of dogs. I. Clinical and genetical data. *J. Genet.*, **52**, 425.

STARTUP, F. G. (1960) Diseases of the canine eye. Part III. *Vet. Rec.*, **72**, 724.
—— (1966) Congenital abnormalities of the iris of the dog. *J. small Anim. Pract.*, **7**, 99.
SZCZUDLOWSKI, K. (1958) Szczatkowa blona zreniczna u psa. (Persistent pupillary membrane in a dog.) *Med. weteryn.*, **14**, 359.
TEICHERT, G. (1963) Freie Vorderkammerzysten bei einem Hund. (Free cysts in the anterior chamber of a dog.) *Kleintier-Prax.*, **8**, 106.
ÜBERREITER, O. (1957) Membrana pupillaris cornea adherens persistens beim Hunde. *Dtsch. tierärztl. Wschr.*, **64**, 507.
—— (1959) Die Kammerwasservenen beim Hunde. (The aqueous veins of the dog.) *Wien. tierärztl. Mschr.*, **46**, 721.
—— (1967) Retinochorioiditis maculosa disseminata beim Hund. *Proc. XVIIIth World Vet. Congr., Paris.* p. 479.
VERWER, M. A. J. & TEN THIJE, P. A. (1967) Tumour of the epithelium of the ciliary body in a dog. *J. small Anim. Pract.*, **8**, 627.
WARREN, A. G. (1946) Persistent pupillary membrane in the dog. *Vet. Rec.*, **58**, 504.
WHITFORD, E. L. (1965) Lymphocytic lymphosarcoma of the canine eye. *J. Amer. vet. med. Ass.*, **147**, 837.
ZIETZSCHMANN, O. (1906) Die Akkomodation und die Binnenmuskulatur des Auges. (Accommodation and the internal musculature of the eyes.) *Schweiz. Arch. Tierheilk.*, **48**, 442.

The Anterior Chamber

BÁRÁNY, E. & WIRTH, A. (1954) An improved method for estimating rate of flow of aqueous humour in individual animals. *Acta Ophthal.*, **32**, 99.
BELLHORN, R. W. (1967) Diagnosis and management of glaucoma. *Mod. vet. Pract.*, **48** (5), 42.
—— (1967) Diagnosis and management of glaucoma. *Proc. Amer. anim. Hosp. Ass.*, 34th Ann. Meeting. 197.
DARRASPEN, E. & FLORIO, R. (1938) Des hydrophtalmies chez le chien. *Rev. Méd. Vét.*, **90**, 5.
—— & LESCURE, F. (1960) A propos d'un cas d'hémorragie endoculaire. Relation possible avec une dysprotéinémie. (Intraocular haemorrhage and its possible relationship to dysproteinaemia.) *Ibid.*, **111**, 275.
—— (1960) A propos de l'hydrophtalmie, dite primitive, du chien. (The early stages of glaucoma in the dog.) *Ibid.*, **111**, 877.
DEMONT, G. A. (1930) Contribution a l'étude du glaucome chez le chien. Dissertation, Paris.
FLORIO, R. & JOUBERT, L. (1946) Contribution a l'étude de la pathogénie et du traitement des hydrophtalmies, chez le chien. *Rev. Méd. Vét.*, **97**, 567.
FREMMING, B. D. (1960) A method for treatment of glaucoma in the dog. *Mod. vet. Pract.*, **41** (3), 50.
GANDOLFO, C. (1942) Untersuchungen über die normale Augenspannung beim Hund. *Nuovo. Vet.*, **47**, 53.
GLEESON, L. N. (1965) Two cases of ophthalmic surgery. *Irish vet. J.*, **19**, 81.
GRIEDER, H. (1920) Untersuchungen über Glaucom und Hydrophthalmus. *Schweiz. Arch. Tierheilk.*, **62**, 269.
HEIDRICH, H-D. (1954) Zur Glaukomdiagnostik beim Hund. (The diagnosis of glaucoma in the dog.) *Mh. Vet.-Med.*, **7**, 154.
HENRY, A. & LESBOUYRIES, G. (1927) Strongle des vaisseaux dans l'oeil d'un chien. *Bull. Soc. cent. Med. Vét.*, **80**, 263.
HOLT, J. R. (1960) The treatment of glaucoma in the dog. *Advances in Small Animal Practice*, Vol. 2. Oxford: Pergamon. p. 82.
ISHIKAWA, F. (1930) Experimentelles Glaucom beim Hund mit besonderer Rücksicht auf Sehnervenerkrankungen. (Experimental glaucoma in the dog, with special reference to optic nerve damage.) *Albrecht v. Graefes Arch. Ophthal.*, **124**, 387.
JOURDAN, R. H. (1950) Pathogenesis of canine glaucoma. *J. Amer. vet. med. Ass.*, **117**, 419.
LIVESEY, G. H. (1905) A contribution to the study of the diseases of the eye in the dog. *J. comp. Path.*, **18**, 31.
LOVEKIN, L. G. (1964) Primary glaucoma in dogs. *J. Amer. vet. med. Ass.*, **145**, 1081.
MAGRANE, W. G. (1957) Canine glaucoma. I. Methods of diagnosis. *J. Amer. vet. med. Ass.*, **131**, 311.

—— (1957) Canine glaucoma. II. Primary classification. *Ibid.*, **131**, 372.

—— (1957) Canine glaucoma. III. Seconday classification. *Ibid.*, **131**, 374.

—— (1957) Canine glaucoma. IV. Treatment. *Ibid.*, **131**, 456.

—— (1959) Canine glaucoma. *Proc. Amer. Soc. Vet. Ophthal.*

——(1961) Canine glaucoma. *Advances in Small Animal Practice.* Vol. 3. Oxford: Pergamon. p. 104.

—— (1967) Iridencleisis using electrocautery. *Proc. Amer. anim. Hosp. Ass.*, 34th Ann. Meeting. 193.

McCunn, J. (1934) Observations on a few equine and canine diseases. *Vet. Rec.*, **14**, 599.

Petrovic, D. (1955) Die Reaktion des Hundeauges auf die experimentell aseptisch eingetragenen Fremdkorper in die vordere Augenkammer. (The reaction of the dog's eye to sterile experimental foreign bodies in the anterior chamber.) *Acta vet. Acad. Sci. hung.*, **5**, 4.

Roberts, S. R. (1967) Recognizing glaucoma—the appearance, course and effects of the disease in clinical veterinary practice. *Proc. Amer. Soc. vet. Ophthal.*, 8.

Rouquette, V. (1937) Contribution a l'hydrophtalmie chez le chien. *Dissertation*, Toulouse.

Rubin, L. F. (1967) Treatment of glaucoma—an up-to-date evaluation of medical management of the disease in veterinary medicine. *Proc. Amer. Soc. vet. Ophthal.*, 13.

Schnelle, G. B. & Jones, T. C. (1945) Dirofilaria immitis in the eye and in an inter-digital cyst. *J. Amer. vet. med. Ass.*, **107**, 14.

Schwartzman, R. M. (1956) A surgical correction of glaucoma in the dog—a case report. *J. Amer. vet. med. Ass.*, **128**, 18.

Sédan, J. (1966) A propos de nos incursions dans l'ophtalmologie vétérinaire. (Experiences in veterinary ophthalmology.) *Arch. port. Oftal.*, **18** (Suppl.), 287.

Zhivotovsky, D. S. (1967) Intraocular pressure standards in dogs. (In Russian.) *Vestn. Oftal.*, **80**, 37.

Stack, W. F. (1960) Posterior sclerotomy—a surgical procedure for treatment of glaucoma. *J. Amer. vet. med. Ass.*, **136**, 453.

Troncoso, M. U. (1947) *Gonioscopy.* Philadelphia: Davis.

Überreiter, O. (1939) Glaukom beim Hunde. *Arch. wiss. prakt. Tierheilk.*, **74**, 235.

Vainisi, S. J. (1967) Understanding glaucoma: anatomy, physiology and pathology. *Proc. Amer. Soc. vet. Ophthal.*, 1.

Vierheller, R. C. (1967) Surgical treatment of glaucoma—a reappraisal of recommended operative techniques in veterinary practice. *Proc. Amer. Soc. vet. Ophthal.*, 20.

Weadon, M. (1940) Surgical technics in glaucoma. *J. Amer. vet. med. Ass.*, **96**, 107.

—— (1942) Glaucoma in dogs. *Ibid.*, **100**, 344.

Whiteford, R. D. (1963) Anatomical considerations in canine glaucoma. *Auburn Vet.*, **19**, 67.

The Lens

Adler, S. (1967) Surgical treatment of dislocated lenses. *Brit. J. Ophthal.*, **51**, 73.

Anderson, A. C. & Shultz, F. T. (1958) Inherited (congenital) cataract in the dog. *Amer. J. Path.*, **34**, 965.

Barraquer, J. (1958) Zonulolysis Enzymatica. *Rep. to the Roy. Soc. Med., Barcelona,* April.

Bartholomew, A. C. (1936) Removal of the lens in small animals. *Vet. J.*, **92**, 262.

Beamer, R. J. (1959) Diseases of the canine crystalline lens. *Mod. vet. Pract.*, **40** (20), 38.

—— (1959) Diseases of the canine crystalline lens. *Mod. vet. Pract.*, **40** (24), 30.

Berlin, R. (1887) Beobachtungen über Staar und Staaroperationen bei Tieren. (Observations on cataract and cataract operations in animals.) *Z. Augenheilk.*, **5**, 59.

Bordet, R. (1961) Quelques particularités de la chirurgie oculaire vétérinaire. *Bull. Soc. franç. Ophtal.*, **74**, 460.

Carbo, M. Luera. (1967) Extraccion intracapsular del cristalino del perro,mediante el empleo de bajas temperaturas, utilizando el cryoextractor de Duch. *Proc. XVIIIth World Vet. Congr., Paris.* p. 487.

Carter, J. D. (1961) Cataract extraction using chymotrypsin for zonulolysis. *Missouri Vet.*, **10** (3), 11.

Catford, G. V. & Millis, E. (1967) Clinical experience in the intra-ocular use of acetylcholine. *Brit. J. Ophthal.*, **51**, 183.

24

COATS, G. (1914) Two cases of congenital abnormality in the dog. I. Congenital central cataract in two fox terriers belonging to one litter. *Roy. Lond. ophthal. Hosp. Rep.*, **19**, 385.

COGAN, J. E. H. (1958) Enzymatic zonulolysis. *Proc. roy. Soc. Med.*, **51**, 927.

—— (1959) Intracapsular cataract extraction using alphachymotrypsin. *Brit. J. Ophthal.*, **43**, 193.

CONDEMINE, R. (1939) Contribution a l'étude de la cataracte chez chien. Thesis. Paris: Vigot.

CONWAY, J. (1965) Preliminary report of cataract extraction by freezing. *Brit. J. Ophthal.*, **49**, 141.

DARRASPEN, E. et al. (1961) Technique de l'opération de la cataracte chez le chien. *Bull. Soc. franç. Ophtal.*, **74**, 521.

DAVIES, T. G. (1965) Intracapsular cataract extraction using low temperature. *Brit. J. Ophthal.*, **49**, 137.

DOBREE, J. H. (1957) Principles of cataract surgery in the human subject. *Vet. Rec.*, **69**, 317.

D'OMBRAIN, A. (1961) Canine cataract. *Med. J. Aust.*, **1**, 906.

DORE, J. L. (1963) Eye conditions in aged dogs. *J. S. Afr. vet. med. Ass.*, **34**, 163.

ESPOSITO, A. C. (1962) The Esposito erisophake and cataract extraction. *Brit. J. Ophthal.*, **46**, 697.

FASANELLA, R. M. (1963) *Modern Advances in Cataract Surgery*. London: Pitman.

FILE, T. M. (1961) Studies on the use of antihistamines in cataract surgery. *Amer. J. Ophthal.*, **51**, 1240.

FORMSTON, C. (1945) Observations on subluxation and luxation of the crystalline lens in the dog. *J. comp. Path.*, **55**, 168.

—— (1966) The clinical aspects of cataract in animals. *Aspects of Comparative Ophthalmology*. Oxford: Pergamon. p. 121.

GALLI, A. (1930) La cura medica nella cateratta incipiente. *Nuovo Ercol.*, **35**, 301.

GARBUTT, R. J. (1950) An aid to cataract surgery. *Vet. Med.*, **45**, 242.

GELATT, K. N. (1966) Selection and preparation of the patient for cataract surgery. *Proc. Amer. Soc. vet. Ophthal.*, 1.

GRAY, H. (1932) Some medical and surgical conditions in the dog. *Vet. Rec.*, **12**, 1.

GREAUD, R. (1950) Contribution au traitement chirurgical de la cataracte chez le chien. *Thesis*. Paris: Foulou.

HIPPEL, E. (1930) Embryologische Untersuchungen über Vererbung angeborener Katarakt, über Schichstar des Hundes sowie über eine besondere Form von Kapselkatarakt. (Embryological investigations on inherited congenital cataract, lamellar cataract in the dog, and a special form of capsular cataract.) *Albrecht v. Graefes Arch. Ophthal.*, **124**, 300.

HØST, P. & SVEINSON, S. (1936) Arvelig katarakt hos hunder. (Congenital cataract in dogs). *Norsk. Vet. Tidsskr.*, **48**, 244.

HUMPHRISS, D. (1950) Bunty. (A report of bilateral lens luxation, lendectomy and the fitting of spectacles.) *S. Afr. Optom.*, **17**, 67.

IVY, A. C. et al. (1959) Therapeutic improvement in canine cataract. *Vet. Med.*, **54**, 205.

JACOB, H. (1919) De cataracta senilis van den hond. (Senile cataract in the dog.) *T. Diergeneesk.*, **46**, 387.

—— (1922) Die cataracta senilis des Hundes, ein Masstab der Altersschätzung. (Senile cataract in dogs, a method of age estimation.) *Arch. wiss. prakt. Tierheilk.*, **47**, 6.

KLEBERGER, K. E. (1967) An ophthalmological evaluation of DMSO. *Ann. N.Y. Acad. Sci.*, **141**, 381.

KNIGHT, G. C. (1957) The extraction of the dislocated and the cataractous crystalline lens of the dog with the object of preserving some useful vision. *Vet. Rec.*, **69**, 318.

—— (1958) The extraction of the dislocated and of the cataractous lens in the dog. *Proc. Brit. Small Anim. Vet. Ass. Congr.* p. 33.

—— (1960) Canine intraocular surgery. *Vet. Rec.*, **72**, 642.

—— (1962) The indications and technique for lens extraction in the dog. *Ibid.*, **74**, 1065.

—— (1966) The cataractous lens of the dog and its extraction. *Aspects of Comparative Ophthalmology*. Oxford: Pergamon. p. 145.

KOCH, S. A. & RUBIN, L. F. (1967) Probable nonhereditary congenital cataracts in dogs. *J. Amer. vet. med. Ass.*, **150**, 1374.

KRWAWICZ, T. (1961) Intracapsular extraction of intumescent cataract by application of low temperature. *Brit. J. Ophthal.*, **45**, 279.

—— (1961) Further results in intumescent cataract extraction done with the cryo-extractor. *Klin. oczna*, **31**, 201.

—— (1963) Further experience with intracapsular cataract extractions by application of low temperature. *Brit. J. Ophthal.*, **47**, 36.

KROTOVA, S. I. (1963) Age peculiarities of the eye in dogs. *Byull. éksp. Biol. Med.*, **55**, 52. (In Russian.)

LAIGNIOR, — & TAILLANDIER, — (1950) Contibution a la recherche d'une technique de l'operation de la cataracte chez le chien. *Rec. Méd. Vét.*, **126**, 602.

LAPOLLA, L. (1930) La jonoforesi oculare nella cura cateratta del cane. *Nuovo Ercol.*, **35**, 383.

—— & MASTRONARDI, M. (1962) Cataract in young dogs. *Acta med. vet. (Napoli)*, **8**, 311.

LAVIGNETTE, A. M. (1966) Cataract surgery in dogs: technique. *Proc. Amer. Soc. vet. Ophthal.*, **11**.

LETTOW, E. et al. (1966) Spontane Cataracta tetanica bei einem Hund. (Spontaneous tetanic cataract in a dog.) *Berl. Münch. tierärztl. Wschr.*, **79**, 445.

LURIE, L. (1961) Cataract extraction by expression. *Brit. J. Ophthal.*, **45**, 133.

MAGRANE, W. G. (1953) Extracapsular cataract extraction by suction. *Proc. Amer. Vet. Med. Ass.*, **207**.

—— (1954) Rationale of cataract surgery. *N. Amer. Vet.*, **35**, 759.

—— (1961) Cataract extraction; an evaluation of 104 cases. *J. small Anim. Pract.*, **1**, 163.

—— (1967) Cryosurgical lens extraction; Uses and limitations. *Proc. XVIIIth World Vet. Congr., Paris.* p. 475.

—— (1968) Cryosurgical lens extraction: Uses and limitations. *J. small Anim. Pract.*, **9**, 71.

MAJILTON, E. A. (1959) Early surgical removal of canine cataract. *Mod vet. Pract.*, **40** (3), 53.

MALEVAL, M. (1904) Un cas curieux d'hérédité de la cataracte chez le chien. *Rec. Méd. vét.*, **81**, 360.

MEANS, T. I. (1942) The simplified cataract operation in the dog. *J. Amer. vet. med. Ass.*, **100**, 151.

MÖLLER, H. (1886) Casuistiche Mitteilungen über das Vorkommen und die operative Behandlung des grauen Stares beim Hunde. (Case report of cataract and its operative treatment in a dog.) *Z. Augenheilk.*, **4**, 138.

MOORE, J. G. (1967) Simplified cataract extraction. *Brit. J. Ophthal.*, **51**, 339.

MORGAN, O. G. (1952) Ocular conditions in animals. *Vet. Rec.*, **64**, 49.

—— (1952) Ocular conditions in animals. *Guy's Hosp. Rep.*, **66**, 154.

NIEMEYER, K. H. (1962) Use of a zonulolytic agent in the canine eye. *Small anim. Clin.*, **2**, 446.

PADADOPOULOS, P. & FORMSTON, C. (1966) Observations on the reclination of the crystalline lens in the dog by means of the intra-vitreal injection of alphachymotrypsin and on the effect of this agent on the ocular tissues with special reference to the retina. *Aspects of Comparative Ophthalmology.* Oxford: Pergamon. p. 329.

PARK, E. G. et al. (1959) Coloured photography of cataractous lens. *Vet. Med.*, **54**, 268.

PELLATHY, A. (1929) Pathologische Anatomie der experimentellen Tetanie-Katarakt bei Hunden. (Pathology of experimental tetanic cataract in the dog.) *Klin. Mbl. Augenheilk.*, **83**, 438.

PERRY, C. S. (1941) Intracapsular cataract operation in the dog. *J. Amer. vet. med. Ass.*, **98**, 45.

POULOS, P. (1966) Selenium-Tocopherol treatment of senile lenticular sclerosis in dogs. (Four case reports.) *Vet. Med.*, **61**, 986.

RATIGAN, W. J. (1928) Needling cataracts. *Vet. Med.*, **23**, 358.

REIHART, O. F. (1933) A new method of treating corneal opacities and cataract. *N. Amer. Vet.*, **14** (10), 47.

RIBELIN, W. E. et al. (1967) Development of cataracts in dogs and rats from prolonged feeding of Sulfaethoxypyridazine. *Toxicol. appl. Pharmacol.*, **10**, 557.

RUBIN, L. F. & BARNETT, K. C. (1967) Ocular effects of oral and dermal application of Dimethyl sulphoxide. *Ann. N.Y. Acad. Sci.*, **141**, 333.

—— & GELATT, K. N. (1968) Spontaneous resorption of the cataractous lens in dogs. *J. Amer. vet med. Ass.*, **152**, 139.

—— & MATTIS, P. A. (1966) Dimethyl sulphoxide: lens changes in dogs during oral administration. *Science*, **153**, 83.

RUBINSTEIN, K. (1967) Complications of cryoextraction of cataracts. *Brit. J. Ophthal.*, 51, 178.

SIMPSON, H. D. (1956) Intraocular plastic lens implantation in canine cataract surgery. *N. Amer. Vet.*, 37, 573.

SMITH, E. R. et al. (1967) The influence of Dimethyl sulphoxide on the dog with emphasis on the ophthalmological examination. *Ann. N.Y. Acad. Sci.*, 141, 386.

SMYTHE, R. H. (1957) Some observations on the surgery of the eye in aminals. *Vet. Rec.*, 69, 322.

STARTUP, F. G. (1960) Enzymatic zonulolysis as an aid to cataract surgery in the dog. *Vet. Rec.*, 72, 245.

—— (1963) Observations on the technique of cataract surgery in the dog. Ph.D. Thesis, University of London.

—— (1965) Low temperature cataract extraction. *Vet. Rec.*, 77, 978.

—— (1966) The luxated lens of the dog and its extraction. *Aspects of Comparative Ophthalmology.* Oxford: Pergamon. p. 151.

—— (1967) Cataract surgery in the dog. I. History and review of the literature. *J. small Anim. Pract.*, 8, 667.

—— (1967) Cataract surgery in the dog. II. Published results. *Ibid*, 8, 671.

—— (1967) Cataract surgery in the dog. III. Factors responsible for failure. *Ibid.*, 8, 675.

—— (1967) Cataract surgery in the dog. IV. General considerations. *Ibid.*, 8, 681.

—— (1967) Cataract surgery in the dog. V. Pre-operative preparation. *Ibid.*, 8, 685.

—— (196) Cataract surgery in the dog. VI. Enzymatic zonulolysis. *Ibid.*, 8, 689.

—— (196) Cataract surgery in the dog. VII. Cryoextraction. *Ibid.*, 8, 693.

—— (196) Cataract surgery in the dog. VIII. Vitreous loss. *Ibid.*, 8, 697.

TEUNISSEN, G. & BLOK-SCHURING, P. (1966) Diabetes mellitus bei Hund und Katze. *Schweiz. Arch. Tierheilk.*, 108, 409.

VIERHELLER, R. C. (1957) Canine cataract surgery: suggested technique for the occasional operator. *Vet. Med.*, 52, 487.

—— (1962) Cataract surgery in the dog. *Mod. vet. Pract.*, 43 (7), 43.

—— (1962) Cataract surgery in the dog. *Ibid.*, 43 (8), 39.

VLADUTIU, O. & IONESCO, Gh. (1967) L'aerosol-ionotherapie dans les affections oculaires chez les animaux. *Proc. XVIIIth World Vet. Congr., Paris.* p. 488.

WEADON, M. (1947) Surgical relief of lenticular cataract in the dog. *N. Amer. Vet.*, 28, 600.

WESTHUES, M. (1926) Der Schichstar des Hundes. (Lamellar cataract of the dog.) *Arch. wiss. prakt. Tierheilk.*, 54, 32.

—— (1937) Die Luxatio lentis anterior beim Hunde und ihre operative Behandlung. (Anterior lens luxation in the dog and its operative treatment.) *Münch. tierärztl. Wschr.*, 88, 121.

WILKINSON, J. S. (1960) Spontaneous Diabetes mellitus. *Vet. Rec.*, 72, 548.

WOLLENSAK, J. (1963) The behaviour of the Zonule of Zinn. *Öst. ophthal. Ges.*, 7th Ann. Meeting, June 1962. p. 43.

WYMAN, M. (1966) Cataract surgery in dogs: post-operative care and complications. *Proc. Amer. Soc. vet. Ophthal.*, 21.

—— et al. (1966) Cataract surgery in the dog. *Mod. vet. Pract.*, 47 (9), 30.

ZORAB, E. C. (1961) Survey of cataract surgery technique in the United Kingdom. *Brit. J. Ophthal.*, 45, 614.

The Vitreous Humour

DELAHUNT, C. S. & ANDERSON, J. (1963) Spontaneous intraocular haemorrhage in Beagle dogs. *Lab. anim. Care*, 13, 542.

REESE, A. B. (1955) Persistent hyperplastic primary vitreous. *Amer. J. Ophthal.*, 40, 317.

RUBIN, L. F. (1963) Asteroid hyalosis in the dog. *Amer. J. vet. Res.*, 24, 1256.

The Retina and Optic Nerve

—— (1963) Detachment of retina in Collies. *J. small Anim. Pract.*, 4, 128.

—— (1967) Inherited defects in dogs and cats in Australia. *Aust. vet. J.*, 43, 221.

AJMERITO, G. C. (1957) Le alterazioni del fondo dell'occhio rilevabili oftalmoscopicamente nelle nefropatie croniche del cane. (Ophthalmoscopic alterations in the fundus of the eye in chronic nephritis in the dog.) *Atti soc. ital. Sci. vet.* 11, 958.

ARASIMOWICZ, C. & CHWIROT, R. (1959) Operativer Zugang zum Sehnerven beim Hunde. (Operative approach to the optic nerve in the dog.) *Ophthalmologica (Basle)*, **138**, 381.

BARNETT, K. C. (1962) Hereditary retinal atrophy in the Poodle. *Vet. Rec.*, **74**, 672.

—— (1963) Progressive retinal atrophy. *J. small Anim. Pract.*, **4**, 465.

—— (1964) Abnormalities and defects in pedigree dogs. IV. Progressive retinal atrophy. *Advances in Small Animal Practice*. Vol. 5. Oxford: Pergamon. p. 53.

—— (1965) Canine retinopathies. I. History and review of the literature. *J. small Anim. Pract.*, **6**, 41.

—— (1965) Canine retinopathies. II. The Miniature and Toy Poodle. *Ibid.*, **6**, 93.

—— (1965) Canine retinopathies. III. The other breeds. *Ibid.*, **6**, 185.

—— (1965) Canine retinopathies. IV. Causes of retinal atrophy. *Ibid.*, **6**, 229.

—— (1965) Retinal atrophy. *Vet. Rec.*, **77**, 1543.

—— (1965) Two forms of hereditary and progressive retinal atrophy in the dog. *Anim. Hosp.* **1**, 234.

—— (1966) Primary tapeto-retinal degenerations in dogs. *Aspects of Comparative Ophthalmology*. Oxford: Pergamon. p. 77.

—— (1967) Factors influencing official control of hereditary defects in dogs—Ophthalmological aspects. *Proc. XVIIIth World Vet. Congr., Paris.* p. 491.

—— (1967) The diagnosis of central progressive retinal atrophy in the Labrador Retriever. *J. small Anim. Pract.*, **8**, 631.

—— & KEELER, C. R. (1967) Fundus photography. *Vet. Rec.*, **80**, 624.

—— (1968) Retinal photography in animals. *Brit. J. Ophthal.*, **52**, 200.

BEEHLER, C. C. et al. (1964) Retinal detachment in adult dogs resulting from oxygen toxicity. *Arch. Ophthal.*, **71**, 665.

BUDINGER, J. M. (1961) Diphenylthiocarbazone blindness in dogs. *Arch. Path.*, **71**, 304.

DE CARVALHO, C. M. F. (1963) Fundo de ōlho normal do cāo e alteracōes que nēle ocurrem em algumas doenças. (The normal ocular fundus of the dog and lesions in some diseases). *Archos. Esc. Sup. vet. Est. Minas. Gerais.*, **15**, 205.

CATCOTT, E. J. (1950) An illustrated study of the ocular fundus of normal and diseased dogs. Ph.D. Thesis, Ohio State University.

CHEVKI, A. (1928) Über ein intrabulbares Gliom biem Hund. *Berl. tierärztl. Wschr.*, **44**, 856.

COGAN, D. G. & KUWABANA, T. (1965) Photoreceptive abiotrophy of the retina in the Elkhound. *Path. vet.*, **2**, 101.

DARRASPEN, E. et al. (1961) Le fond d'oeil du chien (Aspects normaux). (The fundus of the dog. Normal aspects.) *Bull. Soc. Ophtal. Fr.*, **4**, 198.

DONOVAN, E. F. & WYMAN, M. (1964) Fundus photography of the dog and cat by means of the Noyori hand fundus camera. *Amer. J. vet. Res.*, **25**, 865.

—— (1965) Ocular fundus anomaly in the Collie. *J. Amer. vet. med. Ass.*, **147**, 1465.

ENGERMAN, R. L. & BLOODWORTH, J. M. B. (1965) Experimental diabetic retinopathy in dogs. *Arch. Ophthal.*, **73**, 205.

—— et al. (1965) Vascular system of the dog retina; light- and electron-microscopic studies. *Exp. Eye Res.*, **5**, 296.

FANKHAUSER, R. (1965) Degenerative, lipoidiotische Erkrangung des Zentralnervensystems bei zwei Hunden. *Schweiz. Arch. Tierheilk.*, **107**, 73.

FREEMAN, H. M. et al. (1966) Retinal detachment, chorio-retinal changes and staphyloma in the Collie. I. Ophthalmoscopic findings. *Arch. Ophthal.*, **76**, 412.

GRICE, H. C. & HUTCHISON, J. A. (1960) Retinoblastoma in a dog. *J. Amer. vet. med. Ass.*, **136**, 444.

HAGEN, O. (1953) Lipid dystrophic changes in the central nervous system in dogs. *Acta path. microbiol. scand.*, **33**, 22.

HAUSLER, H. R. et al. (1964) Retinopathy in a dog following diabetes induced by growth hormone. *Diabetes*, **13**, 122.

HODGMAN, S. F. J. (1962) Abnormalities of possible hereditary origin in dogs. *Vet. Rec.*, **74**, 1239.

—— et al. (1949) Progressive retinal atrophy in dogs. The disease in Irish Setters (red). *Ibid.*, **61**, 185.

HUBER, E. (1937) Fondo de ojo normal del perro. Ratinogramas obtenidos con el retinografo de Norderson. *Rev. Med. vet. (B. Aires)*, **19**, 643.

IKEDA, H. (1966) Electroretinograms in experimental animals. *Aspects of Comparative Ophthalmology.* Oxford: Pergamon. p. 27.

JOSHUA, J. O. & OTTAWAY, C. W. (1947) A case of cranial nerve tumour with acquired hydrocephalus in the dog. *Vet. Rec.*, **59**, 649.

KANBAI, G. G. (1961) Changes of the fundus oculi in canine distemper. *Veterinariya*, **38** (6), 46.

KEEN, H. (1960) Spontaneous diabetes in man and animals. *Vet. Rec.*, **72**, 555.

KEEP, J. M. (1962) Hereditary retinal atrophy in the Poodle. *Vet. Rec.*, **74**, 1193.

KOPPAND, N. (1960) Lipodystrofi i sentralnervesystemet hos hund. (Lipodystrophy in the central nervous system of dogs.) *Nord. Med.*, **63**, 821.

KRAMER, V. O. (1960) Über Farbanomalien im Augenhintergrund von Haustieren. (Colour anomalies of the fundus of the eye in domestic animals.) *Schweiz. Arch. Tierheilk.*, **102**, 501.

KRISHNAMURTY, D. (1949) Cysticercus cellulosae; their incidence in canines. *Indian vet. J.*, **25**, 367.

DeLAHUNTA, A. & CUMMINGS, J. F. (1967) Neuro-ophthalmologic lesions as a cause of visual defect in dogs and horses. *J. Amer. vet. med. Ass.*, **150**, 994.

LEONARDI, E. (1930) Fondo oculare del cane. *Ann. Ottal.*, **58**, 18.

LESBOUYRIES, — & CHARTON, — (1943) Décollement bilatéral de la rétine chez le chien. (Bilateral retinal detachment in the dog.) *Bull. Acad. vét. Fr.*, **16**, 40.

LUCAS, D. R. (1954) Retinal dystrophy in the Irish Setter. I. Histology. *J. exp. Zool.*, **126**, 537.

LUGINBÜHL, H. (1958) Die farbphotographische Darstellung des Augenhintergrundes bei verschiendenen Haustieren. *Schweiz. Arch. Tierheilk.*, **100**, 187.

MAGNUSSON, H. (1909) Om nattblindhet hos hund såsom fölid af släktskapsafvel. *Svensk. vet. Tidskr.*, **14**, 462.

—— (1911) Über Retinitis pigmentosa und Konsanquinitat beim Hunde. (Retinitis pigmentosa and blood relationship in dogs.) *Arch. vergl. ophthal.*, **2**, 147.

—— (1917) Noch ein Fall von Nachblindheit beim Hunde. (Another case of night blindness in the dog.) *Albrecht v. Graefes Arch. Ophthal.*, **93**, 404.

MAGRANE, W. G. (1953) Congenital anomaly of the optic disc in Collies. *N. Amer. Vet.*, **34**, 646.

—— (1955) Progressive retinal atrophy and associated blindness; breed incidence. *Ibid.*, **36**, 743.

MANDELLI, G. & TRADATI, F. (1965) Osservazioni cliniche ed anatomopatologiche su di un caso di cecità del cane. (Pathological and clinical findings in a case of progressive blindness in an adult male dog.) *Clin. vet. (Milano)*, **88**, 33.

MENNER, E. (1939) Vergleichende Untersuchungen über die Retina wildebender und domestizierter Caniden. (Comparative investigations on the retina of wild and domestic dogs.) *Z. Naturf.*, **93**, 77.

MUTLU, F. & LEOPALD, I. H. (1964) Structure of the retinal vascular system of the dog, monkey, rat, mouse and cow. *Amer. J. Ophthal.*, **58**, 261.

OKUN, E. et al. (1961) Retinal breaks in the senile dog. *Arch. Ophthal.*, **66**, 702.

PARRY, H. B. (1951) Recent advances in canine medicine, with particular regard to blindness, viral hepatitis and post-infective neurological disorders. *Vet. Rec.*, **63**, 323.

—— (1953) Degenerations of the dog retina. I. Structure and development of the retina of the normal dog. *Brit. J. Ophthal.*, **37**, 385.

—— (1953) Degenerations of the dog retina. II. Generalised progressive atrophy of hereditary origin. *Ibid.*, **37**, 487.

—— (1953) Degenerations of the dog retina. III. Retinopathy secondary to glaucoma. *Ibid.*, **37**, 670.

—— (1954) Degenerations of the dog retina. IV. Retinopathies associated with dog distemper-complex virus infections. *Ibid.*, **38**, 295.

—— (1954) Degenerations of the dog retina. V. Generalised progressive atrophy of uncertain origin. *Ibid.*, **38**, 545.

—— (1954) Degenerations of the dog retina. VI. Central progressive atrophy with pigment epithelial dystrophy. *Ibid.*, **38**, 653.

—— (1955) Degenerations of the dog retina. VII. Central non-progressive degeneration due to an anomaly of ganglion cells and their axons. *Ibid.*, **39**, 29.

—— (1955) Degeneration and pigment cell dystrophies of the dog retina. *Excerpta Med. Sect. VIII. Neurol. and Psychiat.*, **8**, 866.

—— et al. (1951) The electroretinogram in the normal dog. *J. Physiol. (Lond.)*, **115**, 47P.

—— (1951) An objective test for hereditary night blindness in Irish Setters. *Ibid.*, **115**, 48P.

—— (1953) The electroretinogram of the dog. *Ibid.*, **120**, 28.

—— (1955) Electroretinogram during development of hereditary retinal degeneration in the dog. *Brit. J. Ophthal.*, **39**, 349.

PATTERSON, D. F. & MEDWAY, W. (1966) Hereditary diseases of the dog. *J. Amer. vet. med. Ass.*, **149**, 1741.

PATZ, A. & MAUMENCE, A. E. (1962) Studies on diabetic retinopathy. I. Retinopathy in a dog with spontaneous diabetes mellitus. *Amer. J. Ophthal.*, **54**, 532.

—— et al. (1965) Studies on diabetic retinopathy. II. Retinopathy and nephropathy in spontaneous canine diabetes. *Diabetes*, **14**, 700.

PESCE, P. A. (1953) La retinite pigmentosa o retinite atrofica, malattia ereditaria del cane. (Atrophy of the retina, an hereditary disease in dogs.) *Veterinaria (Milano)*, **2** (4), 24.

RIBELIN, W. E. & KINTNER, L. D. (1956) Lipodystrophy of the central nervous system in a dog. A disease with similarities to Tay-Sachs disease of man. *Cornell Vet.*, **46**, 532.

ROBERTS, S. R. (1959) Detachment of the retina in animals. *J. Amer. vet. med. Ass.*, **135**, 423.

—— (1964) Posterior ectasia syndrome. *Vet. Disp.*, **6** (4), 1.

—— (1966) Collie ectasia syndrome. *Proc. Amer. anim. Hosp. Ass.*, 33rd Ann. Meeting. 71.

—— (1967) Color dilution and hereditary defects in Collie dogs. *Amer. J. Ophthal.*, **63**, 1762.

—— et al. (1966) The Collie ectasia syndrome: Pathology of eyes of pups one to fourteen days of age. *Amer. J. Ophthal.*, **61**, 1458.

—— (1966) The Collie ectasia syndrome: Pathology of young and adult dogs. *Ibid.*, **62**, 728.

ROHEN, J (1954) Sperrarterien in der Aderhaut und am Sehnerventritt beim Hund. (Arterial constriction in the choroid and optic disc in the dog.) *Albrecht v. Graefes Arch. Ophthal.*, **156**, 90.

RUBIN, L. F. (1963) Hereditary retinal detachment in Bedlington Terriers. *Small anim. Clin.* **3**, 387.

—— (1966) Preretinal arteriolar loops in the dog. *J. Amer. vet. med. Ass.*, **148**, 150.

—— (1967) Clinical electroretinography in dogs. *J. Amer. vet. med. Ass.*, **151**, 1456.

—— (1968) Heredity of retinal dysplasia in Bedlington Terriers. *J. Amer. vet. med. Ass.*, **152**, 260.

—— & SAUNDERS, L. Z. (1965) Intraocular larva migrans in dogs. *Path. vet.*, **2**, 566.

—— et al. (1967) Hemeralopia in dogs; heredity of hemeralopia in Alaskan Malamutes. *Amer. J. vet. Res.*, **28**, 355.

SAUNDERS, L. Z. (1952) Congenital optic nerve hypoplasia in Collie dogs. *Cornell Vet.*, **42**, 67.

—— (1960) The clinical appearance and pathology of some congenital ocular defects in Collie dogs. *Proc. Amer. Soc. vet. Ophthal.*

SAURER, H. (1947) Beitrag zur Photographie des Augenhintergrundes bei Haustieren. *Schweiz. Arch. Tierheilk.*, **89**, 199.

SCHAFFRINNA, J. (1956) Zwei Fälle von Retinitis anaemica beim Hund. (Two cases of anaemic retinitis in dogs.) *Mh. Vet.-Med.*, **11**, 370.

SCHNELLE, B. G. (1952) Progressive retinal atrophy in a dog. *J. Amer. vet. med. Ass.*, **121**, 177.

SEBRUYNS, M. (1941) Het tapetum cellulosum bij de roofdieren (hond en kat). (The tapetum lucidum of the dog and cat.) *Vlaams diergeneesk. T.*, **10**, 121.

SEIFERLE, E. (1949) Über Nachblindheit beim Hund. *Dtsch. tierärztl. Wschr.*, **56**, 42.

SIBAY, T. M. & HAUSLER, H. R. (1967) Eye findings in two spontaneously diabetic related dogs. *Amer. J. Ophthal.*, **63**, 289.

SILVA, A. G. (1949) Contribuicão ao conhecimento do fondo do ôlho normal do cão. (Contribution to the knowledge of the normal ocular fundus of the dog.) *Rev. Fac. Med. vet. Univ. S. Paulo*, **4**, 197.

SMYTHE, R. H. (1963) Progressive retinal atrophy in the dog. *Mod. vet. Pract.*, **44** (8), 61.

STEELE, J. D. et al. (1953) Retinopathy in dogs. *Aust. vet. J.*, **29**, 104.

TANSLEY, K. (1954) Inherited retinal degenerations in animals. *Proc. XVIII int. Cong. Ophthal.*

TOLENTINO, F. I. et al. (1965) Biomicroscopy of the vitreous in Collie dogs with fundus abnormalities. *Arch. Ophthal.*, **73**, 700.

TRADATI, F. et al. (1959) Su di un caso di retinopatia nel cane. *Atti. Soc. ital. Sci. vet.*, **13**, 663.

USHER, D. H. (1924) A note on the dog's tapetum in early life. *Brit. J. Ophthal.*, **8**, 357.

VAINISI, S. J. (Editor) (1966) Canine and feline ocular fundus. *Amer. Anim. Hosp. Ass.*

VIERNEISEL, H. & RITTENBACH, P. (1962) Klinische und pathologisch-anatomische Untersuchungen zweier Glioblastome beim Hunde. (Clinical and histopathological findings in two glioblastomata in dogs.) *Berl. Münch. tierärztl. Wschr.*, **75**, 88.

WEITZEL, G. et al. (1955) Struktur der im Tapetum lucidum von Hund und Fuchs enthaltenen Zinkverbindung. (Structure of the tapetum lucidum in the dog and fox containing zinc compounds.) *Z. physiol. Chem.*, **299**, 193.

WHITEHEAD, J. (1964) Hereditary defects of the ocular fundus in Collies. *N.Y.C. Vet.*, **7** (6), 7.

WILLIAMS, J. O. et al. (1961). Glioma of the optic nerve of a dog. *J. Amer. vet. med. Ass.*, **138**, 377.

WILSON, F. D. (1962) Cystophlegia due to Cysticercus cellulosae in the brain of a dog. A case report. *Indian vet. J.*, **39**, 393.

WYMAN, M. (1963) A case report of bilateral retinal detachment. *Speculum*, **16** (2), 32.

—— & Donovan, E. F. (1965) The ocular fundus of the normal dog. *J. Amer. vet. med. Ass.*, **147**, 17.

YOUNG, G. B. (1955) Inherited defects of dogs. *Vet. Rec.*, **67**, 15.

Infectious Diseases

BARRON, C. N. & SAUNDERS, L. Z. (1959) Ein Fall von intraoculärer Toxoplasmose beim Hunde. (A case of intraocular toxoplasmosis in a dog.) *Schweiz. Arch. Tierheilk.*, **101**, 349.

BASSON, P. A. et al. (1966) Nosematosis: Report of a canine case in the Republic of South Africa. *J. S. Afr. vet. med. Ass.*, **37**, 3.

CARMICHAEL, L. E. (1964). The pathogenesis of ocular lesions of Infectious Canine Hepatitis. I. Pathology and virological observations. *Path. Vet.*, **1**, 73.

—— (1965) The pathogenesis of ocular lesions of Infectious Canine Hepatitis. II. Experimental ocular hypersensitivity produced by the virus. *Ibid.*, **2**, 344.

CELLO, R. M. (1960) Ocular manifestations of Coccidioidomycosis in a dog. *Arch. Ophthal.*, **64**, 897.

CHUNG, H. L. et al. (1940) Histopathological observations in twelve cases of canine leishmaniasis in Peiping. *Chin. med. J.*, **3** (suppl.), 212.

COHRS, P. (1951) Toxoplasmose-Encephalitis des Hundes. (Toxoplasmosis and encephalitis in dogs.) *Dtsch. tierärztl. Wschr.*, **58**, 161.

DARRASPEN, E. et al. (1961) Manifestations oculaires d'une neuro-infection virale; la rhino-amygdalite contagieuse du chien. (Ocular manifestations of a viral neuro-infection; rhino-tonsillitis in the dog.) *Bull. Soc. Ophtal. Fr.*, **4**, 204.

—— (1961) Manifestations oculaires d'une infection virale; la rhino-amygdalite contagieuse du chien. *Bull. Soc. franç. Ophtal.*, **74**, 471.

—— & LESCURE, F. (1962) Manifestations oculaires de la rhino-amygdalite contagieuse du chien. *Rev. Méd. vét.*, **113**, 22.

ERNØ, H. (1963) Diagnosticering af hundesyge ved påvisning af cytoplasmatiske inklusions-legemer intra vitam. (Cytoplasmic inclusions in the third eyelid as an aid to the clinical diagnosis of distemper.) *Nord. Vet.-Med.*, **15**, 11.

FAURE-BRAC, G. (1936) La leishmaniose canine. *Biol. méd. (Paris)*, **26**, 113.

GROULADE, P. et al. (1956) Formes cliniques de la toxoplasmose chez les carnivores domestiques. *Bull. Acad. vét. Fr.*, **29**, 49.

HAGER, G. & MOCHMANN, H. (1958) Leptospirosen und Uveaerkrankungen. (Leptospirosis and uveal disease.) *Z. ärztl. Fortbild.*, **52**, 579.

HEELEY, D. M. (1963) Toxoplasmosis. *J. small Anim. Pract.*, **4**, 128.

—— (1963) Toxoplasmosis. *Advances in Small Animal Practice.* Oxford: Pergamon. Vol. 5. p. 23.

HODGMAN, S. F. J. (1955) Canine Virus Hepatitis (Rubarth's Disease). *Vet. Rev.*, **6**, 67.

JASPER, D. E. (1951) Toxoplasmosis in the dog. Report of a new case. *J. Amer. vet. med. Ass.*, **118**, 22.

JUBB, K. V. et al. (1957) The intraocular lesions of canine distemper. *J. comp. Path.*, **67**, 21.

LEMAINE, G. et al. (1914) Spécificité de la kératite observée chez les chiens atteints de leishmaniose naturelle. *Bull. Soc. Path. exot.*, **7**, 193.

MADDY, K. T. (1958) Disseminated coccidioidomycosis of the dog. *J. Amer. vet. med. Ass.*, **132**, 483.

MANSI, W. (1953) Rubarth's disease (canine virus hepatitis). I. Reaction of dogs to the conjunctival installation of the virus. *J. comp. Path.*, **63**, 236.

MENGES, R. W. (1960) Blastomycosis in animals. A review of an analysis of 116 canine cases. *Vet. Med.*, **55**, 45.

METELKIN, A. I. (1928) K voprosu o diagnosticheskom znachenii keratita i kon'yunktivita pri leishmanioze sobak. (The diagnostic significance of keratitis and conjunctivitis in canine leishmaniasis.) *Vestnik sovrem. Vet.*, **4**, 498.

NICOLAU, S. & PÉRARD, C. (1936) Étude histo-physio-pathologique de l'oeil et du système nerveux dans la leishmaniose généralisée du chien. *Ann. Inst. Pasteur*, **57**, 463.

PLOWRIGHT, W. (1952) An encephalitis-nephritis syndrome in the dog, probably due to congenital encephalitozoon infection. *J. comp. Path.*, **62**, 83.

PRICE, R. A. & POWERS, R. D. (1967) Cryptococcosis in a dog. *J. Amer. vet. med. Ass.*, **150**, 988.

QUEIROZ, J. M. (1959) Lesões do globo ocular e anexos no calazar canino. (Lesions of the eyeball and adnexa in canine Kala-Azar.) *Rev. Ass. méd. bras.*, **5**, 304.

ROBBINS, E. S. (1954) North American blastomycosis in the dog. *J. Amer. vet. med. Ass.*, **125**, 391.

ROBIN, V. (1930) Les accidents oculaires dans la leishmaniose du chien. *Bull. Soc. Ophtal. Paris*, **42**, 463.

ROSSI, P. et al. (1953) Leptospiroses et lésions oculaires chez le chien. *Bull. Acad. vét. Fr.*, **26**, 451.

RUBIN, L. F. & CRAIG, P. H. (1965) Intraocular cryptococcosis in a dog. *J. Amer. vet. med. Ass.*, **147**, 27.

SALFELDER, K. et al. (1965) Experimental ocular histoplasmosis in dogs. *Amer. J. Ophthal.*, **59**, 290.

SELBY, L. A. et al. (1964) Clinical observations on canine blastomycosis. *Vet. Med.*, **59**, 1221.

SESHADRI, V. K. (1955) Surra in dogs. *Indian vet. J.*, **32**, 146.

TRAUTWEIN, G. & NIELSEN, S. W. (1962) Cryptococcosis in two cats, a dog and a mink. *J. Amer. vet. med. Ass.*, **140**, 437.

TREVIÑO, G. S. (1966) Canine blastomycosis with ocular involvement. *Path. Vet.*, **3**, 652.

WILKINS, J. H. et al. (1967) A new canine disease syndrome. *Vet. Rec.*, **81**, 57.

WOLF, G. F. et al. (1958) Blastomycosis in the dog. Two cases with ocular manifestations. *Vet. Med.*, **53**, 595.

—— (1967) Tropical canine pancytopaenia. (Singapore haemorrhagic syndrome.) *Anim. Health*, No. 6. Nov. 1967.

Wherever possible the abbreviations of titles of periodicals are those listed in *World Medical Periodicals*, 3rd Edition, 1961, published by the World Medical Association, New York.

BREEDS MENTIONED IN THE TEXT

INDEX

Abducent nerve, 9
Aberration, optical, 2
  spherical, 2
Ablation, of eye, 135
Ablepharon, 79
Accommodation, 3, 209, 248
Acetazolamide, use of, 42
Acetylcholine, effect on pupil, 212
  in cataract surgery, 295
  use of, 40
Acrylic lens implants, 309
Acuity, visual, development of, 33
  tests for, 31
Adrenaline, effect on pupil, 212
  subconjunctival, 49
  use of, 40
Advancement flaps, in entropion, 86
Aesthesiometry, corneal, 151
After-cataract, 256
Agenesis, 142
Albinism, retinal, 327
  uveal, 214
Alpha-chymotrypsin, 41
  in cataract surgery, 290
  intravitreal injection, 291
Amaurosis, 343
Amblyopia, 343
  ex anopsia, 263
Amethocaine, use of, 38
Ametropia, 4
Amphotericin, 43
Ampicillin, 43
Amsler's needle, 29
Anaesthesia, auriculopalpebral block,
    73
  general, 73
  local, 70
  premedication, 74
  retrobulbar, 71
  topical, 70
Anaesthetics, local, 38
Anatomy, ocular, 5

Angiostrongylus vasorum, 231
Angle, filtration, 229
Aniridia, 214
Anisocoria, 212
Ankyloblepharon, 79, 91
Anophthalmos, 128
Anterior chamber, 228
  implant, 309
  irrigation, 67
  opening, in cataract surgery, 270
  parasites, 231
  puncture, 29
Antibiotics, 43
  subconjunctival administration, 46
Anticoagulants, use of, 41
Antifungal drugs, 43
Antihistaminics, in cataract surgery,
    265
  use of, 38
Antiseptics, types, 37
Antiviral drugs, 45
Aphakia after cataract extraction, 260
Aphakic crescent, 312
  penumbra, 313
  vision, 260
Applications, anaesthesia, 70
  external, 34
Aqueous flare, 181
Aqueous humour, 228
  chemical composition, 228
  formation, mechanism of, 229
  osmotic pressure, 230
  outflow, 229
  plasmoid, 228
Area, centralis, 325
  cribrosa, 10
Argyrol, 37
Argyrosis of cornea, 37
Ariboflavinosis, effect on cornea, 180
Arteries, central retinal, 341
  ciliary, 8, 9
  ethmoidal, 8